NEOADJUVANT CHEMOTHERAPY – CURRENT APPLICATIONS IN CLINICAL PRACTICE

Edited by **Oliver F. Bathe**

Neoadjuvant Chemotherapy – Current Applications in Clinical Practice
Edited by Oliver F. Bathe

Published by InTech
Janeza Trdine 9, 51000 Rijeka, Croatia

Publishing Process Manager Niksa Mandic

Technical Editor Teodora Smiljanic

Cover Designer InTech Design Team

Additional hard copies can be obtained from orders@intechopen.com

Neoadjuvant Chemotherapy – Current Applications in Clinical Practice,
Edited by Oliver F. Bathe
p. cm.
ISBN 978-953-307-994-3

For EU product safety concerns:
IN TECH d.o.o., Prolaz Marije Krucifikse Kozulić 3, 51000 Rijeka, Croatia,
info@intechopen.com or visit our website at intechopen.com.

Meet the editor

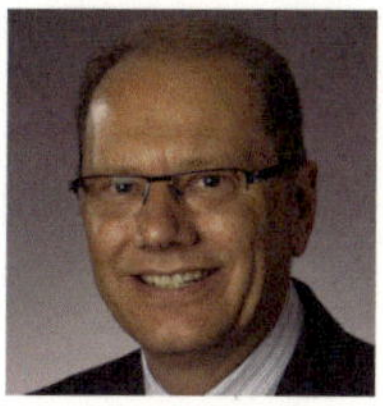

Dr Oliver Bathe is associate professor of surgery and oncology at the University of Calgary. He practices as a surgical oncologist with a special interest in hepatobiliary, pancreatic and gastrointestinal tumors. He implemented one of the first trials investigating the role of neoadjuvant chemotherapy in the context of colorectal liver metastases. As a result of his long-standing interest in the multimodality approach to treating colorectal liver metastases, he has served in a leadership role in the NCIC Clinical Trials Group Gastrointestinal Tumor Group, as well as other cooperative clinical trials groups. Bathe also directs a basic and translational research program. Using annotated clinical samples encountered in clinical practice, he and his group have successfully identified biomarkers that refine the diagnosis of gastrointestinal and pancreatic tumors and that facilitate the personalization of clinical management.

Contents

Preface

It was not so long ago that the therapeutic mainstays for solid tumors consisted of surgery and radiation. The discovery that nitrogen mustard and antifolates (methotrexate) could be used to induce remissions in childhood leukemia (Farber & Diamond, 1948; Goodman, Wintrobe et al., 1946) heralded a new therapeutic approach. Since then, the most significant therapeutic advances in oncology have been related to the discovery of novel systemic agents. In the context of solid tumors, systemic chemotherapy has allowed the oncologist to address the systemic nature of cancer, which has frequently metastasized by the time it has manifested clinically.

But with progress, new questions arise. As more agents become available, the most efficacious agents or combinations must be defined. Optimal treatment algorithms also involve minimizing toxicity and maximizing quality of life. And how should chemotherapy be administered in conjunction with surgery?

It is known, based on animal studies and the "cell kill" hypothesis proposed by Skipper and co-workers, i.e. a given dose of chemotherapy kills a constant fraction of tumor cells (Skipper, Schabel & Wilcox, 1964; Wilcox, Griswold, Laster, Schabel & Skipper, 1965), that cytotoxic drugs are most effective when used for smaller tumors. Therefore, there is a strong rationale for administering chemotherapy on an adjuvant basis, after surgical removal of gross disease, for treatment of any remaining microscopic disease. Indeed, this strategy has been shown effective in clinical studies, through the pioneering efforts of such investigators as Emil Frei (for osteosarcoma), Bernard Fisher, Gianni Bonadonna and Umberto Veronesi (for breast cancer), as well as a number of cooperative groups for colorectal cancer (Bonadonna et al., 1976; Gastrointestinal Tumor Study Group, 1984; Higgins, Amadeo, McElhinney, McCaughan, & Keehn, 1984; Jaffe, Frei, Traggis, & Bishop, 1974; Panettiere et al., 1988; Wolmark et al., 1988). As a result of early successes, the majority of clinical trials investigating the combination of surgery and systemic therapy have involved the adjuvant approach.

The rationale for administration of chemotherapy prior to surgery – neoadjuvant chemotherapy – is very different. Indeed, there is little evidence so far that it improves survival over adjuvant chemotherapy. In general, neoadjuvant chemotherapy provides early treatment of systemic and micrometastatic disease. Many patients who have had surgery do not recover sufficiently to receive adjuvant chemotherapy; therefore, giving it before surgery ensures delivery of systemic therapy to a larger proportion of individuals. Administration of chemotherapy in the presence of gross, measurable disease provides information on the sensitivity of a given tumor to a particular chemotherapeutic regimen, perhaps guiding the choice of agents postoperatively (when disease is no longer visible). In some instances, downstaging may reduce disfigurement, dysfunction and morbidity associated with extensive resections, such as in rectal cancers, vulvar carcinomas and penile carcinomas. Downstaging with neoadjuvant chemotherapy may also convert an unresectable cancer to a resectable cancer, such as in colorectal liver metastases. Neoadjuvant chemotherapy may facilitate selection of candidates for surgery: it may be argued that individuals who have progression on chemotherapy or who cannot tolerate chemotherapy would not fare well with aggressive locoregional treatments. Finally, some systemic agents (most notably angiogenesis inhibitors) are not known to be effective in the adjuvant setting (Kemeny et al.; Van Cutsem, Lambrechts, Prenen, Jain, & Carmeliet). Therefore, administration prior to surgery may enhance delivery in conditions where they are effective.

As with any treatment strategy, neoadjuvant chemotherapy also has some potential disadvantages. If progression occurs, a previously resectable tumor may become unresectable. Toxicities, including thromboembolic complications and lasting organ toxicity may increase the risk of subsequent surgery. To detractors, such outcomes would represent a disadvantage. Moreover, there is the problem of surgical planning following a complete response. Therefore, there is a need to seriously study the role of neoadjuvant chemotherapy in each specific instance, where different chemotherapeutic regimens are utilized for various types of cancer.

In general, data supporting the role of neoadjuvant chemotherapy are more plentiful for the more common tumors. For example, data related to neoadjuvant chemotherapy for breast cancer, rectal cancer and metastatic colorectal cancer are accumulating rapidly, and the role of this treatment approach is slowly becoming elucidated. For less common tumors, very few data are available to support the role of neoadjuvant chemotherapy, and research on this treatment approach is just beginning. In such instances, the experiences related to more common tumor types may inform trials on these more rare clinical entities.

Interest in neoadjuvant chemotherapy also intensifies with the availability of more effective systemic agents. For example, in the case of extremity sarcoma, while neoadjuvant chemotherapy may reduce locoregional recurrence, the paucity of systemic agents with a high response rate may limit its utility for limb salvage, limiting its application outside of clinical trials. As systemic agents are developed that reliably shrink sarcomas, it can be expected that the interest in a neoadjuvant approach will increase. Certainly, this was the case for gastrointestinal stromal tumors once imitinib became available; the interest in neoadjuvant chemotherapy for colorectal liver metastases has similarly surged since the availability of more effective chemotherapies.

This book represents an assembly of the current knowledge related to neoadjuvant chemotherapy in various types of cancers. The authors are experts in their respective clinical fields, from very disparate institutions around the world. Each chapter presents the most current information related to neoadjuvant chemotherapy in a particular clinical situation. Together, these works are complementary, as discoveries made on any particular tumor type may have implications on other tumor types where there is a relative paucity of experience with neoadjuvant chemotherapy.

But this is a rapidly changing field. Therefore, while the experiences described by each of the experts should be considered state of the art, they may also be viewed as a starting point for future work. The reader may see opportunities for biomarker development. New agents are rapidly becoming available, even for previously resistant tumor types, perhaps enhancing the prospects for new applications of the neoadjuvant approach. And with more liberal application of the neoadjuvant approach using more effective agents, there may be instances when the role of surgery falls into question. Certainly there is precedent for this, as in gastric lymphoma, testicular cancer and anal carcinomas, where surgery has been largely supplanted by chemotherapy or chemoradiation (Einhorn, Williams, Mandelbaum, & Donohue, 1981; Koch et al., 2005; Nigro et al., 1983). Only with the courageous and scientific investigation of the neoadjuvant approach will such paradigm shifts be possible. This combined work should represent a springboard for such future investigation.

Oliver F. Bathe
University of Calgary
Canada

References

Bonadonna, G., Brusamolino, E., Valagussa, P., Rossi, A., Brugnatelli, L., Brambilla, C., et al. (1976). Combination chemotherapy as an adjuvant treatment in operable breast cancer. *N Engl J Med, 294*(8), 405-410.

Einhorn, L. H., Williams, S. D., Mandelbaum, I., & Donohue, J. P. (1981). Surgical resection in disseminated testicular cancer following chemotherapeutic cytoreduction. *Cancer, 48*(4), 904-908.

Farber, S., & Diamond, L. K. (1948). Temporary remissions in acute leukemia in children produced by folic acid antagonist, 4-aminopteroyl-glutamic acid. *N Engl J Med, 238*(23), 787-793.

Goodman, L. S., Wintrobe, M. M., & et al. (1946). Nitrogen mustard therapy; use of methyl-bis (beta-chloroethyl) amine hydrochloride and tris (beta-chloroethyl) amine hydrochloride for Hodgkin's disease, lymphosarcoma, leukemia and certain allied and miscellaneous disorders. *J Am Med Assoc, 132*, 126-132.

Gastrointestinal Tumor Study Group (1984). Adjuvant therapy of colon cancer--results of a prospectively randomized trial. Gastrointestinal Tumor Study Group. *N Engl J Med, 310*(12), 737-743.

Higgins, G. A., Jr., Amadeo, J. H., McElhinney, J., McCaughan, J. J., & Keehn, R. J. (1984). Efficacy of prolonged intermittent therapy with combined 5-fluorouracil and methyl-CCNU following resection for carcinoma of the large bowel. A Veterans Administration Surgical Oncology Group report. *Cancer, 53*(1), 1-8.

Jaffe, N., Frei, E., 3rd, Traggis, D., & Bishop, Y. (1974). Adjuvant methotrexate and citrovorum-factor treatment of osteogenic sarcoma. *N Engl J Med, 291*(19), 994-997.

Kemeny, N. E., Jarnagin, W. R., Capanu, M., Fong, Y., Gewirtz, A. N., Dematteo, R. P., et al. Randomized phase II trial of adjuvant hepatic arterial infusion and systemic chemotherapy with or without bevacizumab in patients with resected hepatic metastases from colorectal cancer. *J Clin Oncol, 29*(7), 884-889.

Koch, P., Probst, A., Berdel, W. E., Willich, N. A., Reinartz, G., Brockmann, J., et al. (2005). Treatment results in localized primary gastric lymphoma: data of patients registered within the German multicenter study (GIT NHL 02/96). *J Clin Oncol, 23*(28), 7050-7059.

Nigro, N. D., Seydel, H. G., Considine, B., Vaitkevicius, V. K., Leichman, L., & Kinzie, J. J. (1983). Combined preoperative radiation and chemotherapy for squamous cell carcinoma of the anal canal. *Cancer, 51*(10), 1826-1829.

Panettiere, F. J., Goodman, P. J., Costanzi, J. J., Cruz, A. B., Jr., Vaitkevicius, V. K., McCracken, J. D., et al. (1988). Adjuvant therapy in large bowel adenocarcinoma: long-term results of a Southwest Oncology Group Study. *J Clin Oncol, 6*(6), 947-954.

Skipper, H. E., Schabel, F. M., Jr., & Wilcox, W. S. (1964). Experimental Evaluation of Potential Anticancer Agents. Xiii. On the Criteria and Kinetics Associated with "Curability" of Experimental Leukemia. *Cancer Chemother Rep, 35*, 1-111.

Van Cutsem, E., Lambrechts, D., Prenen, H., Jain, R. K., & Carmeliet, P. Lessons from the adjuvant bevacizumab trial on colon cancer: what next? *J Clin Oncol, 29*(1), 1-4.

Wilcox, W. S., Griswold, D. P., Laster, W. R., Jr., Schabel, F. M., Jr., & Skipper, H. E. (1965). Experimental evaluation of potenital anticancer agents. XVII. Kinetics of growth and regression after treatment of certain solid tumors. *Cancer Chemother Rep, 47*, 27-39.

Wolmark, N., Fisher, B., Rockette, H., Redmond, C., Wickerham, D. L., Fisher, E. R., et al. (1988). Postoperative adjuvant chemotherapy or BCG for colon cancer: results from NSABP protocol C-01. *J Natl Cancer Inst, 80*(1), 30-36.

1

Neoadjuvant Systemic Therapy in Breast Cancer

Vladimir F. Semiglazov[1] and Vladislav V. Semiglazov[2]
[1]*Petrov Research Institute of Oncology, St. Petersburg*
[2]*St.-Petersburg Pavlov Capital Medical University*
Russia

1. Introduction

Neoadjuvant systemic therapy (NST) has become a frequently used option for systemic therapy in primary operable breast cancer. All patients with a clear indication for adjuvant systemic treatment can be offered systemic therapy preoperatively. These recommendations focus on early response to NST and on tailoring therapy to response and biological and histological markers.

Three main goals for NST in operable breast cancer were defined:

- To reduce mortality from breast cancer with reduced toxicity.
- To improve surgical options.
- To acquire early information on response and biology of the disease.

A recent Oxford meta-analysis (EBCTCG, 2005) of randomized studies of more than 4000 women, comparing postoperative and neoadjuvant chemotherapy for operable breast cancer, demonstrated equivalent overall survival rates with a hazard ratio of 0.98 ($p = 0.67$). Neoadjuvant chemotherapy was associated with fewer adverse effects, and associated with a higher rate of breast conserving surgery ($p < 0.001$). In addition, patients who achieved a pCR had a better survival than those who had residual disease in the breast and lymph nodes. Neoadjuvant chemotherapy is associated with a small increase in the risk of loco-regional recurrence in patients who went on to receive radiotherapy without surgery as local therapy

2. Neoadjuvant systemic therapy

2.1 Neoadjuvant chemotherapy

Some early nonrandomized and randomized trials suggested that neoadjuvant chemotherapy might result in improved disease-free survival rates compared with standard adjuvant treatment (Scholl et al., 1994; Semiglazov et al. 1994), but some of these trials were not designed as a direct comparison of preoperative and postoperative chemotherapy. In 1998, the National Surgical Adjuvant Breast and Bowel Project (NSABP) reported the result of a large prospective randomized trial (Protocol B- 18) that compared 4 cycles of doxorubicin and cyclophosphamide (AC) given preoperatively to the same dose of AC given postoperatively (Fisher et al., 1998; Wolmark et al., 2001). The disease-free survival and overall survival rates for the 2 treatment arms of this trial were almost identical. B-18 demonstrated that clinical and pathologic tumor response were predictors of overall survival. Similar to other reports, despite a 36% clinically complete response (cCR) rate, only 13% of all patients had a pathologically complete response (pCR), defined as the absence of invasive tumor in the breast. A meta-analysis of 9 randomized studies (not involving taxanes) demonstrated the equivalence of neoadjuvant and adjuvant treatments for breast cancer in terms of survival, disease progression, and distant recurrence and showed that an increased risk of locoregional disease recurrence is associated with neoadjuvant treatment, especially when primary systemic treatment is not accompanied by any surgical intervention (eg, radiation therapy alone) (Mauri et al., 2005).

Preoperative neoadjuvant chemotherapy with agents such as doxorubicin and taxanes is an effective treatment for patients with breast cancer and leads to an increased rate of successful breast- conserving surgery and a decreased proportion of patients with metastatic involvement of the axillary lymph nodes (Kaufmann et al., 2006). Neoadjuvant chemotherapy also provides an opportunity to assess potential responses of the tumor to a given agent, which is an important consideration in selecting postoperative (adjuvant) therapy. Data from large phase 2 and phase 3 chemotherapy trials have shown that 3 to 4 months of preoperative treatment can be given without compromising either locoregional control or long-term survival (Bonadonna et al., 1998; Smith et al., 2002).

The NSABP Protocol B-27 was designed to determine the effect of adding docetaxel after 4 cycles of preoperative doxorubicin and cyclophosphamide on clinical and pathological response rates and on disease-free survival and overall survival of women with operable breast cancer. There were trends toward improved disease-free survival with the addition of docetaxel. Preoperative docetaxel, but not postoperative docetaxel, significantly improved disease-free survival in patients who had a clinical partial response after doxorubicin and cyclophosphamide. Pathologic complete response, which was doubled (from 13% to 26%) with preoperative docetaxel, was a significant predictor of overall survival regardless of treatment (Bear et al., 2006).

European Cooperative Trial in Operable Breast Cancer (ECTO) was designed to assess the effects of adding paclitaxel to an anthracycline- based regimen in patients with operable breast cancer, and to compare the same regimen given preoperatively and postoperatively (Gianni et al., 2009).

The ECTO study found a significant improvement in distant recurrence free survival (DRFS) in patients with operable early-stage breast cancer when paclitaxel was incorporated into a sequential adjuvant regimen of noncross-resistant chemotherapies that was originally pioneered by the Milan group (Gianni et al., 2009). This advantage was also seen in women with node-negative disease who constituted 40% of patients enrolled in the adjuvant arms. Comparison of the same paditaxel/doxorubicin/CMF regimen given preoperatively instead of postoperatively resulted in similar DRFS but a significantly higher percentage of patients were able to undergo breast-conserving surgery without a detrimental effect on local recurrence or survival.

The ECTO study recruited a typical and representative sample of patients and its findings are consistent with a recent meta-analysis from the Early Breast Cancer Trialists Group, which showed that taxane-based adjuvant regimens are superior to anthracycline-based regimens in terms of recurrence rate (Peto, 2007). Pooled data from another meta-analysis also showed that incorporation of taxanes into anthracycline-based regimens significantly improved both disease-free (DFS) and overall survival (OS) in patients with early-stage breast cancer (De Laurentiis et al., 2008).

2.2 Duration and sequence of neoadjuvant chemotherapy

The superior outcomes of patients who achieved favorable responses in the breast had led investigators to question whether using in-breast response as an *in vivo* chemosensitivity test and tailoring therapy accordingly may improve outcomes. GeparTrio was one of the studies that set out to answer this question. In this multicenter German study, all 2,090 patients received an initial 2 cycles of neoadjuvant TAC chemotherapy (docetaxel 75 mg/m^2, doxorubicin 50 mg/m^2, and cyclophosphamide 500 mg/m^2 every 21 days). Patients were then divided on the basis of sonographic evaluation into responders (tumor size decreased by > 50%) and nonresponders (tumor size decreased by < 50%). A third group, patients whose tumors increased in size by 25% or more, was removed from the study and treated at the discretion of their oncologist. The study continued in two parts, one evaluating a change of therapy for nonresponders, and one evaluating the optimal duration of therapy in the responders (Von Minckwitz et al., 2008).

In the first part, the 622 patients who did not respond to the initial 2 cycles of TAC chemotherapy were randomly assigned to four more cycles of TAC chemotherapy or four 21-day cycles of an NX regimen (vinorelbine 25 mg/m^2 on days 1 and 8 and capecitabine [Xeloda] 1,000 mg/m^2 orally twice daily on days 1-14). Sonographic response rate was chosen as the primary endpoint, and it should be noted that the statistical plan was based on a hypothesis of non-inferiority (rather than superiority) of NX compared to TAC. There was no difference in sonographic response rates for the two regimens, confirming the non-inferiority of NX. The rates of pCR were low for both NX and TAC, at 6.0% and 5.3%, respectively. It must be emphasized that this study did not set out to demonstrate an improvement in outcome for switching to a non- cross-resistant chemotherapy regimen, nor did it show such a difference. In the second part of the GeparTrio study, the 1,390 patients who responded to an initial 2 cycles of neoadjuvant TAC chemotherapy were randomized to either 4 or 6 further cycles of TAC pre-operatively, ie, 6 versus 8 cycles in total. The primary aim of this part of the study was to detect an increased pCR rate of 26% versus 20% in the I group receiving a longer duration of therapy. There were no significant differences in the rates of pCR (8 cycles 23.5% vs 6 cycles 21.0%, P = 0.27) or BCS (67.5% vs 68.5%, P = .68) (von Minckwitz et al., 2008). Thus, the knowledge of chemotherapy sensitivity does not appear to predict a greater benefit for more of what was already proven effective (TAC, in this case).

The Aberdeen study also assessed the potential benefit of switching chemotherapy regimens in the neoadjuvant setting, but in this case the randomization between "sticking or switching" occurred in the responders rather than the nonresponders (Smith et al., 2002). In this study, 162 patients were enrolled and received four 21-day cycles of an anthracycline chemotherapy regimen (CVAP: cyclophosphamide 1,000 mg/m^2, vincristine 1.5 mg/m^2, doxorubicin 50 mg/m^2, and prednisolone 40 mg for 5 days). The 104 patients classified as responders by clinical assessment were randomized to 4 cycles of CVAP or 4 cycles of docetaxel (100 mg/m^2 every 21 days). All 55 nonresponders received 4 cycles of docetaxel. Intention-to-treat (ITT) analysis showed that the addition of docetaxel significantly enhanced cRR in the responders, compared to continuation of CVAP (85% vs 64%, P =0 .03). The pCR rate was also superior in the docetaxel group (ITT analysis, 31% vs 15%, P =0 .06; for patients completing 8 cycles, 34% vs 16%, P =0.04). In addition, updated follow-up at 3 years indicated improved survival in the docetaxel arm, although this was not a primary endpoint of the study design and was not incorporated into statistical plan (Heys et al.,

2002). However, nonresponders also benefited from switching to docetaxel, with over half (55%) of these patients going on to achieve clinical responses, and a small proportion (2%) achieving pCRs. Neither the GeparTrio nor the Aberdeen studies therefore provide evidence of a convincing role for response (or lack thereof) to neoadjuvant chemotherapy as an *in vivo* tool for chemotherapy selection, but they suggest that most patients may benefit from exposure to a varied chemotherapy approach in the neoadjuvant setting.

2.3 Neoadjuvant endocrine therapy

A useful strategy to improve knowledge about treatment effects is the early identification of features, which are associated with response or resistance to primary therapy. Previously published studies indicated that pathological complete remission (pCR) rate was significantly higher following preoperative chemotherapy for patients whose tumors did not express estrogen receptor (ER) and progesterone receptor (PgR), compared with the receptor- positive cohort (Ring et al., 2004; Colleoni et al., 2004). Despite the significantly higher incidence of pCR achieved by preoperative chemotherapy for patients with endocrine-nonresponsive disease, the disease-free survival (DFS) was significantly worse for this cohort compared with the ER positive expression cohort in several studies (Colleoni et al., 2008).
More recently neoadjuvant endocrine therapy has emerged as an attractive alternative in postmenopausal women with large or inoperable hormone receptor positive breast cancers. Although there have been no large randomized trials comparing surgery with neoadjuvant endocrine therapy, there have been a series of studies using aromatase inhibitors (AIs) which have produced promising results. A number of large randomized trials have compared various AIs directly with tamoxifen. An important endpoint in each of these studies has been the rate at which breast conservation has been achieved. There are a number of benefits to using neoadjuvant therapy compared with primary surgery. The most obvious benefit is that women with large operable or locally advanced breast cancers can be downstaged allowing them to become operable or more suitable for less extensive surgery (Dixon & Macaskill, 2009). For instance, those who originally would have required mastectomy can often be converted to breast-conserving surgery. This is an advantage because studies have demonstrated that breast-conserving surgery followed by radiotherapy has significant psychological benefits, better cosmetic outcomes, and comparable disease control rates compared to mastectomy. There are as yet limited long-term data on patients who have had breast-conserving surgery after neoadjuvant therapy, but the results to date are reassuring. The majority of patients who are spared mastectomy with neoadjuvant endocrine therapy are elderly, but studies have shown that even in older women, if they are given the choice, they are no more likely to choose mastectomy than younger women. Neoadjuvant endocrine therapy is also an excellent treatment for older patients with estrogen receptor cancers who are unfit for surgery because of significant comorbidities. For these patients, shrinkage can allow resection under local anesthesia, or for a select group with short life expectancy, treatment with endocrine therapy can provide long-term disease control for the rest of their lives.

2.3.1 Letrozole compared with tamoxifen

The first endocrine neoadjuvant study was the P024 trial and included 337 postmenopausal women with large operable or locally advanced ER-positive and PR-positive breast cancers (Eiermann et al., 2001). All patients required mastectomy at diagnosis or were inoperable. In this study patients were randomly selected to receive 4 months of letrozole or 4 months of tamoxifen. Objective response rates (ORR) by palpation, mammography, and ultrasound were all significantly higher in the letrozole treated group. There was also a significantly higher rate of breast-conserving surgery for patients randomly assigned to receive letrozole (45% vs. 35% in the tamoxifen group; p = 0.022).

2.3.2 Anastrozole compared with tamoxifen

Two large randomized studies have compared anastrozole with tamoxifen. In the Immediate Preoperative Arimidex, Tamoxifen or Combined with Tamoxifen (IMPACT) trial, 330 patients from the UK and Germany were randomly selected to receive anastrozole alone, tamoxifen alone, or a combination for 3 months before surgery (Smith et al., 2005). The study differed from P024 in that patients who were suitable for breast-conserving surgery at the outset were enrolled. There was no significant difference seen in ORRs between the three treatments as measured by calipers and ultrasound. There was a subgroup of 124 patients who were considered to require mastectomy at baseline. Although there remained no difference in this group in ORR, a significantly higher number of women were deemed suitable for breast-conserving surgery following treatment with anastrozole, compared with tamoxifen (46% vs. 22%; p = 0.03).

In the Preoperative Arimidex Compared with Tamoxifen trial, the entry criteria was similar to the IMPACT trial, although this study also included patients who were inoperable (Cataliotti et al., 2006). This study also differed in that it included a group of patients who were given concurrent neoadjuvant chemotherapy. Randomisation was to the 202 patients treated with anastrozole alone or the 201 patients treated with tamoxifen alone for 3 months. There was no significant difference in ORR by ultrasound or caliper measurements between the different treatment arms, although there was a trend in favor of anastrozole for those patients treated with neoadjuvant endocrine therapy alone. There was a significantly higher ORR in the anastrozole group for patients whose tumors were initially assessed as requiring mastectomy or were inoperable.

A combined analysis of the two anastrozole studies included 535 patients and again failed to show any difference between treatments (Smith, 2004). There was again an overall improvement in ORR in favor of anastrozole in the subgroup of patients who were deemed to require mastectomy or be inoperable at the outset. Both were assessed by calipers (47% vs. 35%; p = 0,026) and ultrasound (36% vs. 26%; p = 0.048). A significant change in both feasible and actual surgery in favor of anastrozole was also evident for those patients who required a mastectomy or were inoperable at diagnosis.

2.3.3 Exemestane compared with tamoxifen

Several recent studies support the use of aromatase inhibitors as neoadjuvant therapy for hormone-responsive breast cancer. For example, we reported the results of a study comparing the efficacy of exemestane and tamoxifen as neoadjuvant therapy (Semiglazov et al., 2005). In that study, 151 postmenopausal women with ER-positive and/or PgR-positive breast cancer were randomly assigned to receive exemestane or tamoxifen for 3 months. Neoadjuvant treatment with exemestane significantly improved clinical objective response (76% vs 40%; P = .05) and the rate of breast-conserving surgery (37% vs 20%; P =0.05), but it did not result in any significant differences in objective response as determined by mammogram or ultrasound. Thus, exemestane is more effective than tamoxifen as a neoadjuvant treatment option for postmenopausal women with ER-positive disease.

2.3.4 Hormonal versus chemotherapy in the neoadjuvant treatment

Duration of neoadjuvant hormonal treatment for breast cancer in most studies was 3-6 months. The few studies that investigated prolonged treatment with neoadjuvant endocrine therapy suggest that a further reduction in tumour size can be achieved and that even surgery can be withheld for elderly women on continuing hormonal treatment. However, the optimum duration of neoadjuvant endocrine therapy has to be established.

For many years, primary systemic (neoadjuvant) therapy has been given before local treatment for women with locally advanced breast cancer in an effort to make such disease operable. Chemotherapy has been the mainstay of this approach, but more recently neoadjuvant endocrine therapy has emerged as an attractive alternative in post-menopausal women with large hormone receptor positive breast cancers. A number of randomized trials (like P024, IMPACT, PROACT) have compared various aromatase inhibitors directly with tamoxifen. An important endpoint in each of these studies has been the rate at which breast conservation has been achieved. The presence of steroid hormone receptors (ER and/or PR) are target for endocrine therapy. Preoperative chemotherapy may be less effective in postmenopausal patients with ER-positive and/or PR-positive tumors at least with respect to doxorubicin-containing or taxane-containing regimens. Pathological complete response (pCR) rates after chemotherapy were significantly higher among patients with tumors that were both ER-negative and PR-negative compared with patients whose tumors had any (even low) expression of steroid hormone receptors (Colleoni et al. 2004, 2008). In the ECTO I trial, pCR after neoadjuvant chemotherapy was observed in 42% of women with ER-negative tumors, compared with 12% in the ER-positive group (Gianni et al. 2009). In the NSABP B-27 study, ER-negative tumors had higher rates of pCR than ER-positive tumors when treated with neoadjuvant AC, as well as when treated with AC followed by docetaxel (Bear ., et al. 2006). Before our trial there were few, if any, direct comparisons of primary neoadjuvant endocrine therapy with primary neoadjuvant chemotherapy in patients with hormone-responsive breast cancer.

This was an open-label, randomized phase 2 trial of once-daily endocrine therapy (exemestane or anastrozole) or chemotherapy (doxorubicin and paclitaxel, every 3 week for 4 cycles) in postmenopausal women with primary ER-positive breast cancer. A total of 239 patients with ER-positive and/or PgR-positive breast cancer (T2N1-2, T3N0-1, T4N0M0) were randomly assigned to receive neoadjuvant endocrine therapy (ET) [anastrazole 1 mg/day or exemestane 25 mg/day for 3 months, 121 patients] or chemotherapy (CT) [doxorubicin 60 mg/m2 with paclitaxel 200 mg/m2, four 3-week cycles, 118 patients]. All patients were considered to be ineligible for breast-conserving surgery (BCS) at enrollment. After BCS all patients received radiotherapy (50 Gy in 25 fractions). The median follow-up time was 5.6 years.

The primary efficacy end point was already reported (Semiglazov et al., 2007). Overall response (OR=CR+PR) was similar in the endocrine therapy group (65.5%) compared with chemotherapy group (63.6%; $p>0.5$).

Interim analysis of this trial showed similar objective response in patients who were receiving exemestane and in patients who were receiving anastrazole. It allowed us to review and to analyze dates on all patients who were receiving aromatase inhibitors in the endocrine therapy group.

There was a trend toward higher overall rates of OR and breast-conserving surgery among patients with tumors expressing high levels of ER (Allred score ≥6) in the endocrine therapy compared with the chemotherapy group (43% vs 24%, $p=0.054$; Table 1).

	Endocrine Therapy	Chemotheapy	
Response, n (%)	(n=70)	(n=63)	P Value
Clinical objective response	49 (70)	38(60)	0.068
Mammography	46 (66)	38 (60)	0.088
Breast-conserving surgery	30(43)	15 (24)	0.054

*High levels of estrogen receptor expression are defined as ≥6 Allred score or ≥120 fmol/g.

Table 1. Overall Objective Response in Patients With High Levels of Estrogen Receptor Expression*

After completing neoadjuvant treatment, 31 patients (13%) did not undergo surgical resection: 12.3% of patients who were receiving endocrine therapy and 13.5% of patients who were receiving chemotherapy. Twenty-two patients did not receive surgery because of disease progression. These patients were switched to the other study therapy: patients initially treated with endocrine therapy received chemotherapy, and patients treated with chemotherapy received endocrine therapy. Progressive disease was observed in 9% of patients who were receiving endocrine therapy and 9% of patients who were receiving chemotherapy (P>0.5). Stable disease was seen in 21% of patients who were receiving endocrine treatment and 26% of patients who were receiving chemotherapy.

Analysis of BCS rates according to pretreatment characteristics showed a non-significant trend towards increased BCS in patients with clinical stage T2, ER+/PgR+, 70 years and older (p=0.054- 0.088) receiving neoadjuvant endocrine therapy.

The rate of BCS was particularly marked in patients receiving endocrine therapy, who achieved a clinical response. There was no significant difference between endocrine therapy (ET) and chemotherapy (CT) relative to the incidence of locoregional recurrences and distant metastases (8.2% and 7.6%, p=0.99; 14.8% and 15.2%, p=0.83, respectively). There was no significant difference in DFS through 5 years of follow up between the 121 patients who received neoadjuvant endocrine therapy and 118 women who received chemotherapy: 71.0% and 67.7% (p>0.5). After a median follow up of 5.6 years 35 events had been reported in the endocrine group (24 in 66 patients who underwent mastectomy and 11 in 40 patients who underwent BCS). 5-year DFS was 63.6% after mastectomy and 72.5% after BCS (p=0.076). The incidence of commonly reported adverse events was higher in patients receiving chemotherapy. No serious adverse events were reported in patients receiving endocrine therapy. Six patients receiving chemotherapy experienced febrile neutropenia leading to treatment interruption. No deaths occurred during the preoperative therapy.

Our trial has shown that preoperartive endocrine therapy with aromatase inhibitors offers the same rate of overall objective response, breast-conserving surgery, 5-years DFS as chemotherapy in postmenopausal patients with ER-positive tumors. The frequency of adverse events was higher among patients who were receiving chemotherapy. Endocrine treatment was well tolerated. Preoperative endocrine therapy with aromatase inhibitors is a reasonable alternative to preoperative chemotherapy for postmenopausal women with ER-positive disease in clinical situation in which the low toxicity of the regimen is considered an advantage. According St.Gallen recommendation (Goldhirsch et al., 2009) neoadjuvant endocrine therapy without chemotherapy was considered reasonable for postmenopausal patients with strongly receptor-positive disease. If used, such treatment should be considered for a duration of 5-8 months or until maximum tumour response.

2.4 Neoadjuvant therapy in HER2+ breast cancer

Amplification or overexpression, or both, of human epidermal growth factor receptor-2 (HER2, also known as ERBB2), a transmembrane receptor tyrosine kinase, is present in around 22% of early breast cancers, 35% of locally advanced and metastatic tumours, and 40% of inflammatory breast cancers, and is associated with aggressive disease and poor prognosis (Ross et al., 2009). Patients with HER2-positive locally advanced or inflammatory breast cancer are therefore in particular need of effective treatment. Trastuzumab (Herceptin, Roche, Basel, Switzerland), a recombinant humanized monoclonal antibody that targets HER2, has efficacy as monotherapy (Baselga et al., 2005) and improves results of chemotherapy in patients with HER2-positive metastatic (Slamon et al., 2001; Marty et al., 2005) and early operable breast cancer (Smith et al., 2007; Romond et al., 2005; Slamon et al., 2005). It is widely approved for use as monotherapy and in combination with chemotherapy or hormone therapy in these patients, but not specifically in those with locally advanced or inflammatory breast cancer. In a pilot study, anthracycline and paclitaxel were successfully combined with trastuzumab in patients with metastastic disease (Bianchi et al., 2003). To reduce the risk of cardiac toxic effects, only three cycles of doxorubicin were given in the pilot study, which corresponds to a cumulative dose of 180 mg per m^2 of body surface area (Gianni et al., 2009). No patient developed symptomatic cardiac dysfunction, although four patients (of 16) had reversible asymptomatic decreases in left ventricular ejection fraction to 50% or lower.

The neoadjuvant Herceptin (NOAH) study was designed to assess efficacy of neoadjuvant chemotherapy with trastuzumab followed by adjuvant trastuzumab versus neoadjuvant chemotherapy alone in patients with HER2-positive locally advanced or inflammatory breast cancer. The NOAH study randomized 228 patients with centrally confirmed HER2+ locally advanced breast cancer to a chemotherapy regimen consisting of 3 cycles of doxorubicin plus paclitaxel (AT); 4 cycles of paclitaxel (T); and 3 cycles of cyclophosphamide, methotrexate, and fluorouracil (CMF), with and without trastuzumab. The addition of trastuzumab significantly improved overall response rate (81% vs 73%, P =0. 18) and pCR rates (43% vs 23%, P =0 ,002) (Gianni et al., 2010).

The primary objective was to compare event-free survival, which was defined as time from randomization to disease recurrence or progression (local, regional, distant, or contralateral) or death from any cause, in patients with HER2-positive disease treated with and without trastuzumab.

Trastuzumab significantly improved event-free survival in patients with HER2-positive breast cancer (3-year event-free survival 71% [95% CI 61-78; n=36 events] with trastuzumab, *vs* 56% [46-65; n-51 events] without; hazard ratio 0.59 [95% CI 0-38-0-90]; p-0.013). Trastuzumab was well tolerated and, despite concurrent administration with doxorubicin, only two patients (2%) developed symptomatic cardiac failure. Both responded to cardiac drugs.

The results of the NOAH study have shown that in patients with HER2-positive locally advanced or inflammatory breast cancer, addition of 1 year of trastuzumab (starting as neoadjuvant and continuing as adjuvant therapy) to neoadjuvant chemotherapy improved overall response rates, almost doubled rates of pathological complete response, and reduced risk of relapse, progression, or death compared with patients who did not receive trastuzumab. Investigators recorded a benefit of trastuzumab in all subgroups tested, including women with inflammatory disease (27% of HER2- positive patients) who benefited substantially from trastuzumab.

The results of the NOAH study consolidate those of other studies of trastuzumab in the neoadjuvant setting. In these mainly non-randomised studies, pathological complete response rates (variously defined) ranged from 17% to 73%, and were better than they were in historical' or concurrent HER2-negative controls (Gluck et al., 2008; Untch et al., 2008). One randomised trial in patients with operable non-inflammatory disease was stopped early when the pathological complete response rate in the trastuzumab group was more than twice as high as that of the control group (65% *vs* 26%) (Buzdar et al., 2005). Patient numbers in this study were small, but preliminary results from another randomized study also show a doubling in pathological complete response rate in the trastuzumab group. These response rates to primary systemic therapy are a surrogate for relapse-free and overall survival in patients who were unselected for HER2 status.

Despite concurrent use of doxorubicin, paclitaxel, and trastuzumab in the NOAH trial, incidence of symptomatic cardiac failure was low (<2%) and less than was expected (2.8-4.1%) on the basis of adjuvant trials in which trastuzumab was given concurrently with paclitaxel after completion of doxorubicin and when trastuzumab was given as monotherapy after completion of a range of cytotoxic regimens (2%). These findings support the accumulating evidence that trastuzumab can be given concurrently with anthracyclines with a low frequency of symptomatic cardiac dysfunction, provided that low cumulative doses or less cardiotoxic anthracyclines are used, and careful cardiac monitoring is done.

The addition of trastuzumab to neoadjuvant sequential anthracycline-taxane chemotherapy (with and without capecitabine) was also investigated in the phase III GeparQuattro study, and led to a doubling of pCR rates (31.8% vs 15.4%, P <0.001) (Von Minckwitz et al., 2008). With the emergence of lapatinib (Tykerb), a dual tyrosine kinase inhibitor against HER1 and HER2, the CALGB is conducting a randomized phase III trial to evaluate paclitaxel with trastuzumab or lapatinib, or both in the preoperative setting. Several other trials are ongoing to evaluate these 2 drugs in the neoadjuvant setting, including Neo-ALTTO (Neoadjuvant Lapatinib and/or Trastuzumab Treatment Optimization) in phase III and CHERLOB in phase II.

Trastuzumab (H) in combination with chemotherapy improves outcomes in patients with HER2-positive breast cancer and is integral to the standards of care for these patients. However, in some patients disease progression still occurs. Pertuzumab (P) and trastuzumab (H) target different epitopes of HER2, and their use in combination has demonstrated improvement in response rates. NEOSPHERE study (Gianni et al., 2011) assessed the efficacy and safety of pertuzumab added to trastuzumab-based neoadjuvant chemotherapy in women with HER2-positive operable, locally advanced/inflammatory breast cancer who had not received prior cancer therapy.

Patients (n = 417) with HER2-positive (IHC3+ or IHC2+ and FISH/CISH+) breast cancer were randomized 1:1:1:1 to receive 4 neoadjuvant cycles of docetaxel (T) plus H, THP, HP or TP. Pertuzumab (P) was given at a loading dose of 840 mg and 420 mg maintenance, trastuzumab (H) at a loading dose of 8mg/kg and 6 mg/kg maintenance, and docetaxel (T) at 75 mg/m^2 with escalation to 100 mg/m^2 if tolerated in a 3weekly schedule. The primary endpoint was pCR in the breast.

About 40% of patients had locally advanced/inflammatory breast cancer and approximately 50% were ER/PR negative. THP combination (docetaxel + trastuzumab + pertuzumab) significantly improved the pCR rate compared with TH (docetaxel + trastuzumab) alone: 45.8% (95% CI 36.1-55.7) vs 29.0% (95% CI 20.6-38.5), p = 0.0141. Patients receiving THP (docetaxel + trastuzumab + pertuzumab) had the highest pCR rate regardless of ER/PR status, although the greatest treatment benefit in all 4 arms was observed in ER/PR-neg patients. The chemotherapy-free HP (trastuzumab+pertuzumab) arm achieved a pCR rate of 16.8%. THP (docetaxel + trastuzumab + pertuzumab) had a similar safety profile to TH. The incidence of AEs was lowest in the HP (trastuzumab+pertuzumab) arm.

Thus, the addition of pertuzumab to trastuzumab-based neoadjuvant chemotherapy resulted in a significant improvement of the pCR rate with no new safety signals of concern. Pertuzumab and trastuzumab have complementary mechanisms of action as pertuzumab inhibits HER2:HER3 heterodimerisation, thereby providing a potential mechanism to overcome tumour escape. These results support the rationale for a planned Phase III, double-blind, placebo-controlled trial evaluating pertuzumab added to standard trastuzumab-based therapy in women with HER2- positive breast cancer.

Despite the dramatic improvement in the outcome of HER2+ breast cancers since the widespread use of HER2-directed therapies, such as trastuzumab, patients continue to develop recurrences and disease progression. The mechanisms of intrinsic and acquired resistance to trastuzumab are likely multifactorial and are being exploited by the use of novel targeted agents in clinical development. The phosphoinositide-3-kinase (PI3K) pathway plays a key role in resistance to trastuzumab through increased signaling through upstream growth factor receptors, PTEN mutations, and other mechanisms, and therefore, is an excellent target for drug development in patients with trastuzumab-resistant, HER2+ breast cancers. Available clinical trials demonstrate encouraging activity of mTOR inhibitors in combination with trastuzumab monotherapy or trastuzumab-based chemotherapy in patients with $HER2^{+}$ metastatic breast cancer pretreated with trastuzumab with or without lapatinib. The results of early-stage clinical trials are currently being confirmed in 2 large phase III trials (Brachman et al., 2009; Vazguez-Martin et al., 2009). Other agents, targeting the PI3K pathway, are in early clinical development for HER2+ breast cancers.

Cross-talk between the estrogen receptor (ER) and the phosphoinositide-3-kinase (PI3K)/Akt/mammalian target of rapamycin (mTOR) pathways is a mechanism of resistance to endocrine therapy, and blockade of both pathways enhances antitumor activity in preclinical models. Study of Baselga et al.(2009) explored whether sensitivity to letrozole was enhanced with the oral mTOR inhibitor, everolimus (RAD001). Response rate by clinical palpation in the everolimus arm was higher than that with letrozole alone (ie, placebo; 68.1% v 59.1%), which was statistically significant at the preplanned, one-sided, α=0.1 level (P=0.062). Marked reduction in progesterone receptor and cyclin D1 expression occurred in both treatment arms, and dramatic downregulation of phosphor-S6 occurred only in the everolimus arm. An antiproliferative response, as defined by a reduction in Ki67 expression to natural logarithm of percentage positive Ki67 of less than 1 at day 15, occurred in 52 (57%) of 91 patients in the everolimus arm and in 25 (30%) of 82 patients in the placebo arm (P<0.01).

The exact mechanism by which mTOR inhibitors appear to reverse resistance to trastuzumab remains unclear. Future clinical trials should attempt to delineate these mechanisms so that patients can be selected appropriately for these therapeutic approaches.

2.5 Triple-negative breast cancer

Triple-negative (ER-negative, PgR-negative, and HER2 receptor-negative) breast cancers (TNBC) account for approximately 15% of all breast cancers and, though in and of itself it is a heterogeneous group, it often exhibits an aggressive phenotype with a generally poor prognosis. Unlike HER2+ or hormone receptor- positive breast cancers, triple-negative tumors lack an established therapeutic target and though initially responsive to many standard treatment regimens, progression and recurrence can be rapid and refractory to alternative approaches. Loss or inactivation of breast cancer type 1 (***BRCA1***) leads to defects in certain DNA repair pathways. Most ***BRCA1*** mutant breast cancers lack ER, PgR, and HER2 expression, and this association has raised the question of defective ***BRCA1*** function in sporadic (non-familial) TNBC (Sorlie et al., 2003). This led to the hypothesis that triple-negative tumors may be more sensitive to DNA damaging agents, such as platinums. A retrospective analyses of patients with triple-negative breast cancer who received taxane/ platinum-based primary chemotherapy demonstrated an overall response of 39% (Uhm et al., 2009), while studies of platinum monotherapy or combinations in the neoadjuvant setting have produced pCR rates of 22%-50% (Garber et al., 2006; Chang et al., 2008).

To exploit the defective DNA repair mechanisms in triple-negative and BRCA-deficient breast cancers, recent trials investigated the effect of interfering further with DNA repair through the use of novel small molecule inhibitors of poly-ADP ribose polymerase (PARP). This is a critical enzyme in cell proliferation and DNA repair. Results from several preliminary trials have been reported. The first was a phase II trial which evaluated the oral PARP inhibitor, olaparib, as a single agent as second- or later-line therapy in 54 patients with locally advanced or metastatic BRCA-deficient breast cancer (Tutt et al., 2009). Despite this use of olaparib as a single agent in a pretreated population, a response rate of41% was reported for patients receiving the higher of 2 evaluated doses.

One of the key issues related to interpretation of trials investigating triple-negative breast cancer is the heterogeneity of this tumor subtype. Although most basal-like tumors are also triple-negative, there is discordance between triple-negative designation on clinical assays and basal-like breast cancer on gene expression arrays (Schneider et al., 2008). There is also heterogeneity within triple-negative breast cancer regarding expression of p53, *BRCA1*, and other relevant genes. Thus, there is danger in making clinical decisions based on cross- trial comparisons, as the patient populations are not identical and the definition of triple-negative breast cancer or basal-like breast cancer differs across studies. Additionally, subset analyses with non-centralized review of tumor markers should be interpreted with caution since a substantial percentage of patients may not have triple-negative disease based on incorrect classification. Prospective trials with carefully defined triple-negative status using validated biomarker analysis are necessary to optimize the use of targeted therapy in this patient population.

2.6 Molecular profiling in prognosis and patient selection for neoadjuvant systemic therapy

Gene expression profiling with the use of DNA microarrays has added valuable information to our understanding of breast cancer biology. In the seminal work of Perou et al. (2011) the ability to interrogate thousands of genes at the same time was translated into a "molecular portrait" of each tumor sample studied, and the concomitant analysis of the individual molecular portraits of breast cancer tumor samples made the definition of molecular subtypes of breast cancer possible (Perou et al., 2011). In order to analyze this large quantity of information (thousands of genes per sample evaluated), a hierarchical clustering method was used to group genes according to similar patterns of expression. The proposed molecular classification of breast cancer was divided into five classes: luminal-A, luminal-B, basal-like, HER2-positive and normal-like tumors (Sotiriou et al., 2003; Sorlie et al., 2003). Subsequently, the correlation between molecular subtypes and clinical data have shown a significant difference in overall survival between the subtypes.

Despite this progress, the clinical applicability of molecular classification is limited by the tight correlation between the molecular subtypes and currently available immunohistochemical markers (ER, PR, HER2, Ki67) (Sotiriou & Pusztai, 2009). For example, the molecular subtype HER2-positive is clinically detected by IHC or fluorescent in situ hybridization (FISH) according to published guidelines (Sauter et al., 2009). Although a good correlation has been established between the molecular subtype HER2 and clinically assessed HER2-positive breast cancer, the opposite is not true, because 30% of HER2-positive breast cancers are molecularly characterized as luminal-B (Cheang et al., 2009). Luminal-A and luminal-B molecular subtypes are, by definition, hormone receptor positive tumors, but the distinction between these two subtypes is controversial.

One of the proposed clinical definitions characterizes luminal-A and luminal-B tumors using hormone receptor status, HER2 status and the Ki67 index (percentage of Ki67-positive nuclei by IHC). Luminal-A is defined as being ER- and/or PR-positive, HER2-negative and Ki67-low (Ki67 index < 14%). Luminal-B is defined as ER- and/or PR- positive, HER2-negative and Ki67-high (Ki67 index > 14%). Another luminal-B subtype has also been proposed, namely luminal HER2 enriched, with tumors being ER- and/or PR- positive, HER2-positive and Ki67-high (ki67 index > 14%) (Perou, 2011).

Study Jinno et al (2011) was to evaluate the clinical utility of breast cancer intrinsic subtypes in the prediction of pathological complete response (pCR) in a cohort of breast cancer patients receiving neoadjuvant chemotherapy.

Patients with stage II/III breast cancer received 4 cycles of chemotherapy XT (capecitabine 1650mg/m^2 on days 1-14 and docetaxel 60mg/m on day 8 every 3 weeks), followed by 4 cycles of FEC (fluorouracil 500 mg/m^2, epirubicin 90mg/m^2, cyclophosphamide 500mg/m^2). Immunohistochemical (IHC) analysis of ER, PgR, HER2. EGFR, cito-ceratine 5/6. and Ki67 was performed in core needle biopsy samples at baseline. Tumors were classified as luminal A (ER+ and/or PgR+, and Ki67<20%), Luminal B (ER+ and PgR+, and Ki67 > 20%). Luminal-HER2 (ER+ and/or PgR+, and HER2+), HER2-enriched (ER- PgR-, and HER2+), or triple-negative (ER-, PgR-, and HER2-). Triple-negative tumors with and without EGFR+ and/or cito-ceratine 5/6+ were further classified as basal-like and non-basal-like TN (NBTN), respectively. Pathologic complete response (pCR) was defined as no microscopic evidence of residual viable tumor cells, invasive or noninvasive, in all resected specimens of the breast. Twenty-six (31.3%) patients were classified as luminal A, 12 (14.5%) were luminal B, 15 (18.1%) were luminal-HER2, 9 (10.8%) were HER2, 10 (12.0%) were basal-like, and 11 (13.3%) were NBTN. The overall response rate was 90.4%, including a complete response in 30 patients and a partial response in 45 patients. The overall pCR rate was 15.5% (12/83). The highest pCR rate (40.0%) was observed in patients with basal- like tumors. In triple-negative patients, basal-like patients showed significantly higher pCR rate than NBTN patients (40.0% vs. 9.1%. p = 0.01). There were no cases with pCR in a cohort of luminal-

HER2 subtype patients. A higher proportion of luminal B patients had pCR than luminal A patients (25.0% vs. 3.8%, p = 0.01). Data indicate that breast cancer subtypes are useful predictive biomarkers of pCR in breast cancer patients treated with neoadjuvant systemic chemotherapy.

Despite advances, 20% to 30% of patients with early breast cancers will experience relapse with distant metastatic disease. Risk of recurrence is influenced by stage at initial presentation and the underlying biology of the tumor. Tumor size, nodal involvement, grade, lymphovascular invasion, and estrogen receptor (ER) and human epidermal growth factor receptor 2 (HER2) status are all independent risk factors for relapse (Chia et al., 2008). However, we do not have a comprehensive understanding of the patterns of spread and specific sites of recurrence.

The objectives of the study by Kennecke et al. (2010) were to determine the influence of breast tumor molecular subtypes on site of metastatic disease and to define the associated patient outcomes using a large validated tissue microarray (TMA) of primary invasive breast cancer specimens. Ten-year survival estimates were significantly different (P <0.001) among subgroups; 70% of patients with luminal A tumors were alive at 10 years compared with 54.4% of luminal B, 46.1% of luminal/ HER2, 48.1% of HER2-enriched, 52.6% of basal-like, and 62.6% of nonbasal triple negative (TN) patients. Median duration of survival from time of first distant metastasis also differed significantly, with luminal A patients achieving the longest survival (2.2 years) followed by luminal B (1.6 years), luminal/HER2+ (1.3 years), HER2-enriched (0.7 years), basal- like (0.5 years), and triple-negative (TN) nonbasal patients (0.9 years; P <0 .001). These differences in relapse according to subtype were maintained with 15-year distant relapse rates for luminal A (27.8%), luminal B (42.9%), luminal/HER2 (47.9%), HER2-enriched (51.4%), basal-like (43.1%) and TN nonbasal (35.1%) subgroups.

The study by Kennecke et al. (2010) demonstrates important differences in metastatic behavior between the breast cancer subtypes as defined by a panel of immunohistochemical markers and contributes to an expanding knowledge of prognostic and predictive markers that will allow individualized therapy for advanced breast cancer similar to current approaches in development for early-stage disease.

In the article by Voduc et al. (2010) a six-marker immunohistochemical panel (ER, PR, HER2, epidermal growth factor receptor, CK 5/6, and Ki-67) was used to classify nearly 3,000 patients treated with breast conserving surgery (BCS) and radiation therapy (RT) or mastectomy as luminal-A, luminal-B, luminal-HER2, HER2-enriched, basal-like, and triple-negative nonbasal. The intrinsic molecular subtype was successfully determined in 2,985 tumors. The median follow-up time was 12 years, and there have been a total of 325 local recurrences and 227 regional lymph node recurrences. Luminal A tumors (ER or PR positive, HER2 negative, Ki-67 < 14%) had the best prognosis and the lowest rate of local or regional relapse. For patients undergoing breast conservation, HER2-enriched and basal subtypes demonstrated an increased risk of regional recurrence, and this was statistically significant on multivariable analysis. After mastectomy, luminal B, luminal-HER2, HER2-enriched, and basal subtypes were all associated with an increased risk of local and regional relapse on multivariable analysis.

In a second important study assessing molecular profiling using an alternative classification scheme for risk assessment of locoregional relapse (LRR) in breast cancer, Mamounas et al. (2010) evaluated the 21-gene profile (Oncotype DX), in more than 1,500 patients with node-negative ER-positive disease from National Surgical Adjuvant Breast and Bowel Project studies treated by breast-conserving surgery (BCS) plus radiotherapy (RT) or mastectomy without RT. In the patients treated with mastectomy, a high recurrence score (RS) was associated with a significantly higher risk of local-regional recurrence (LRR). The results demonstrated that patients with node-negative ER- positive disease and a high 21 -gene recurrence score, particularly those patients younger than 50 years, had a relatively high risk of LRR with mastectomy without radiotherapy (RT), suggesting that the 21-gene profile test may identify a cohort of patients with lymph node-negative disease who may potentially benefit from postmastectomy RT. Given that this study was a retrospective analysis, it will be important to validate these data in another data set before changing standard treatment recommendations. In contrast, it appears that the low LRR rate in ER-positive patients with a low 21-gene recurrence score is comparable to the low LRR rate in the luminal-A group identified in the Voduc et al. (2010) study and it is likely that a majority of these patients with low recurrence scores have tumors that would be categorized as luminal-A tumors.

In addition to larger validation studies and companion molecular protocols linked to clinical trials evaluating molecular profiling in locoregional management of breast cancer, there is a need for additional basic research to identify molecular profiles that consistently predict for locally aggressive disease. It should be noted that both classification schemes (the 21-gene recurrence score and the luminal/HER2/basal scheme) are derived from years of research demonstrating the potential of these markers in risk assessment for metastasis and overall survival. While locoregional relapse and systemic metastasis are clearly linked, risk factors and potential molecular profiles, which best predict for locoregional relapse, may be quite different from those molecular profiles that predict for systemic metastasis.

It appears from both the Voduc et al. (2010) study and the Mamounas et al. (2010) study that patients with favorable luminal-A tumors or those with a low 21-gene recurrence score are at low risk for both local relapse and systemic disease. Patients with basal-like tumors, which are clearly at high risk for systemic metastasis, may also have an increased risk for local-regional recurrence (LRR) after surgical and radiotherapy (RT) treatment.

Although the proposed classification allows for broader application, due to the widespread use of IHC, some inherent limitations raise concern: IHC evaluation is limited by interobserver variability, qualitative readouts and technical reproducibility (Oyama et al., 2007).

2.7 Prognostic utility of multigene assays

The 21-gene recurrence score (RS) assay and 70-gene signature demonstrated prognostic utility in patients with both node-negative and node-positive early-stage, hormone receptor-positive breast cancer (Sotiriou & Pusztai, 2009). Neither assay has been validated nor demonstrated prognostic utility in hormone receptor-negative breast cancer. Both the 21-gene and 70-gene assays also provide additional information for treatment decision-making beyond algorithms based on standard clinicopathologic criteria such as Adjuvant-Online (Albain et al., 2009). Although the original validation of the 21-gene RS assay established its prognostic ability in patients treated with adjuvant tamoxifen, a recent study demonstrated similar prognostic ability in patients who received an aromatase inhibitor as upfront adjuvant therapy (Dowsett et al., 2008). For both prognosis and prediction, only the 21-gene RS assay has been studied with specimens from phase III adjuvant therapy trials (Albain et al., 2009, 2010).

The ability of Genomic Grade Index (GGI) to predict response to neoadjuvant chemotherapy was evaluated in 229 tumor samples collected before neoadjuvant chemotherapy with paclitaxel, fluorouracil, doxorubicin and cyclophosphamide (T/FAC) (Liedtke et al., 2009). In general, pathologic complete response (pCR) is associated with better disease outcome regardless of hormone receptor status (Guarneri et al., 2006). Histologic grade is known to be a predictor of pathologic complete response, but inherent limitations to histological grade assessment limits its applicability.

In the evaluation of GGI as a predictor of response, a more precise method for evaluating pathologic response called residual cancer burden (RCB) was used as a comparator (Symmans & Peintiger, 2007). RCB better defines different ranges of pathologic response after neoadjuvant chemotherapy. It is calculated as continuous variable, using pathologic measurements of the primary tumor and nodal metastases. In post-treatment surgical resection specimens a bidimensional diameter of primary tumor bed and the proportion of invasive tumor cells in the same area are measured. The number of nodes containing metastases and the diameter of the large lymph node metastases are also components of RCB. The prognostic information obtained with RCB was evaluated in 382 patients treated with neoadjuvant chemotherapy. In a multivariate analysis containing age, clinical stage, hormone receptor status, hormone treatment and pathologic response (pCR versus residual disease), RCB was an important prognostic factor associated with distant relapse-free survival (HR = 2.50; 95% CI 1.70-3.69; $p < 0.001$). Minimal residual cancer burden (RCB-I) and pCR (RCB-0) were associated with similar favourable long-term relapse-free prognosis. RCB adds to a better understanding of response to primary chemotherapy.

In the evaluation of GGI compared to RCB to predict chemotherapy response, a data set comprising 229 samples from 132 ER-positive and 97 ER-negative patients was used. All patients had HER2 non-amplified tumors, which avoided the interference of chemotherapy and trastuzumab response. Pathologic response was assessed as follows: RCB- 0 indicating pCR, and RCB-I, RCB-II, RCB-III for minimal, intermediate and extensive residual disease respectively. GGI was assessed for each tumor sample and assigned as low or high risk, as in the original publication, but also as a continuous variable. The GGI evaluation characterized 84.6% of grade 1 tumors as low risk and 88.3% of grade 3 as high risk. The histological grade 2 group was divided into 62.7% low risk and 37.3% high risk. For the ER-positive and ER-negative subgroups, 44.8% and 89.6% respectively were assigned to the GGI high-risk category. For the overall group treated with neoadjuvant T/FAC, high-risk GGI was associated with higher response than low-risk GGI (40% versus 12%; $p < 0.001$). A positive correlation was observed between GGI high-risk category and the level of observed response to neoadjuvant chemotherapy, with 85.8% of patients with RCB-0 or RCB-I, characterized as GGI high-risk (Metzger et al., 2010).

The similar outcome predictions between the different signatures motivated a search for underlying biologic processes that could be represented by different genes in non-overlapping signatures. A large meta-analysis of publicly available breast cancer gene expression and clinical data evaluated the contribution of known biological processes to the performance of different gene signatures. "Coexpression modules" for ER signaling, ERBB2 amplification and proliferation were generated, putting together a comprehensive list of genes with highly correlated expression (Metzger et al., 2010). The meta-analysis was able to confirm in 2833 patients that the initial classification of breast cancer molecular subtypes was highly conserved, with the exception of normal-like breast cancer, which could not be identified.

In all breast cancer subtypes (HER2, basal-like, luminal-A, luminal-B) the coexpression module proliferation was the most important determinant of prognosis. Although the coexpression module HER2 could be identified in the subtype HER2, the prognostic information was mainly driven by genes related to proliferation. HER2 and basal-like subtypes were consistently characterized as high proliferative tumors. In the luminal subtypes, the module of genes related to proliferation could divide this group into a low-proliferative subtype (A) with better prognosis and a highly proliferative group with poorer prognosis (B). The evaluation of clinical variables demonstrated that tumor size and nodal status still have independent prognostic value and need to be evaluated together with the information obtained from gene-signatures.

Understanding breast cancer molecular heterogeneity has made it possible to develop gene signatures that can be applied to predict prognosis and response to therapies in daily practice. The superiority of gene signatures to classic histopathologic variables is related to their ability to better define a greater proportion of low-risk patients that do not need to be treated with systemic neoadjuvant and adjuvant therapy, while still correctly identifying those patients who fall into a high-risk group. Clinical variables related to the measurement of tumor progression such as tumor size and nodal involvement remain significantly associated with prognosis and should therefore continue to be evaluated in conjunction with gene signatures.

3. Conclusion

Neoadjuvant systemic therapy is an appropriate management strategy in certain well-defined patient cohorts, namely those in whom surgery is not feasible due to locally advanced disease at presentation; patients with large tumors requiring mastectomy, but wishing for breast conservation; and patients participating in clinical trials. Neoadjuvant therapy does not improve the outcomes in terms of disease-free survival or overall survival (OS), compared with adjuvant systemic treatment, and should not be chosen with this intent. There is currently no evidence to support deviating from a planned neoadjuvant regimen by changing drugs based on the observed response.

Advances in the understanding of breast cancer tumor biology have greatly increased the assessment of patient prognosis, as well as which patients most benefit from neoadjuvant chemotherapy or endocrine therapy. The current challenge is how to best merge multigene assays with clinical biologic variables to achieve classifiers with even greater predictive utility. The enhanced knowledge of breast cancer biologic heterogeneity has also led to the development and clinical investigation of novel therapeutics aimed at cell function and essential signaling pathways. These agents are already producing survival benefits in patients with early-stage or advanced disease. However, many questions remain regarding the appropriate use of these compounds, including optimal patient selection, preventing and overcoming resistance, and management of associated toxicities. Furthermore, there is increased attention to the need to block multiple targets simultaneously to optimize response and overcome resistance that results from signaling pathway cross-talk.

Finally, multiple biomarkers of response have been evaluated and show promise, but are not yet ready for routine clinical use.

4. Acknowledgment

We thank Dr. Garik Dashan for the preparation of the references.

5. References

Albain, K., Paik, S. & van't Veer, L. (2009). Prediction of adjuvant chemotherapy benefit in endocrine responsive, early breast cancer using multigene assays. *Breast;* Vol. 18 (suppl 3), pp.141-145, ISSN 0960-9766.

Albain, K., Barlow, W. & Shak, S. (2010). Prognostic and predictive value of the 21-gene recurrence score assay in postmenopausal women with node-positive, oestrogen-receptor-positive breast cancer on chemotherapy: a retrospective analysis of a randomized trial. *Lancet Oncol,* Vol. 11, pp. 55-65, ISSN 1470-2045.

Albain, K., Carey, L., Gradishar, W., Gralow, J. & Lipton, A. (2010). Proceedings of the First Global Workshop on Breast Cancer : Pathways to the Evalution and Clinical Development of Novel Agents for Breast Cancer. *Clinical Breast Cancer,* Vol. 10 (N6 December), pp. 421 - 439, ISSN 1526-8209.

Baselga, J., Carbonell, X. & Castaneda-Soto, N. (2005). Phase II study of efficacy, safety, and pharmacokinetics of trastuzumab monotherapy administered on a 3-weekly schedule. *J Clin Oncol,* Vol. 23, pp. 2162-2171, ISSN 0732-183x

Baselga, J., Semiglazov, V., Van Dam, P., Manikhas, A. & Bellet, M. (2009). Phase II Randomized Study of Neoadjuvant Everolimus Plus Letrozole Compared With Placebo Plus Letrozole in Patients With Estrogen Receptor-Positive Breast Cancer. *Journal of Clinical Oncology,* Vol 27, No 16 (June 1), pp. 2630-2637, ISSN 0732-183x

Bear, H., Anderson, S. & Smith, R. (2006). Sequential preoperative or postoperative docetaxel added to preoperative doxorubicin plus cyclophosphamide for operable breast cancer: National Surgical Adjuvant Breast and Bowel Project Protocol B-27. *J. Clin Oncol,* Vol. 24, pp. 2019-2027, ISSN 0732-183x

Bianchi, G., Albanell, J. & Eiermann, W. (2003). Pilot trial of trastuzumab starting with or after the doxorubicin component of a doxorubicin plus paclitaxel regimen for women with HER2-positive advanced breast cancer. Clin. Cancer Res. Vol. 9, pp. 5944-5951, ISSN 1078-0432

Bonadonna, G., Valagussa, P. & Bramilla, C. (1998). Primary chemotherapy in operable breast cancer: eight-year experience at the Milan Cancer Institute. *J Clin. Oncol,* Vol. 16, pp. 93-100, ISSN 0732-183x

Brachmann, S., Hofmann, I. & Schnell, C. (2009). Specific apoptosis induction by the dual PI3K/mTOR inhibitor NVP-BEZ235 in HER2 amplified and PIK3CA mutant breast cancer cells. *Proc Natl Acad Sci USA,* Vol. 106, pp. 22299-22304, ISSN 0027-8424

Buzdar, A.; Ibrahim, N., Francis, D., Booser, D., Thomas, E. & Theriault, R. (2005). Significantly higher pathological complete remission(PCR) rate after neoadjuvant therapy with trastuzumab, paclitaxel and epirubicin chemotherapy: Results of a randomized trial in human epidermal growth factor receptor 2–positive operable breast cancer. *J.Clin Oncol.* Vol. 23. pp.3676–3685, ISSN 0732-183x

Cataliotti, L., Buzdar, A. & Noguchi, S. (2006). Comparison of Anastrozole versus Tamoxifen as Preoperative Therapy in Postmenopausal Women with Hormone Receptor-Positive Breast Cancer: The Pre-operative «Arimidex» Compared to Tamoxifen (PROACT) Trial. *Cancer.* Vol. 106, №10, pp. 2095-2103, ISSN 0008-543x

Chang, H., Slamon, D. & Gornbein, J. (2008). Preferential pathologic complete response (Pcr) by triple-negative (-) breast cancer to neoadjuvant docetaxel (T) and carboplatin (C.). *J. Clin. Oncol.*, Vol. 26 (15 suppl), p 31s (abstract 604), ISSN 0732-183x

Cheang, M., Chia, S. & Voduc, D. (2009). Ki67 Index, HER2 Status, and Prognosis of Patients with luminal B Breast Cancer. *J Natl Cancer Inst*, Vol. 101, pp. 736-50, ISSN 0027-8874

Chia, S., Norris, B. & Speers, C. (2008). Human epidermal growth factor receptor 2 overexpression as a prognosis factor in a large tissue microarray series of node-negative breast cancers. *J. Clin. Oncol*, Vol. 26, pp. 5697-5704, ISSN 0732-183x

Colleoni, M., Viale, G. & Zahrieh, D. (2004). Chemotherapy is more effective in patients with breast cancer not expressing steroid hormone receptors: a study of preoperative treatment. *Clin Cancer Res*, Vol. 10, pp. 6622-6628, ISSN 1078-0432.

Colleoni, M., Viale, G., Zahrieh, D., Bottiglieri, L., Gelber, R., Veronesi, P., Balduzzi, A., Torrisi, R., Luini, A., Intra, M., Dellapasqua, S., Cardillo, A., Ghisini, R., Peruzzotti, G. & Goldhirsch, A. (2008). Expression of ER, RgR, HER1, HER2, and response: a study of preoperative chemotherapy. *Ann. of Oncology*, Vol. 19, N.3. (March 2008), pp. 465-472, ISSN 0923-7534.

De Laurentis, M., Cancello, G. & D'Agostino, D. (2008). Taxane-based combinations as adjuvant chemotherapy of early breast cancer: a meta-analysis of randomized trials. *J. Clin Oncol*, Vol. 26, pp. 44-53, ISSN 0732-183x

Dixon, M. & Macaskill, J. (2009). Neoadjuvant Endocrine Therapy. *ASCO educational book*, 2009. pp. 39-43

Dowsett, M., Cuzich, J. & Wales, C. (2008). Risk of distant recurrence using Oncotype-DX in postmenopausal primary breast cancer patients treated with anastrazole or tamoxifen: a TransATAC study. *Presented at: the San Antonio Breast Cancer Symposium*. Abstract 53.

Early Breast Cancer Trialists' Collaborative Group (2005). Effects of chemotherapy and hormonal therapy for early breast cancer on recurrence and 15-year survival: an overview of the randomized trials. *Lancet*, Vol. 365, pp. 1687-1717, ISSN 0140-6736.

Eiermann, W., Paepke, S. & Appfelstaedt, J. (2001). Preoperative treatment of postmenopausal patients with letrozole: a randomized double-blind multicenter study. *Ann Oncol*, Vol. 12, pp. 1527-1532, ISSN 0923-7534

Fisher, B., Bryant, J. & Wolmark, N. (1998). Effect of preoperative chemotherapy on the outcome of women with operable breast cancer. *J Clin Oncol*, Vol. 16, pp. 2672-2685, ISSN 0732-183x

Garber, JE., Richardson, A. & Harris, L. (2006). Neo-adjuvant cisplatin (CDDP) in «triple-negative» breast cancer (BC). *Breast Cancer Res Treat*, Vol. 100 (suppl 1), S 149 (abstract 3074), ISSN 0167-6806.

Gianni, L., Baselga, J., Eiermann, W., Porta, J. & Semiglazov, V. (2009). Phase III trial evaluating the addition of paclitaxel to doxorubicin followed by cyclophosphamide, metotrexate and fluorouracil as adjuvant or primary systemic therapy: European Cooperative Trial in Operable Breast Cancer. *J Clin Oncol*, Vol 27, No 15 (May 2009), pp 2474-2481, ISSN 0732-183X

Gianni, L., Eiermann, W., Semiglazov, V., Manikhas, A. & Lluch, A. (2010). Neoadjuvant chemotherapy with trastuzumab, followed by adjuvant trastuzumab versus neoadjuvant chemotherapy alone, in patients with HER-positive, locally advanced breast cancer (the NOAH trial): a randomized controlled superiority trial with a parallel HER2-negative cohort. *The Lancet*, Vol 375, pp 377-384, ISSN 0140-6736

Gianni, L., Pienkowski, T., Roman, L., Tseng, L. & Liu, M. (2011). Addition of pertuzumab (p) to trastuzumab (H)-based neoadjuvant chemotherapy significantly improves pathological complete response in women with HER2-positive early breast cancer: result of a randomized phase II study (NEOSPHERE). *The Breast*. Vol 20, suppl 1 (March 2011), pp. 573, ISSN 0960-9776

Gluck, S., McKenna, E. Jr & Royce, M. (2008). Capecitabine plus docetaxel, with or without trastuzumab, as preoperative therapy for early breast cancer. *Int J Med Sci*. Vol 5, pp. 341-346. ISSN 1449-1907

Goldhirsch, A., Ingle, J., Gebber, R., Coates, A., Thurlimann, B. & Senn, H. (2009). *Annals of Oncology*, Vol. 20, N 4 (June 2009), pp 1133-1144, ISSN 0923-7534

Guaneri, V., Brogilio, K. & Kau, S. (2006). Prognostic value of pathologic complete response after primary chemotherapy in relation to hormone receptor status and other factors. *J Clin Oncol*, Vol. 24, pp. 1037-1044, ISSN 0732-183x

Heys, S., Hutcheon, A. & Sarkar, T. (2002). Neoadjuvant docetaxel in breast cancer: 3-year survival results from the Aberdeen trial. *Clin Breast Cancer*, Vol. 3, Suppl 2, pp. 69-74, ISSN 1526-8209

Jinno, H., Matsuda, S., Sakata, M., Hayashida, T., Takahashi, M. & Hirose, S. (2011). Differential pathologic response from primary systemic chemotherapy across breast cancer intrinsic subtypes. *The Breast*, Vol. 20, suppl 1. (March 2011), p. 39, ISSN 0960-9776.

Kaufmann, M., Hortobagyi, G. & Goldhirsch, A. (2006). Recommendations from an international expert panel on the use of neoadjuvant (primary) systemic treatment of operable breast cancer: an update. *J Clin. Oncol.* Vol. 24, pp. 1940-1949, ISSN 0732-183x

Kennecke, H., Yerushalmi, R., Woods, R., Chon, U., Cheang, R. & Voduc, D. (2010). Metastatic Behavior of Breat Cancer Subtypes. *J. Clin. Oncol.*, Vol. 28, N.20 (July 2010), pp. 3271-3272, NSSN 0732-183X

Liedtke, C., Hatzic, C. & Symmans, W. (2009). Genomic Grade Index is associated with response to chemotherapy in patients with breast cancer. *J.Clin.Oncol.*, Vol. 27, N 19 (Jul 1), pp. 3185-3191, ISSN 0732-183x

Mamounas, E., Tang, G. & Fisher, B. (2010). Association between the 21-gene recurrence score assay and risk of locoregional reccurrence in node negstive estrogen receptor positive breast cancer Results from NSAB B14 and NSABP B 20. *J Clin Oncol*, Vol. 28, pp. 1677 1683, ISSN 0732-183x

Marty, M., Cognetti, F. & Maraninchi, D. (2005). Randomized phase II trial of the efficacy and safety of trastuzumab combined with docetaxel in patients with human epidermal growth factor receptor 2-positive metastatic breast cancer administered as first-line treatment: the M77001 study group. *J. Clin.Oncol*, Vol. 23, pp. 4265-74, ISSN 0732-183x

Mauri, D., Pavlidis, N. & Ioannidis, JP. (2005). Neoadjuvant versus adjuvant systemic treatment in breast cancer: a meta-analysis. *J.Natl.Cancer Inst.* Vol. 97, N.3 (Feb. 2005), pp. 188-194, ISSN 0027-8874

Metzger, O., Ignatiadis, M. & Sotirion, C. (2010). Genomic Grade Index: an important tool for assessing breast cancer tumor grade and prognosis. *Critical Reviews in Oncology/Hematology*, Vol. 74, pp. 1-10, ISSN 1040-8428.

Oyama, T., Isshikawa, Y. & Hayashi, M. (2007). The effects of fixation, processing and evalution criteria on immunohistochemical detection of hormone receptors in breast cancer. *Breast Cancer*, Vol 14, pp. 182-188, ISSN 1340-6868

Perou, C. (2011). Molecular classification of breast cancer and its emerging clinical relevance. *The Breast*, Vol. 20, Suppl. 1 (March 2011), pp. S2-S3, ISSN 0906-9776

Peto, R (2007). *Plenary Lecture presented at the San Antonio Breast Cancer Conference*, San Antonio. TX. (December 13), http://www.sabcs.org/EnduringMaterials/Index.asp#webcast

Ring, A., Smith, I. & Ashley, S. (2004). Oastrogen receptor status, pathological complete response and prognosis in patients receiving neoadjuvant chemotharapy for early breast cancer. *Br J Cancer*, Vol. 91, pp. 2012-2017, ISSN 0007-0920

Romond, E., Perez, E. & Bryant, J. (2005). Trastuzumab plus adjuvant chemotherapy for operable HER2-positive breast cancer. *N Engl J Med*, Vol. 353, pp. 1673-1684, ISSN 1533-4406

Ross, J., Slodkowska, E., Symmans, W., Pusztai, L., Ravdin, P. & Hortobagyi, G. (2009). The HER- 2 receptor and breast cancer: ten years of targeted anti-HER-2 therapy and personalized medicine. *Oncologist*, Vol. 14, pp. 320-368, ISSN 1083-7159

Sauter, G., Lee, J. & Bartlett, J. (2009) Guidelines for human epidermal growth factor receptor 2 testing biologic and methologic consider ations. *J Clinic Oncol*, Vol. 27, pp. 1323 1333, ISSN 0732-183x

Schneider, B., Winer, E. & Foulkes, W. (2008). Triple negative breast cancer risk factors to protential targets. *Clin Cancer Res*, Vol. 14, pp. 8010-8018, ISSN 1078-0432

Scholl, S., Fourquet, A. & Asselain, B. (1994). Neoadjuvant versus adjuvant chemotherapy in premenopausal patients with tumors considered too large for breast conserving surgery preliminary results of randomised trial S6. *Eur J Cancer*, Vol. 30A, pp. 645-652

Semiglazov, V., Topuzov, E. & Bavli, J. (1994). Primary(neoadjuvant) chemotherapy and radiotherapy compared with primary radiotherapy alone in stage IIb-IIIa breast cancer. *Ann Oncol*, Vol 5, pp. 591-595, ISSN 0923-7534

Semiglazov, V., Kletsel, A. & Semiglazov, V. (2005) Exemestane (E) vs tamoxifen (T) as neoadjuvant endocrine therapy for postmenopausal women with ER+ breast cancer(T2N1-2,T3N0-1,T4N0M0)[abstract]. *J Clin Oncol ASCO Annual Meeting Proceedings [Post- Meeting Edition]*, Vol. 223 (16S), p. 530, ISSN 0732-183x

Semiglazov, V., Semiglazov, V., Dashyan, G., Ziltsova, E. & Ivanov, V. (2007). Phase II randomized trial of primary endocrine therapy versus chemotherapy in postmenopausal patients with estrogen receptor-positiv breast cancer. *Cancer*, Vol. 110, pp. 244-254, ISSN 0008-543x.

Slamon, D., Leyland-Jones, B. & Shak, S. (2001). Use of chemotherapy plus a monoclonal antibody against HER 2 for metastatic breast cancer that over expresses HER2. *N Engl J Med*, Vol. 344, pp. 783-792, ISSN 1533-4406

Slamon, D. & Eiermann, W. (2005). Phase III randomized trial comparing doxorubicin and cyclophophomide followed by docetoxel(FC-T) with doxorubicin and cyclophophomide followed by docetaxel and trastuzumab (AC-TH) with docetoxel,carboplatin and trastuzumab(TCH) in HER2 positive early breast cancer patients: BCIRG 006 study. *Breast cancer Res Treat*, Vol. 94(suppl 1), S5, ISSN 0067-6806

Smith, I., Heys, S. & Hutcheon, A. (2002) Neoadjuvant chemotherapy in breast cancer: significantly enhanced response with docetaxel. *J Clin Oncol.*, Vol. 20, pp. 1456-1466, ISSN 0732-183x

Smith, I. (2004). Anstrozole versus tamoxifen as preoperative therapy for oestrogen receptor-positive breast cancer in postmenopausal women: Combined analysis of the IMPACT and PROACT trials. *Presented at 4th European Breast cancer Conference*, Hamburg, Germany.

Smith, I., Dowsett, M. & Ebbs, S. (2005) Neoadjuvant treatment of postmenopausal breast cancer with anastrazole, tamoxifen, or both in combination: The immediate preoperative anastrazole, tamoxifen, or combined with tamoxifen(IMPACT) multicenter double-blind randomized trual. *J Clin Oncol*, Vol. 23, N 22, pp. 5018-5116, ISSN 0732-183x

Smith, I., Procter, M. & Gelber, R. (2007). For the HERA study team 2 year Follow-up of trastuzumab after adjuvant chemotherapy in HER2 - positive breast cancer. A randomized controlled trial. *Lanset*, Vol. 369, pp. 29-36, ISSN 0140-6736

Sorlie, T., Tibshirani, R. & Parker, J. (2003) Repeated observation of breast tumor subtypes in independent gene expression data sets. *Proc Natl Acad Sci USA*, Vol. 100, pp. 8418-8423, ISSN 0027-8424

Sotiriou, C., Neo, Sy. & McShane, L. (2003) Breast cancer classification and prognosis based on gene expression profiles from a population-based study. *Proc Natl Acad Sci USA*, Vol. 100, pp. 10393-10398, ISSN 0027-8424

Sotiriou, C. & Pusztai, L. (2009). Gene-expression signatures in breast cancer. *N. Engl J Med*, Vol. 360, pp. 790-800, ISSN 1533-4406

Symmans, W. & Peintiger, F. (2007) Measurement of residual breast cancer burden to predict survival afyer neoadjuvant chemotherapy. *J.Clin Oncol*, Vol 25, pp. 4414-4422, ISSN 0732-183x

Tutt, A., Robson, M. & Garber, J. (2009). Phase II trial of the oral PARP inhibitor olaparib in BRCA-deficient advanced breast cancer. *J Clin Oncol*, Vol. 27(suppl) 803s (abstract CRA501), ISSN 0732-183x

Uhm, J., Park, Y. & Yi, S. (2009). Treatment outcomes and clinicopathologic characteristics of triple-negative breast cancer patients who received platinum-containing chemotherapy. *Int J Cancer*, Vol. 124, pp. 1457-1462, ISSN 0020-7136

Untch, M., Rezai, M. & Loibl, S. (2008). Neoadjuvant treatment of HER2 overexpressing primary breast cancer with trastuzumab given concomitantly to epirubicin/cyclophosphamide followed by docetaxel±capecitabine. First analysis of efficacy and safety of the GBG/AGO multicenter intergroup-study "GeparQuattro". *6th European Breast Cancer Conference*. Berlin, Germany, April 15-19. Abstr 1LB

Vazguez-Martin, A., Oliveras-Ferreros, C. & del Barco, S. (2009). m TOR inhibitors and the anti-diabetic biguanide metphormin: new insights into the molecular management of breast cancer resistance to the HER 2 tyrosine kinase inhibitor lapatinib (Tykerb). *Clin Transl Oncol*, Vol. 11, pp. 455-459, ISSN 1699-048x

Voduc, K., Cheang, MCU. & Tyldesley, S. (2010). Breast cancer subtypes and the risk of local and regional relapse. *J Clin Oncol*, Vol. 28, pp. 1684-1691, ISSN 0732-183x

Von Minckiwitz, G., Rezai, M. & Loibl, S. (2008). Effect of trastuzumab on pathologic complete response rate of neoadjuvant EC-docetaxel treatment I HER 2-overexpressing breast cancer: Results of the phase III Gepar-Qattro study (abstract 226) .*ASCO Breast Cancer Symposium*.

Von Minckwitz, G., Kummel, S. & Vogel, P. (2008). Intensified neoadjuvant chemotherapy in early- responding breast cancer: phase III randomized GeparTrio study. *J Natl Cancer Inst*. Vol. 100, pp. 552-562, ISSN 0027-8874

Von Minckwitz, G., Kummel, S. & Vogel, P. (2008). Neoadjuvant vinorelbin- capecitobine versus docetaxel-doxorubicin-cyclophosphimide in rarly nonresponsive breast cancer: phase III randomized Gepar Trio. *J Natl Cancer Inst*. Vol. 100, pp. 542-551, ISSN 0027-8874

Wolmark, N., Wang, J., Mamounas, E., Bryant, J. & Ficher, B. (2001). Preoperative chemotherapy in patients with operable breast cancer: nine year results from National Surgical Adjuvant Breast and Bowel Project B-18. *J Natl Cancer Inst Monogr*. Vol. 30, pp. 96-102, ISSN 0027-8874

2

Neoadjuvant Therapy in Breast Cancer

Angela Lewis Traylor[1], Nathalie Johnson[1] and Esther Han[2]
[1]*Legacy Medical Group – Surgical Oncology, Legacy Cancer Services, Portland, Oregon*
[2]*Oregon Health and Sciences University, Department of Surgery*
Sam Jackson Parkway, Portland, Oregon
USA

1. Introduction

This is an exciting time we live in. As technology has advanced at lightning speed, so has molecular science and knowledge. With the mapping of the genome, a transformation in medical science has followed. Translational application of bench research to the bedside has blossomed also at an unprecedented pace. There are many new targeted agents on the horizon and future discoveries seem limitless. Although we have advanced in technology, in many ways we have not significantly changed our therapeutic treatment approach in breast cancer. The pattern of surgery first and adjuvant therapy next remains mainstream. This chapter will start by delineating traditional thoughts on systemic therapy prior to surgery as it is currently practiced and close with thoughts on where we are headed in the future.

2. Neoadjuvant chemotherapy

Historically, neoadjuvant chemotherapy (NCT) has been used in patients with locally advanced inoperable disease. More commonly, it is used in patients with operable tumors of all stages with promising outcomes. The term "neo" is Greek for new or recent, and "adjuvant" originated from Latin, and means to assist or to help. However, neoadjuvant chemotherapy is more accurately defined as primary systemic therapy. There are advantages afforded by the use of NCT, controversial issues surrounding its use, prognostic indicators of response, and some possible disadvantages.

Several randomized and non-randomized studies have evaluated the efficacy of neoadjuvant chemotherapy (Table 1)[1]. NCT allows "in-vivo" evaluation of tumor biology and an assessment of remission rate, complete response to treatment or complete pathologic response (cPR), tumor progression, and identification of chemo- resistant tumors. Complete pathologic response (cPR) has emerged as a significant predictor of tumor response and may predict long-term outcomes. Further, NCT allows down staging of tumors by decreasing tumor size and extent of tumor mass, thereby facilitating breast conservation therapy (BCT).

Neoadjuvant chemotherapy was first used in 1973 at the Milan Cancer Institute[2,3,4]. Their goal at the time of the study was to achieve prompt tumor response or shrinkage in locally advanced inoperable disease in order to facilitate the delivery of radiation therapy. Jacquillat et al. first used NCT for operable breast cancer in 1980 in Paris, France[5]. Since then there have been multiple non-randomized trials demonstrating variable response rates of

Reference	No. of Patients	Tumour Stage	Chemotherapeutic Regimen	Follow-up (months)	Overall Response (%)	Overall Survival (%)	Disease-free Survival (months)	Breast-conserving surgery (%)	pCR (%)
13	250	I-IIIB	Vinb-thi-met-FU±adr	61	71	58-95	52-100?	–	–
14	536	>2.5cm	Cyc-met-FU, FU-adr-cyc, FU-epi-cyc	96	76	69	55	85	3
15	50	6(3-12)cm*	Infusional FU-adr-cis	–	98	–	–	62#	27
16	88	II,III	Doc	–	68	–	–	72	20
17	126	T1-3, N0-2	Adr-vinc-cys-FU± met		86	–	–	85§	–
18	50	High risk, operable	Dox-vino-cyc-FU	31	88	–	–	78	22
19	100	III + inflammatory	Cyc-met-FU± thi	27	70	43 87**	28 67**	11	–
20	122	IIB-IIIB	Pac + cis	–	91	–	–	–	42

*Values are median (range). §Depending on stage at treatment (I-IIIB); #30 per cent had no surgery; § includes 33 per cent who had radiotherapy only; ¶ non-responders; **responders. pCR, pathological complete response; vinb, vinblastine; thi, thiotepa; met, methotrexate; FU, 5-flourouracil; adr, adriamycin; cyc, cyclophosphamide; epi, epirubicin; cis, ciplatin; doc, docetaxel; dox, doxorubicin; vinc, vincristine; vino, vinorelbine; tam, tamoxifen; pac, paclitaxel.

Table 1. Non-Randomized trials of Neoadjuvant Chemotherapy.[1]

large operable and inoperable tumors to NCT. The reported pCR (complete pathologic response) rates vary from 3 % to 24 %[1]. In multiple randomized clinical trials the pCR observed varies between 4% and 34 %[1].

The largest prospective randomized trial of NCT was the National Surgical Adjuvant Breast and Bowel Project (NSABP) B-18. This trial showed an overall response rate of 79%, and a pCR of 13%[6,7]. 1493 patients with operable breast cancer were stratified by age, clinical tumor size, and clinical nodal status to preoperative versus postoperative administration of Adriamycin/cyclophosphamide (AC) q 21 days x four cycles. Patients older than 50 years old were also given Tamoxifen 10mg BID x 5 years after completion of chemotherapy.

Updated results from B-18 continue to demonstrate the significant correlation between pCR and DFS. The trial also demonstrated the equivalence between preoperative and postoperative chemotherapy. Breast conservation therapy (BCT) rates were 67% versus 60%.

Another landmark trial, NSABP B-27, enrolled 2411 patients in a randomized prospective trial to compare the efficacy of docetaxel in the preoperative versus postoperative setting after neoadjuvant AC x four cycles[7]. The patients were randomized into three groups (Figure 1). All patients received Tamoxifen 20mg PO daily x 5 years.

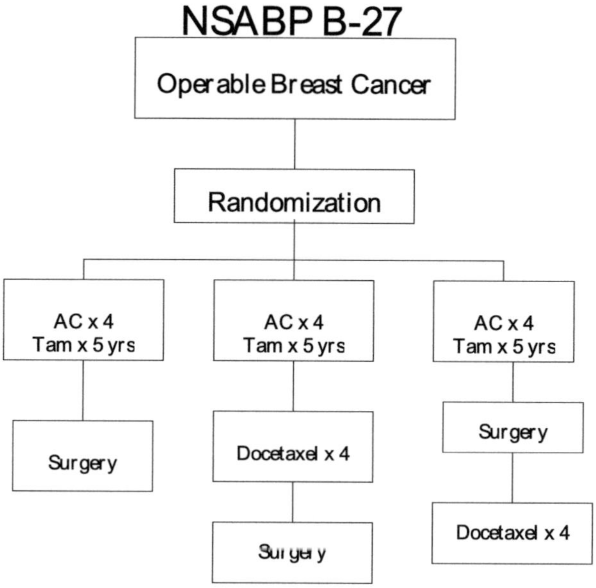

Fig. 1.[7]

The overall response rate was 91 % for those who received preoperative AC and docetaxel vs. 85.7 % for those who received preoperative AC alone ($p < 0.001$). The pCR was 26 % vs. 13.7 % ($p < 0.001$). Preoperative AC-docetaxel also significantly downstaged the axillary lymph nodes. 50.7% of the AC- alone group had negative lymph nodes vs. 58.1 % of the AC-docetaxel group ($p< 0.01$). Both B-18 and B-27 demonstrate tumor response to NCT as a significant predictor of pathologic nodal status.

Studies on tumor growth and kinetics also support the use of neoadjuvant chemotherapy[8]. Several investigators have demonstrated the inhibitory effect that the "in-situ" or undisturbed primary tumor with intact vasculature has on metastatic deposits and the development of spontaneous metastases after removal of the primary tumor[9,10]. In past studies, tumor growth was often measured grossly. However, Gunduz et al. used cytokinetic parameters to evaluate tumor growth[8]. The parameters included: Labeling index, primer-dependent DNA polymerase index or growth fraction, DNA synthesis time, and cell cycle time. It was shown that following tumor removal changes were observed, specifically, accelerated growth in the residual tumor focus within 24hrs. The labeling index and growth fraction were increased with a decrease in tumor doubling time. There was minimal change in DNA synthesis and cell cycle time. Minimal changes in these last two parameters suggest increased growth was not the result of increased DNA synthesis and cell cycle times, but increased growth secondary to conversion of non-cycling cells in G0 phase into proliferation. Could the intact or "in-situ" primary tumor cause quiescence or down regulation of non-cycling cells and thus inhibit metastatic deposits? This is a very interesting question that may be answered in future studies on NCT.

Unfortunately, NCT is not a panacea. There are a small number of patients who will have have disease progression while receiving neoadjuvant therapy. In theory, for this group, NCT may be delaying delivery of effective surgical treatment to those with chemo-resistant tumors. DeLana et al. showed six patients (5.5%) who had disease progression in response to induction chemotherapy. However, the percentage of people with disease progression remains miniscule in most studies. No patients in Jacquillat's study had disease progression[5]. In the current era of thinking of breast cancer as a systemic disease, it also begs the question as to whether or not nonresponders to NCT are a group of biologically more aggressive tumors whose outcome is poor, regardless of pre or post operative therapy.

NCT may also increase local recurrence rates in those treated with BCT. Mauriac et al. demonstrated an initial BCT rate of 63% at 34 months follow-up, which decreased to 45% at 124 months follow-up[1,11]. This effect may be partially due to the non-uniform and varied response patterns of the primary tumor to NCT (Figure 2)[12].

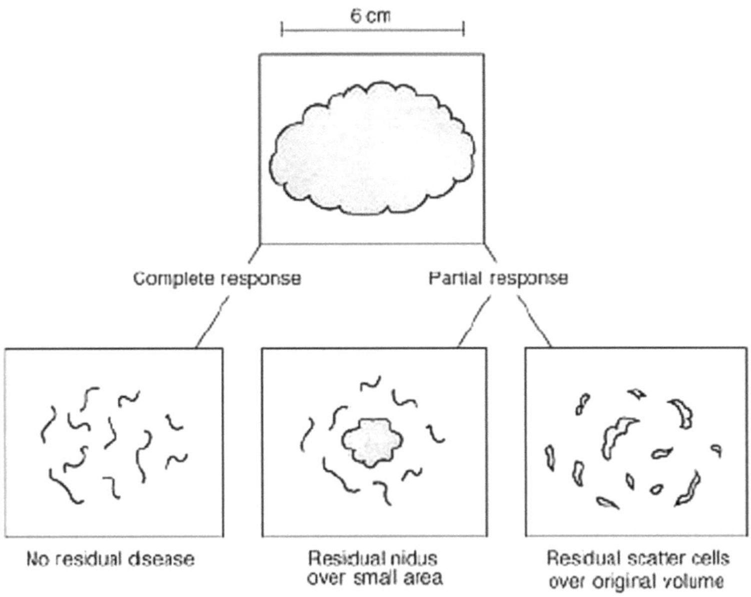

Fig. 2.[2]

Examples of the various pathologic responses observed after neoadjuvant chemotherapy. In some instances, malignant cells are clustered around a residual nidus after disease response. In other cases, residual tumor cells are scattered over the residual volume of disease. A breast-conserving surgical procedure directed toward a central nidus may leave different volumes of residual disease in these two clinical scenarios.

NSABP B-18 showed ipsilateral recurrence rates of 10.7% for NCT versus 7.6% for the adjuvant chemotherapy group. This discrepancy may be attributable to those mastectomy candidates who were converted to BCT candidates after tumor response to NCT. The European Organization for Research and Treatment of Cancer (EORTC) 10902 trial showed no difference in local recurrence rates between NCT and adjuvant chemotherapy[13].

Although NCT has not yet been shown to improve OS or DFS, it has led to the elucidation of pCR as a significant prognostic indicator. Due to the lack of standardization of the definition of pCR, a new measure of response has been proposed, called residual cancer burden (RCB) [14]. This is a calculated index that combines tumor size and cellularity with the size and number of lymph node metastases. RCB may predict recurrence-free survival and identify a group of high-risk patients and those with chemo-resistant tumors.

Current studies in NCT are looking at ways to predict tumor response to chemotherapy. For instance, it is rare that treatment with chemotherapy of a strongly estrogen receptor positive (ER +), progesterone receptor (PR+) ,Her 2 neu negative tumor will result in a cPR. [15] More and more studies are evaluating response to chemotherapy based on multiple identified subtypes. For instance, lobular cancers (loss of e-cahedrin expression) may not respond well to chemotherapy. Luminal A subtypes (strongly ER+ PR+) tumors often express very low growth rate patterns and may also not respond well to chemotherapy. On the other hand, ER+PR- (luminal B) type tumors and ER-PR-Her2neu- (basal type) tumors respond far better to chemotherapy and more often will result in cPR.[15].Novel chemotherapeutic agents such as the antiangiogenic agent, bevacizumab, and monoclonal antibody, trastuzumab, are now being tested in neoadjuvant clinical trials. The future lies in the ability to tailor NCT according to predictable prognostic indicators such as tumor subtype , and molecular therapeutic markers and in the development of specific NCT regimens with individualization based on tumor biology.

3. Neoadjuvant endocrine therapy

Systemic chemotherapy (NCT) was first used in the neoadjuvant setting in trials to downstage locally advanced tumors. Quite naturally it became the popular treatment modality for patients with locally advanced breast cancer considered inoperable or for those with operable breast cancer who desired breast conservation therapy. Since the development of prognostic markers that can be reliably tested the idea of preoperative endocrine therapy based on estrogen and progesterone receptor has also come into question. Initial studies of this approach have been most often performed in postmenopausal women.

A number of clinical trials have compared surgery with primary endocrine therapy in older postmenopausal women with large ER+ tumors destined for mastectomy in whom neoadjuvant chemotherapy was deemed inappropriate due to age and comorbidities. It was clear that many had an initial response to therapy and were able to achieve breast conservation but not all. Unfortunately, some experienced disease progression.

Tamoxifen has for many years been the mainstay of endocrine therapy. Rightfully so, more recent trails have compared Tamoxifen to the newer aromatase inhibitors both in the

adjuvant and neoadjuvant setting. It is clear from the BIG- I 98 (letrazole vs Tamoxifen) and ATAC (Arimidex vs Tamoxifen Alone or in Combination) trials that aromatase inhibitors have slightly superior disease free survival rates (DFS) (about 4-6%) Armed with that knowledge, Ingle et al, recently published a series comparing tamoxifen versus letrazole in the neoadjuvant setting, and found letrazole had superior clinical response rates.[16]
It has, however, become increasingly clear that the strongly ER+PR+HER 2 neu - (luminal A tumors) are the ones that respond best to endocrine therapies. Much energy is now being spent on looking for markers to predict response to endocrine therapy. Multigene prognostic assay tools such as Recurrence Score (Oncotype Dx) and the Amsterdam 70 gene assay (Mammaprint) define a low risk population and also seem to predict response to therapy. Other genomic measurements also hold promise. One is a panel of genes co - expressed with ESR1 that could predict sensitivity to endocrine therapy (SET) and improved relapse free survival.[17] Patients with a high SET had few relapses with Tamoxifen alone.
Another measure of response to endocrine therapy is a decrease in Ki-67 with treatment. Ki-67 is a measure of proliferation and studies are showing that patients who have a decrease in expression of Ki-67 after two weeks of endocrine therapy will go on to have a good response. The American College of Surgeons - Oncology Group study Z 1031 is looking at this measure in post menopausal women with stage 2 or 3 breast cancer be studying it with repeat tumor sampling two weeks after start of therapy for ER+ tumors.
One of the advantages that appear to be offered by neoadjuvant endocrine therapy over chemotherapy is concentric shrinkage of the tumor, thereby making it far more likely to yield negative margins at the time of surgery. This seems to translate into better local control rates with breast conservation therapy and additive radiation.

3.1 Timing of the sentinel node biopsy in the neoadjuvant setting

There is controversy on the timing of the sentinel node biopsy in the setting of neoadjuvant therapy. Should sentinel node (SNB) evaluation occur before or after induction of chemo or endocrine therapy? There are salient points for both sides of this controversy. Lymph node status has been and still is a strong predictor of outcome . However, cPR after neoadjuvant therapy is also a very strong predictor of outcome, even in the setting of positive nodal disease.
One of the concerns with performing the SNB after neoadjuvant treatment is related to the technical ability to find the SNB and its accuracy. Several studies now have demonstrated that, in patients who are clinically node negative at diagnosis, the SN can be identified over 97% of the time with low false negative rates.[17,18] Several studies also support the view that performing the SNB after NCT allows downstaging of the axilla and results in fewer patients being subjected to full axillary node dissection (ALND), with its attendant risk of chronic lymphedema.
Proponents of performing the SNB prior to NCT believe that knowledge of the state of the axilla prior to the initiation of chemotherapy is critical for prognostication. In addition, there are times that knowledge of the number of lymph nodes involved may influence the regimen of chemotherapy delivered or whether radiation is administered after mastectomy. In some cases, only one SN is removed for evaluation and post NCT the SNB technique is repeated. This particular approach (removing only one SN), however, negates the arguments of needing to know number of involved nodes. If only one SN is removed then it is unclear if this was the only involved node. After treatment, it is also unclear whether or

not nodal disease would have cleared with treatment. The authors do not recommend this approach. Instead, if SNB is performed prior to NCT then patients with a positive intraoperative SN should proceed with full axillary evaluation (ALND).

The axilla should be evaluated clinically and if there is any concer, should have axillary ultrasound and needle biopsy of suspicious nodes.

The current recommendation for those with known nodal involvement prior to inception of NCT is to proceed with ALND after chemotherapy.

There are currently trials evaluating the safety of SNB in node positive women who have an excellent response to chemotherapy.

4. The new paradigm

Clinical research in cancer is resulting in a shift towards a new paradigm. In the past, new agents or combinations have been studied in the adjuvant or postoperative setting. The tumor has been removed and the only way to measure success or failure of a treatment is to wait years to document treatment failures. Any studies that were performed prior to tumor extirpation required that all patients, regardless of tumor response, were to receive the same chemotherapeutic drugs. Recently, there has been recognition that performing drug studies prior to removal of the tumor provides instant feed back on response to therapy.

Tumor regression in response to therapy can be gauged by examination of the tumor. In addition, the treatment plan can be altered based on which drugs are eliciting tumor response. The best example of this new change in trial design and concept is seen in the I-SPY 2 trial (**I**nvestigation of **S**erial studies to **P**redict **Y**our Therapeutic **R**esponse with **I**maging **A**nd mo**L**ecular analysis). On this study patients are randomized to standard NCT or investigational drugs with imaging and repeat core biopsies to restudy the tumor molecular changes as treatment progresses. The investigational drugs given in the neoadjuvant setting allows immediate feedback on drug efficacy by measuring tumor response to treatment. This we believe will be the future of cancer clinical trials and will allow us to move forward much more quickly with studies of drug efficacy alone or in combination.

It's a brave new world!

5. References

[1] Charfare, H., Limongelli, S., and Purushotham, A.D. *Neoadjuvant chemotherapy in breast cancer.* British Journal of Surgery 92:14-23, 2005.

[2] De Lena, M., Zucali, R., Viganotti, G., Valagussa, P., and Bonadonna, G. *Combined Chemotherapy-Radiotherapy Approach in Locally Advanced (T3b-T4) Breast Cancer.* Cancer Chemotherapy and Pharmacology 1: 53-59, 1978.

[3] Valagussa, P., Zambetti, P., Bignami, M., De Lena, M., Varini, R., Zucali, R., Rovini, D., and Bonadonna, G. *T3b-T4 Breast Cancer: Factors Affecting Results in Combined Modality Treatments.* Clin. Expl. Metastasis vol 1, No.2:191-202, 1983.

[4] Bonadonna, G., De Lena, M., Brambilla, C., Zucali, R., Uslenghi, C., Valagussa, P., and Veronise, U. *Combination Chemotherapy and Combined Treatment Modality In Disseminated and Locally Advanced Breast Cancer.* Breast Cancer p.437-458, 1977.

[5] Jacquillat, C., et al. *Results of Neoadjuvant Chemotherapy and Radiation Therapy in the Breast-Conserving Treatment of 250 Patients With All Stages of Infiltrative Breast Cancer.* Cancer 66:119-129, 1990.

[6] Fisher, B., et al. *Effect of Preoperative Chemotherapy on the Outcome of Women With Operable Breast Cancer.* Journal of Clinical Oncology vol 16, No. 8:2672-2685,1998.

[7] Mamounas, E., et al. *NSABP Breast Cancer Clinical Trails: Recent Results and Future Directions.* Clinical Medicine and Research vol 1, No. 4:309-326, 2003.

[8] Gunduz, N., et al. *Effect of Surgical Removal on the Growth and Kinetics of Residual Tumor.* Cancer Research 39:3861-3865, 1979.

[9] Ketcham, A.S., et al. *The Development of Spontaneous Metastases after the Removal of a Primary Tumor II. Standardization protocol of five animal tumors.* Cancer 14:875-882, 1961.

[10] Ketcham, A.S., et al. *The effect of removal of a "Primary" tumor on the development of spontaneous metastases I. Development of a standardized experimental technique.* Cancer Research 19:940-944, 1959.

[11] Mauriac, L., et al. *Effect of Primary Chemotherapy in Conservative Treatment of Breast Cancer patients with Operable tumors larger than 3 cm. Results of a randomized trial in a single center.* Annals of Oncology 2:347-354, 1991.

[12] Buchholz, T., et al., *Neoadjuvant Chemotherapy for Breast Cancer. Multidisciplinary Considerations of Benefits and Risks.* Cancer vol 98, No. 6:1150-1160, 2003.

[13] van der Hage, Jos A., et al., *Preoperative Chemotherapy in Primary Operable Breast Cancer:Results from the European Organization for Research and Treatment of Cancer Trial 10902.* Journal of Clinical Oncology vol 19, No. 22:4224-4237, 2001.

[14] Budzar, A., et al., *Preoperative Chemotherapy Treatment of Breast Cancer-A Review.* Cancer vol 110, No. 11:2394-2407, 2007.

[15] Lips, E ,et al, Neoadjuvant chemotherapy in ER+,Her2neu - breast cancer : response predication based on immunohistochemical and molecular characteristics. Breast Cancer Res Treat, DOI 10.1007/s10549-011-1488-0 , on line April 07, 2011

[16] Ingle, J.N. et al, Aromaatase Inhibitors vs Tamoxifen for management of post menopausal breast cancer in the advanced neoadjuvant setting, J Steroid Biochem Mo Biol ,Sept:86(35) 313-9

[17] Chung A., Guiliano A.

[18] Stell V.H., et al, Sentinel Node after neoadjuvant chemotherapy in breast cancer : Breast J 2011 Jan 17(1):71-4

[19] Symmans,W.F., et al ,Genomic index of sensitivity to endocrine therapy for breast cancer,J Clin Oncol,2010 Sept 20:28(27)4101-3

[20] I SPY 2, breast cancer trials. gov web site

3

Surgical Intervention Following Neoadjuvant Chemotherapy in Breast Cancer

Michelle Sowden, Baiba Grube, Brigid Killilea and Donald Lannin
Department of Surgery, Yale University School of Medicine, New Haven
USA

1. Introduction

The concept of pre-operative, or neoadjuvant, chemotherapy for breast cancer initially arose to deal with patients that were deemed non-operable at the time of diagnosis.[1] These were patients with locally advanced disease (usually Stage III) or those with inflammatory breast cancer. As experience in this population grew, it became obvious that many patients who were unresectable at the time of diagnosis were down-staged by chemotherapy. Not only did this improve survival by up to 25%, but it also made many tumors amenable to surgical intervention, usually with a mastectomy.[2, 3]

The first large prospective randomized trial to determine the usefulness of preoperative chemotherapy in women with operable tumors was the NSABP B-18 study that began in 1988. In this study, 1523 women with palpable, biopsy proven breast cancer were randomized to 4 cycles of preoperative or postoperative AC (doxyrubicin 60 mg/m^2 and cyclophosimide 600mg/m^2). [4] The surgical intervention was either a lumpectomy with axillary lymph node dissection or a modified radical mastectomy. The patients who had breast conservation underwent post-operative radiation treatment. The primary endpoints of this trial were overall survival (OS), disease free survival (DFS), and relapse free interval (RFI). The 16 year results of this study were published in 2008.[5] There was no statistically significant difference in OS (P=.90), DFS (P=.27) or RFI (P=.78) between the pre and postoperative chemotherapy groups. The B-18 trial did show a statistically significant improvement in the breast conservation rate following preoperative chemotherapy. That is, lumpectomy was more common in patients receiving preoperative chemotherapy (67% *vs* 60%, P=0.002).

The B-18 trial was followed in 1995 by the NSABP B-27 study. This study evaluated the addition of T (docetaxel 100mg/m^2) to the neoadjuvant regimen. Women were randomized to 1) 4 cycles of preoperative AC followed by surgery 2) 4 cycles of preoperative AC followed by 4 cycles of T then surgery or 3) 4 cycles of preoperative AC, surgery and then 4 cycles of T.[6] While this did show that the addition of docetaxel appeared to increase the number of pathologic complete responses versus AC alone, it did not show an improvement in OS or DFS with the addition of a taxane.[5] Based on the B-18 and B-27 trials, however, neoadjuvant chemotherapy became accepted in a broad population of patients, not just in patients with non-operable tumors.

Neoadjuvant chemotherapy has many additional benefits beyond increased breast conservation rates. The use of preoperative agents allows for in vivo assessment of tumor response. [3] The ability to monitor tumor response allows the clinician to assess effectiveness of an agent against that particular mass. The tumor response to chemotherapy has important prognostic implications. In the B-18 trial, women who had a pathologic complete response (pCR) had superior outcomes compared with women who did not (OS HR=0.32, *P*<.0001; DFS HR=0.47, *P*<.0001).[5] This was again shown in the B-27 trial with pCR improving OS (HR=0.36, *P*<.0001) and DFS (HR=0.49, *P*<.0001).

Another logical and common use of neoadjuvant chemotherapy is for clinical trials. By assessing the in vivo response, researchers are able to get almost immediate feedback on the effectiveness of novel regimens. Doing this in an adjuvant setting would often require large numbers of patients and years of follow-up. In addition, tumor biopsies taken while on trial allow evaluation of biologic correlates and gene expression changes during therapy.

2. Indications for neoadjuvant chemotherapy

Neoadjuvant chemotherapy continues to be the standard of care for patients with locally advanced and inflammatory breast cancers. Locally advanced tumors include those with skin or chest wall involvement and patients with bulky lymphadenopathy. As described previously this therapy can potentially convert those with unresectable tumors into candidates for mastectomy.

Currently the use of neoadjuvant chemotherapy has been expanded to include patients with large tumors that would typically require mastectomy. In these patients the goal of preoperative chemotherapy is to make breast conservation an option. As previously described, the B-18 trial clearly showed that neoadjuvant chemotherapy leads to an increased rate of lumpectomy (67% *v* 60%).[5]

The standard cutoff for use in the setting of large tumor burden is 4 centimeters or greater. However, use in all T2 (2-5cm) lesions is becoming more commonplace. In a study by Christy et. al. it was determined that neoadjuvant chemotherapy significantly reduced the rate of reoperation for positive margins in patients whose tumors measured between 2-4 cm.[7] This study, which was retrospective, evaluated patients with T2 tumors less than 4 cm in size and compared reoperation rates in the pre and postoperative chemotherapy groups. There was a significantly decreased number of positive margins in the patients who received preoperative chemotherapy (10% *v* 32%, *P*=<0.01). This led to a decreased rate of reoperation (3% *v* 35%, *P*=<0.01) and mastectomy (3% *v* 19%, *P*=<0.01). These findings make a compelling argument for use of preoperative chemotherapy in women with T2 tumors who are interested in breast conservation.

An obvious caveat to this recommendation is that patients considered for neoadjuvant chemotherapy must have a clear indication that they would normally receive adjuvant chemotherapy. In other words, the medications must be oncologically indicated, not used simply to decrease the size of the tumor for breast conservation. Most younger patients with tumors larger than 2 cm or node positive disease would fall into the group where chemotherapy is clearly indicated and therefore may be candidates for preoperative treatment.

Another consideration for preoperative chemotherapy is patient age. In the B-18 trial, women under the age of 50 appeared to have the greatest benefit from preoperative therapy. With 16 years of follow-up, that study shows overall survival in women under the age of 50 was slightly better in the preoperative chemotherapy group (61% *vs* 55% (*P*=0.06)).[5] While this finding did not reach statistical significance, it is certainly a compelling trend. This trend was also seen in DFS for this group at 44% *v* 38% (*P*=0.09). Conversely, women over the age of 50 appeared to do better with standard, adjuvant chemotherapy, with OS at 50% in the preoperative group versus 55% in the postoperative group (*P*=. 07) Although these results were of borderline statistical significance, we feel that most women under 50 with larger tumors should at least be considered for neoadjuvant therapy.

3. Surgical considerations after neoadjuvant chemotherapy

Tumor localization

It is imperative that a surgeon be involved in the care of a patient undergoing neoadjuvant chemotherapy from the onset. Surgical planning is best done when the surgeon is able to evaluate the tumor prior to any treatment effect. This allows both the surgeon and the patient to have a reasonable understanding of post-therapy surgical options.

It is also imperative that a radiopaque marker be placed with a core biopsy instrument in the tumor at the time of diagnosis. In a study by Oh et. al. a retrospective review was done of 373 patients undergoing preoperative chemotherapy followed by lumpectomy to evaluate the need for marker placement.[8] Of the 373 patients studied, 145 had radiopaque markers placed and 228 did not. With a follow up of approximately 4 years, the patients with marker placement had an improved rate of local control versus those that did not have a marker placed (98.6% *v* 91.7%, *P*=0.02). This improved rate of local control likely represents a much better ability to accurately localize the site where the tumor was prior to treatment.

The increased use of preoperative chemotherapy in breast cancer prompted a National Institute of Health Conference on local-regional treatment following chemotherapy. This conference held in March, 2007 sought to standardize many aspects of regional treatment after preoperative chemotherapy, including pretreatment clip placement.[9] In the statement from this conference the recommendation is: "*Radiopaque clips should be placed within all abnormalities at the time of biopsy to provide localization for subsequent surgical removal and pathologic assessment of the tumor bed if there is a complete clinical and radiologic response.*" Based on this recommendation it is our practice to place a marker whenever possible.

In addition to radio-opaque marker placement, another novel technique for tumor localization has been recommended by Lannin et. al. This technique involves pretreatment tattooing of the margins of the palpable tumor area by the surgeon (Figure 1).[10] By marking the area of involvement prior to chemotherapy, the surgeon is able to remove the entire area once the treatment is done. This method takes into account the possibility that when the tumor shrinks with chemotherapy it may not shrink concentrically but rather in a honeycomb fashion leading to many microscopic islands of disease within the breast (Figure 2).[11] It is theorized that this honeycomb regression, which can be seen in up to 40% of tumors, may lead to the trend for increased rates of local recurrence that were seen in the B-18 trial (13% *v* 10%, *P*=0.21) and other similar trials.[5, 12] Another benefit of this technique is that the tattooing often obviates the need for needle localization at the time of definitive surgery.

4. How much breast tissue needs to be removed following chemotherapy?

Surgery continues to be the standard of care following neoadjuvant chemotherapy. The down-staging of tumors to make them amenable to breast conservation is one of the primary benefits of preoperative treatment. This benefit, however, presents a conundrum for the surgeon; if the patient appears to have had an excellent clinical response how much breast tissue should be removed?

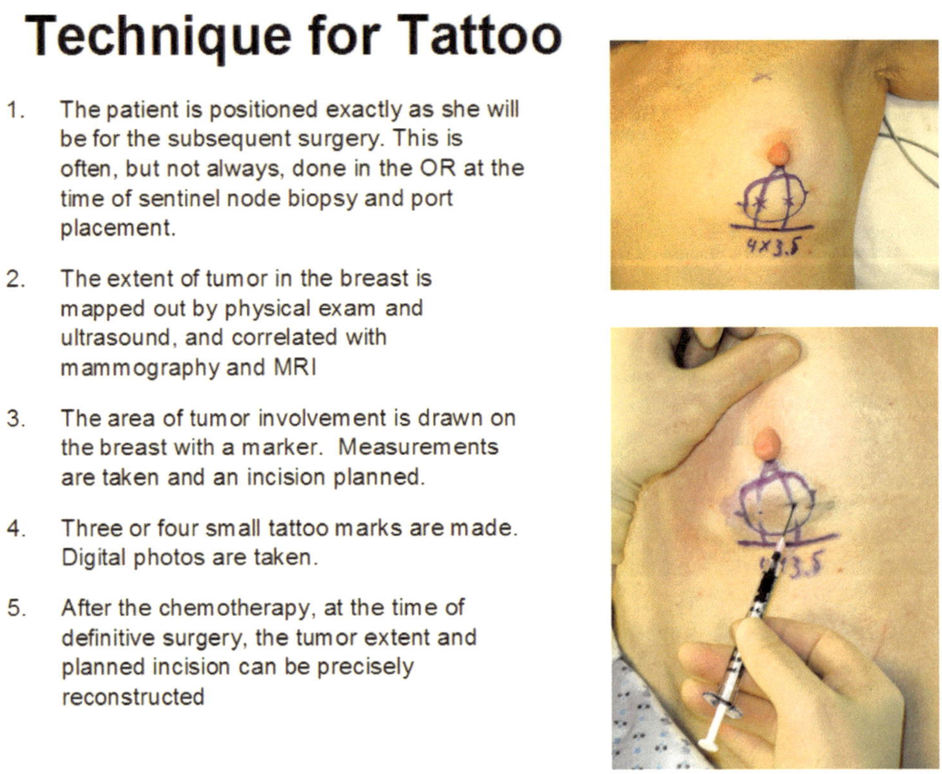

Fig. 1. Technique for placement of tattoos prior to neoadjuvant chemotherapy.

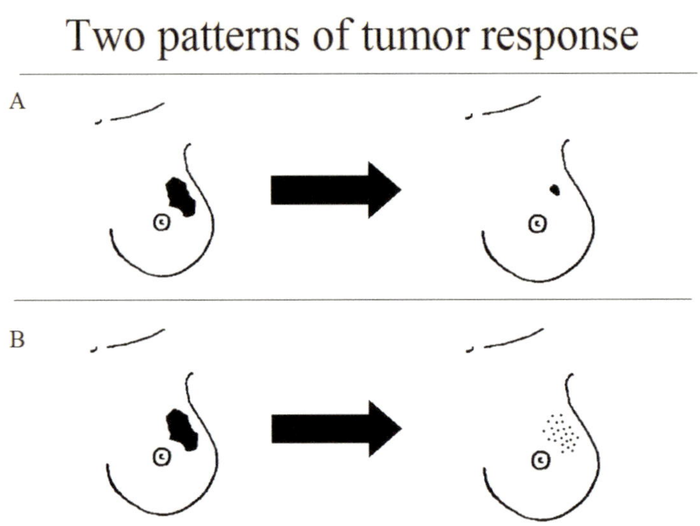

Fig. 2. Types of response to neoadjuvant chemotherapy. Our experience is that about 25% of patients have a complete pathological response and about 5% have no response. The remaining 70% are fairly evenly split between a type A or a type B response, or a combination of both.

This conundrum is exacerbated by the fact that preoperative neoadjuvant chemotherapy followed by breast conservation therapy (BCT) has been found in some studies to lead to an increased rate of local recurrence (LRR). While this was not statistically significant in the B-18 trial, other studies have shown a definitive increase in local recurrence. Mauri et.al. published a meta-analysis of neoadjuvant trials in 2005. This analysis looked at 9 trials comparing adjuvant to neoadjuvant chemotherapy. Encompassing nearly 4000 patients this study showed a 22% increased relative risk of local recurrence in the neoadjuvant treatment arm (P=0.015).[13] While at first blush this number is large enough to make BCT seem implausible, a limitation to this study was the inclusion of trials where radiation was used without surgery. In these trials, as one might expect, there was a substantial increase in LRR. Never the less the trend toward increased LRR does mandate careful surgical planning in order to minimize this risk.

Following chemotherapy, patients need to be evaluated in a multimodal fashion to determine if they are candidates for breast conservation. Breast examination is often done in conjunction with some combination of mammography, ultrasound (US) and magnetic resonance imaging (MRI). Unfortunately there is no one modality that has been shown to have 100% accuracy in the neoadjuvant breast population. In fact, many studies show that each modality is flawed. In a study by Chagpar et. al., 182 patients undergoing neoadjuvant chemotherapy were retrospectively evaluated to assess the accuracy of physical examination, mammography and US for size determination after chemotherapy.[14] Patients were evaluated with all modalities at the time of diagnosis and again prior to surgery, and physical exam and imaging measurements were then compared to the final pathologic measurements. The correlation between pathology and preoperative assessment was moderate at best, with accuracy (+/- 1 cm) at 66% for physical exam, 75% for US and 70% for mammography.

Findings like these have prompted evaluation of MRI in the neoadjuvant population. In a study by Segara et.al., the effectiveness of physical exam and US were compared to MRI at the time of diagnosis and prior to surgery, and again the measurements were compared to final pathology.[15] In this study MRI was slightly superior to the other modalities. They found that the size was accurately predicted (+/- 1cm) in 76% of patients with MRI, 66% with US and 54% with physical exam.

It is clear that no single radiological modality will provide a perfect prediction of residual tumor volume. As a result, it has been suggested that the safest approach following neoadjuvant chemotherapy is to remove the entire volume of breast that was affected by tumor prior to treatment.[16] Advocates of this approach cite the frequency of swiss-cheese-like regression of the tumor and the likelihood of leaving residual tumor cells with lesser resections.[10] While at first glance this appears to negate the benefit of chemotherapy for cytoreduction and breast conservation, this actually is not the case. Figure 3 shows that, for tumors in the 3-5 cm range, the volume of tissue that must be resected to include a 1 cm margin of normal breast tissue around the tumor is actually 3 to 4 times greater than if a very narrow margin is taken. The real value of chemotherapy, therefore, is to allow a pathologically negative margin without removing a wide rim of normal tissue. The goal of surgery after chemotherapy is to resect all of the original tumor and as little as possible of the surrounding normal breast tissue. With the tattoo technique described earlier, the tumor margins are marked and the incision planned prior to the chemotherapy when it can be easily identified by palpation and/or ultrasound. The patient is tattooed and pictures are taken. After the chemotherapy, the original tumor margins can be precisely reconstructed and the exact original tumor volume is resected. (See figure 4)

1 cm margin increases resection volume 3-4 times

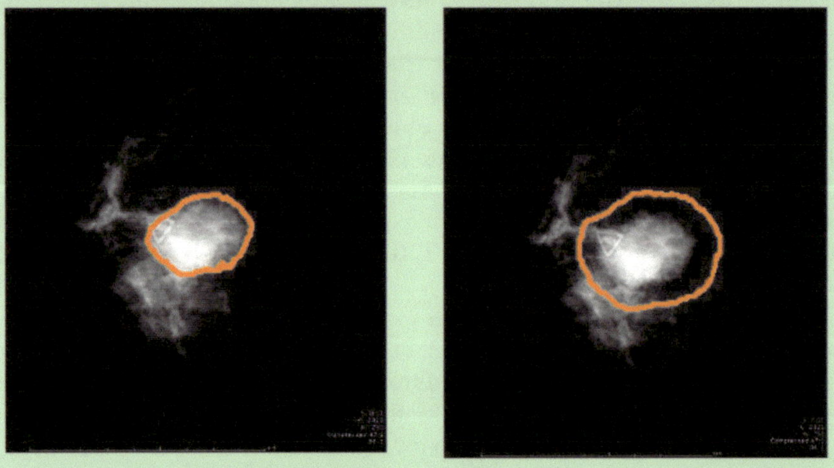

Diameter	Tumor volume	Volume with 1 cm margin
3 cm	14 cm^3	65 cm^3
4 cm	34 cm^3	113 cm^3
5 cm	65 cm^3	180 cm^3

Fig. 3. Calculated volume of a sphere with and without a 1 cm margin for tumors between 3 and 5 cm. This is the mammogram for the patient shown as case number 1 in Figure 4.

Whatever technique is utilized to determine the area of resection, the surgical tenet of clear margins must be adhered to. It is important that the tissue is sent to a pathologist familiar with tissue changes seen after chemotherapy so that an accurate assessment can be made of margins and response. It is also critically important that the pathologist be informed that the patient had preoperative chemotherapy as it can make interpretation of the specimen more difficult. The tissue after chemotherapy will show varying degrees of fibrosis and cell death.

5. Evaluation of sentinel lymph nodes

The timing of sentinel lymph node biopsy in the neoadjuvant breast patient is one of the most controversial topics in surgical oncology. Initial studies regarding the efficacy of sentinel lymph node biopsy after neoadjuvant chemotherapy showed an unacceptably high rate of false negatives. In one small study, up to 30% of patients undergoing sentinel lymph node procedures after chemotherapy had falsely negative nodes. [17]

As experience with sentinel lymph node biopsy increased, the rate of false negatives decreased. The largest study to date dealing with this topic is the NSABP-B27. In this study 428 women had an attempted sentinel lymph node procedure following neoadjuvant chemotherapy. [18] Of these women, 343 had at least one sentinel node identified followed by a completion axillary dissection. In this group of women there were 15 women that had a negative sentinel lymph node with metastatic disease found in at least one non-sentinel lymph node. This led to a false negative rate of 10.7% and an overall success rate of 84.8%. This compared favorably to patients undergoing sentinel lymph node procedures without preoperative chemotherapy. In the NSABP B-32 trial, the rate of false negatives was 9.8% with an overall success rate of 97.2%.[19] While this shows that overall identification rates are lower after neoadjuvant therapy, the false negative rate is acceptable.[20]

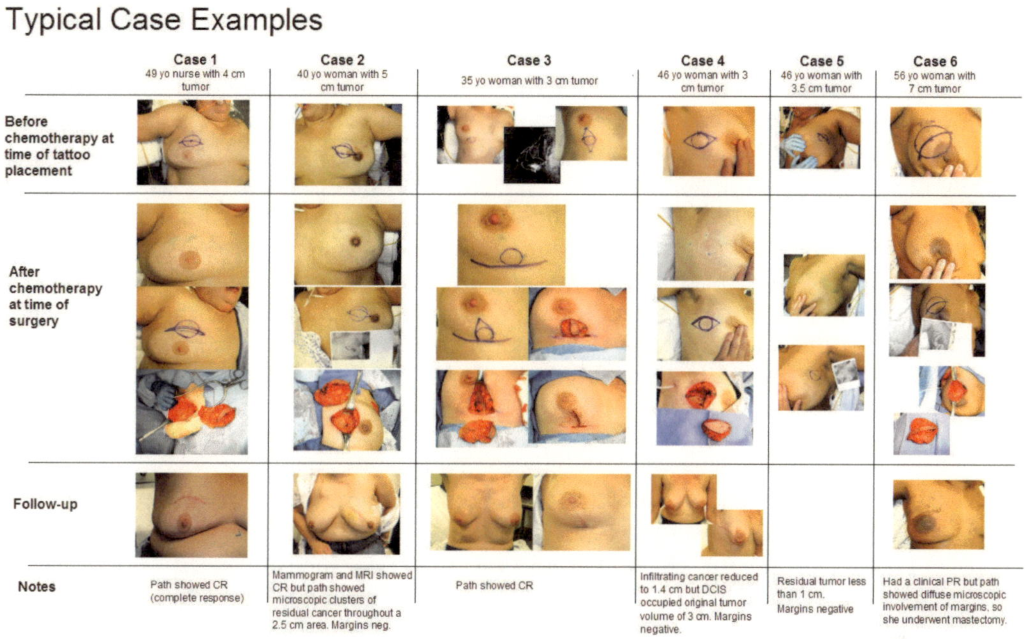

Fig. 4. Representative cases showing pictures before chemotherapy, several months later at the time of surgery, and after several more weeks of follow-up post-operatively.

The advantages and disadvantages of sentinel node biopsy before and after chemotherapy are nicely reviewed in a recent paper by Grube, et al. [21] Sentinel lymph node biopsy performed before chemotherapy has a higher rate of identification (97.2% v 84.8%)[18, 19] This could potentially save a patient from an axillary dissection if a successful sentinel procedure prior to chemotherapy showed a lymph node negative for metastatic disease. While the false negative rates are similar (10.7% v 9.8%) there is a slight advantage in overall accuracy by removing the nodes pre-chemotherapy. The disadvantage of sentinel lymph node biopsy pre-chemotherapy is that up to 30% of patients will have downstaging of their axilla with the preoperative treatment. [22] In these patients, a positive SLNB done before chemotherapy will mandate an unnecessary axillary lymph node dissection after chemotherapy. Doing the sentinel node procedure before chemotherapy also mandates two operations and may delay the onset of chemotherapy.[11]

Advocates of doing the sentinel lymph node procedure after chemotherapy cite the similar false negative rate seen in these patients and feel that this is an oncologically safe procedure.[20] Additionally they cite the potential downstaging of the axilla as a benefit and feel that this may save patients from axillary dissection. The ability to perform just one surgery is also felt to be an advantage. The possible disadvantages include potentially higher false negative rates and lower rates of identification.

6. Conclusions

Neoadjuvant chemotherapy has become much more common in patients treated for breast cancer. Once performed only in patients with locally advanced or inflammatory breast cancers, it is now used in a much wider population of patients. Current evidence would suggest that preoperative chemotherapy should be considered in women with tumors larger than 2 cm who are interested in breast conservation. It should also be considered in women under the age of 50 as there is a trend for survival benefit. Preoperative treatment may also be considered in women who are interested in participating in a clinical trial testing many of the exciting new drugs that are becoming available.

In patients electing neoadjuvant treatment, it is important that surgical input is elicited from the onset. A radiopaque marker should be placed in the tumor at the time of diagnosis to facilitate localization after tumor regression. Tumor tattooing done prior to chemotherapy may assist in post treatment resection and may obviate the need for needle localization. As always, removal of the tumor to clear margins is imperative. Timing of the sentinel lymph node biopsy continues to be controversial and there is no clear consensus whether a pre- or post- chemotherapy protocol is most advantageous.

7. References

[1] Liu SV, Melstrom L, Yao K, Russell CA, Sener SF: Neoadjuvant therapy for breast cancer. *J Surg Oncol* 2010, 101(4):283-291.

[2] Bear HD: Neoadjuvant chemotherapy for operable breast cancer: individualizing locoregional and systemic therapy. *Surg Oncol Clin N Am* 2010, 19(3):607-626.

[3] Gralow JR, Burstein HJ, Wood W, Hortobagyi GN, Gianni L, von Minckwitz G, Buzdar AU, Smith IE, Symmans WF, Singh B *et al*: Preoperative therapy in invasive breast cancer: pathologic assessment and systemic therapy issues in operable disease. *J Clin Oncol* 2008, 26(5):814-819.

[4] Fisher B, Brown A, Mamounas E, Wieand S, Robidoux A, Margolese RG, Cruz AB, Jr., Fisher ER, Wickerham DL, Wolmark N *et al*: Effect of preoperative chemotherapy on local-regional disease in women with operable breast cancer: findings from National Surgical Adjuvant Breast and Bowel Project B-18. *J Clin Oncol* 1997, 15(7):2483-2493.

[5] Rastogi P, Anderson SJ, Bear HD, Geyer CE, Kahlenberg MS, Robidoux A, Margolese RG, Hoehn JL, Vogel VG, Dakhil SR *et al*: Preoperative chemotherapy: updates of National Surgical Adjuvant Breast and Bowel Project Protocols B-18 and B-27. *J Clin Oncol* 2008, 26(5):778-785.

[6] Mamounas EP: NSABP Protocol B-27. Preoperative doxorubicin plus cyclophosphamide followed by preoperative or postoperative docetaxel. *Oncology (Williston Park)* 1997, 11(6 Suppl 6):37-40.

[7] Christy CJ, Thorsteinsson D, Grube BJ, Black D, Abu-Khalaf M, Chung GG, DiGiovanna MP, Miller K, Higgins SA, Weidhaas J *et al*: Preoperative chemotherapy decreases

the need for re-excision of breast cancers between 2 and 4 cm diameter. *Ann Surg Oncol* 2009, 16(3):697-702.

[8] Oh JL, Nguyen G, Whitman GJ, Hunt KK, Yu TK, Woodward WA, Tereffe W, Strom EA, Perkins GH, Buchholz TA: Placement of radiopaque clips for tumor localization in patients undergoing neoadjuvant chemotherapy and breast conservation therapy. *Cancer* 2007, 110(11):2420-2427.

[9] Buchholz TA, Lehman CD, Harris JR, Pockaj BA, Khouri N, Hylton NF, Miller MJ, Whelan T, Pierce LJ, Esserman LJ *et al*: Statement of the science concerning locoregional treatments after preoperative chemotherapy for breast cancer: a National Cancer Institute conference. *J Clin Oncol* 2008, 26(5):791-797.

[10] Lannin DR, Grube B, Black DS, Ponn T: Breast tattoos for planning surgery following neoadjuvant chemotherapy. *Am J Surg* 2007, 194(4):518-520.

[11] Veronesi P, Gentilini O, Fernandez JR, Magnoni F: Breast conservation and sentinel lymph node biopsy after neoadjuvant systemic therapy. *Breast* 2009, 18 Suppl 3:S90-92.

[12] Rajan R, Esteva FJ, Symmans WF: Pathologic changes in breast cancer following neoadjuvant chemotherapy: implications for the assessment of response. *Clin Breast Cancer* 2004, 5(3):235-238.

[13] Mauri D, Pavlidis N, Ioannidis JP: Neoadjuvant versus adjuvant systemic treatment in breast cancer: a meta-analysis. *J Natl Cancer Inst* 2005, 97(3):188-194.

[14] Chagpar AB, Middleton LP, Sahin AA, Dempsey P, Buzdar AU, Mirza AN, Ames FC, Babiera GV, Feig BW, Hunt KK *et al*: Accuracy of physical examination, ultrasonography, and mammography in predicting residual pathologic tumor size in patients treated with neoadjuvant chemotherapy. *Ann Surg* 2006, 243(2):257-264.

[15] Segara D, Krop IE, Garber JE, Winer E, Harris L, Bellon JR, Birdwell R, Lester S, Lipsitz S, Iglehart JD *et al*: Does MRI predict pathologic tumor response in women with breast cancer undergoing preoperative chemotherapy? *J Surg Oncol* 2007, 96(6):474-480.

[16] Christy CJ, Grube, B.J., Lannin, D.R.: Reply to Preoperative Chemotherapy and Potential Impact on Re-excision for Early Breast Cancer. *Ann Surg Oncol* 2009, 16:2958-2959.

[17] Nason KS, Anderson BO, Byrd DR, Dunnwald LK, Eary JF, Mankoff DA, Livingston R, Schmidt RA, Jewell KD, Yeung RS *et al*: Increased false negative sentinel node biopsy rates after preoperative chemotherapy for invasive breast carcinoma. *Cancer* 2000, 89(11):2187-2194.

[18] Mamounas EP, Brown A, Anderson S, Smith R, Julian T, Miller B, Bear HD, Caldwell CB, Walker AP, Mikkelson WM *et al*: Sentinel node biopsy after neoadjuvant chemotherapy in breast cancer: results from National Surgical Adjuvant Breast and Bowel Project Protocol B-27. *J Clin Oncol* 2005, 23(12):2694-2702.

[19] Krag DN, Anderson SJ, Julian TB, Brown AM, Harlow SP, Ashikaga T, Weaver DL, Miller BJ, Jalovec LM, Frazier TG *et al*: Technical outcomes of sentinel-lymph-node resection and conventional axillary-lymph-node dissection in patients with clinically node-negative breast cancer: results from the NSABP B-32 randomised phase III trial. *Lancet Oncol* 2007, 8(10):881-888.

[20] Kelly AM, Dwamena B, Cronin P, Carlos RC: Breast cancer sentinel node identification and classification after neoadjuvant chemotherapy-systematic review and meta analysis. *Acad Radiol* 2009, 16(5):551-563.
[21] Grube BJ, Christy CJ, Black D, Martel M, Harris L, Weidhaas J, Digiovanna MP, Chung G, Abu-Khalaf MM, Miller KD *et al*: Breast sentinel lymph node dissection before preoperative chemotherapy. *Arch Surg* 2008, 143(7):692-699; discussion 699-700.
[22] Kang SH, Kang JH, Choi EA, Lee ES: Sentinel lymph node biopsy after neoadjuvant chemotherapy. *Breast Cancer* 2004, 11(3):233-241; discussion 264-236.

4

Neoadjuvant Chemotherapy in Extra-Pulmonary Neuroendocrine Carcinoma

Halfdan Sorbye
Department of Oncology, Haukeland University Hospital, Bergen
Norway

1. Introduction

Extrapulmonary neuroendocrine carcinoma (EP-NEC) have been found in most organs, but the most common sites are the gastrointestinal tract, cervix uteri and urogenital tract (Strosberg et al., 2010, Walenkamp et al., 2009). Recently it has been defined as a pathological entity in breast cancer (Tavassoli et al., 2003). Additionally, in up to 30% of EP-NEC cases, no primary site can be identified (Kloppel et al., 1996). In the prior 2000 WHO classification, these tumours were known as poorly differentiated endocrine carcinoma (PDEC) (Solcia et al., 2000). In the 2010 WHO GI classification PDEC the nomenclature has been altered, and these tumours are now called neuroendocrine carcinoma (NEC) (Bosman et al., 2010). NEC tumours have a much higher proliferation rate than well-differentiated endocrine tumours. The terms poorly differentiated high-grade and neuroendocrine carcinoma are used synonymously and encompass mainly two histological entities: small-cell neuroendocrine carcinoma (SCNEC) and large-cell neuroendocrine carcinoma (LCNEC) (Bosman et al., 2010). LCNEC is morphologically distinguished from SCNEC by cytological features of a non–small cell carcinoma, including large cell size, low nuclear to cytoplasm volume ratio, coarse chromatin, and frequent nucleoli. They are both characterised by markers of neuroendocrine differentiation with synaptophysin, neuron-specific enolase, chromogranin and CD56 being the primary stains. They are also characterised by a high mitotic rate (defined as >10 mitotic figures per 10 high-power fields or a ki-67 > 20% in the gastrointestinal (GI) tract and other extrapulmonary sites and often with extensive necrosis. Most carcinomas in this family exhibit substantially more mitoses than these thresholds, typically in the range of 40 to 70 mitoses per high-power fields. Up to 40% of NECs contain elements of non-NECs, usually adenocarcinoma or squamous cell carcinoma. Often the diagnosis of a NEC tumor is after surgery on examination of the histological specimen. NECs are characterised by a high proclivity for metastatic dissemination even in patients with clinically localised tumours. This principle is validated by retrospective studies confirming that surgery alone is rarely curative (Brenner et al.,2004a).

In devising treatment strategies for extrapulmonary NEC, many authors refer to the extensive literature surrounding high-grade neuroendocrine carcinoma of the lung (Brenner et al., 2004a, Walenkamp et al., 2009). Several series have, however, questioned the rationale for this, and point out many differences between pulmonary small-cell carcinoma and SCNEC (Brennan et al., 2010, Brenner et al., 2004a, Brenner at al., 2007, Ku et al., 2008). Differences include aetiology (less smoking history in SCNEC), frequency of brain metastases (less in SCNEC), overall survival (superior in SCNEC, and survival may be site specific, i.e. gynaecologic and head and neck cancers may have better outcomes than GI primaries), and molecular differences, e.g. BCl-2 overexpression is more common in lung compared with SCNEC. Guidelines for treating EP- NEC advocate the use of combination chemotherapy with a platinum-based chemotherapy combined with the etoposide (NCCN 2010). No other regimen has consistently shown a benefit over this combination. When a patient has disease limited to the lung, using an aggressive multi-modality therapy including platinum-based chemotherapy and thoracic radiotherapy has showed improved survival. Based on this treatment paradigm for limited-stage small-cell lung cancer, a course of definitive chemotherapy and local therapy (surgery or radiation) can be considered in many patients with loco-regional EP- NEC. Whereas there are no studies examining adjuvant chemotherapy in NEC, their aggressive behaviour warrants consideration of adjuvant therapy in most cases. The North American Neuroendocrine Tumor Society (NANETS) recommend 4-6 cycles of cisplatin or carboplatin and etoposide as adjuvant therapy for resected patients (Strosberg et al., 2010). The use of neoadjuvant chemotherapy has by many been advocated for these patients, as surgery or radiation often has a poor prognosis due to the frequent development of distant metastases. Recently, neoadjuvant chemotherapy for resectable gastric cancer and resectable liver metastasis from colorectal cancer has been shown to increase survival (Cunningham et al., 2006, Nordlinger et al., 2008). Potential advantages to a neoadjuvant approach include; earlier treatment of micrometastatic disease; better compliance to treatment; determination of responsiveness to chemotherapy which can be prognostic and help in planning of postoperative chemotherapy; and avoidance of unnecessary surgery for patients with early systemic disease progression. Potential disadvantages include the risk of missing the window of opportunity for resection because of disease progression. The present paper discuss available literature concerning the use of neoadjuvant chemotherapy for EP-NEC.

2. Gastrointestinal neuroendocrine carcinoma

2.1 Background

Extra-pulmonary neuroendocrine carcinomas can originate anywhere in the gastrointestinal (GI) tract, but are mainly located in the oesophagus, stomach, pancreas and colon (Brenner et al., 2004a). Few data exist about this tumor group as many have been included in the general neuroendocrine tumor group and many are frequently misdiagnosed as poorly differentiated adenocarcinoma. GI primary tumours account for 35-55% of all NEC outside the lung (Galanis et al., 1997, Lee et al., 2007). Approximately 10% of all GI neuroendocrine tumours are NEC. Most GI NEC's are metastatic at the time of diagnosis. In the SEER database, colorectal NEC has an incidence of 2/1,000,000 inhabitants/year, and distant disease at diagnosis was present in 62% of patients (Kang et al., 2007). Median survival from diagnosis in untreated patients is usually 4-6 months, indicating a very rapidly growing tumor. Among 94 GI NEC patients in the National Cancer registry of Spain, 67% presented as distant metastatic disease, median survival was 1.7 months and 39% alive at 5 year (Garcia-Carbonero et al., 2010). Morphologically GI NEC are classified in two types: a small-cell carcinoma, resembling small-cell carcinoma of the lung, and a large-cell pleomorphic carcinoma (Bosman et al., 2010) (Figure 1-2). Small-cell histological preponderance in the squamous GI tract (oesophagus and anus) and large-cell carcinomas in the glandular parts (Shia et al., 2008). Awareness of the latter is essential, as these tumours often are indistinguishable from poorly differentiated non-NET carcinomas.

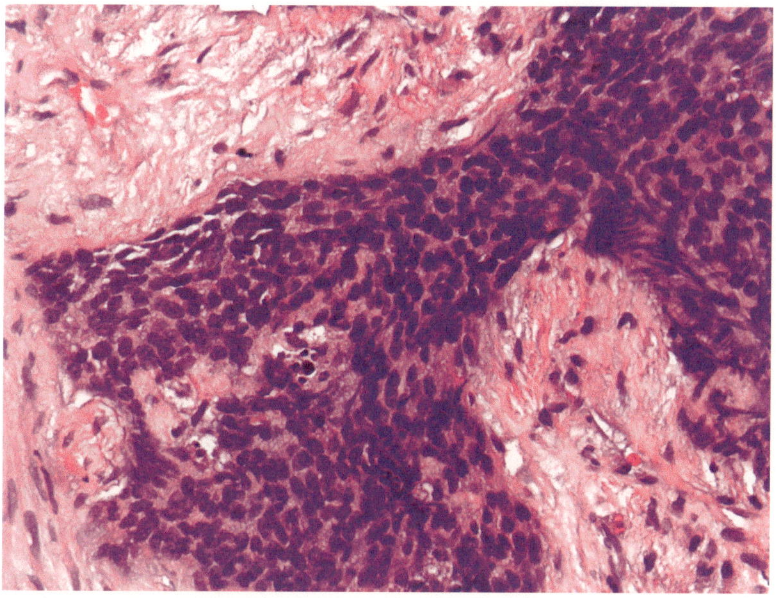

Fig. 1. Small-cell NEC from pancreas.

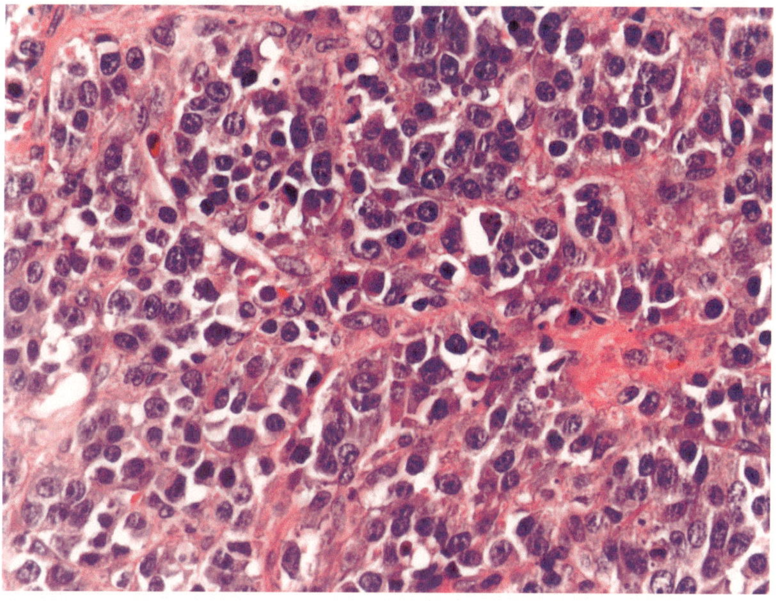

Fig. 2. Large-cell NEC from colon.

Usually synaptophysin will be positive in immunohistochemistry while staining for chromogranin A (CgA) is present at a lower level (Figure 3-4). The presence of CgA indicates a more mature tumor, and the presence of both markers is a good prognostic sign (Faggiano A et al., 2007, Welin et al., 2011). Several pathologists advocate for routine staining with synaptophysin and chromogranin for all tumours initially classified as poorly differentiated gastrointestinal adenocarcinoma.

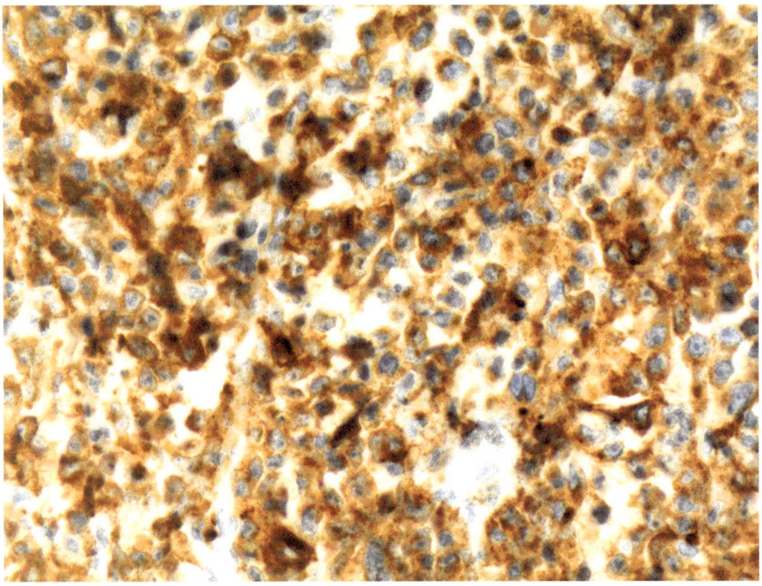

Fig. 3. Synaptophysin positive NEC.

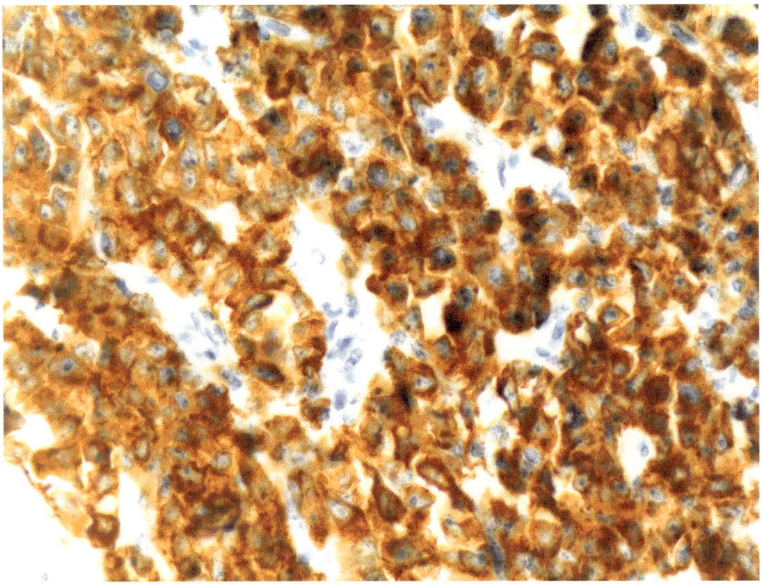

Fig. 4. Chromogranin A positive NEC.

CD56 is another neuroendocrine marker, which can help to classify a tumour. Screening for CgA in serum should be done, but is usually negative and hormonal symptoms are rare (Janson et al., 2010). In most NET guidelines it is stated that somatostatin receptor scintigraphy is usually negative in NEC. A somatostatin receptor scintigraphy should however be performed if ki-67 is below 30-40%, when peptide receptor radionucleotide therapy (PRRT) is a future treatment option. Ki-67 is per definition >20% but is more likely to be between 50 and 100% (Figure 5-6).

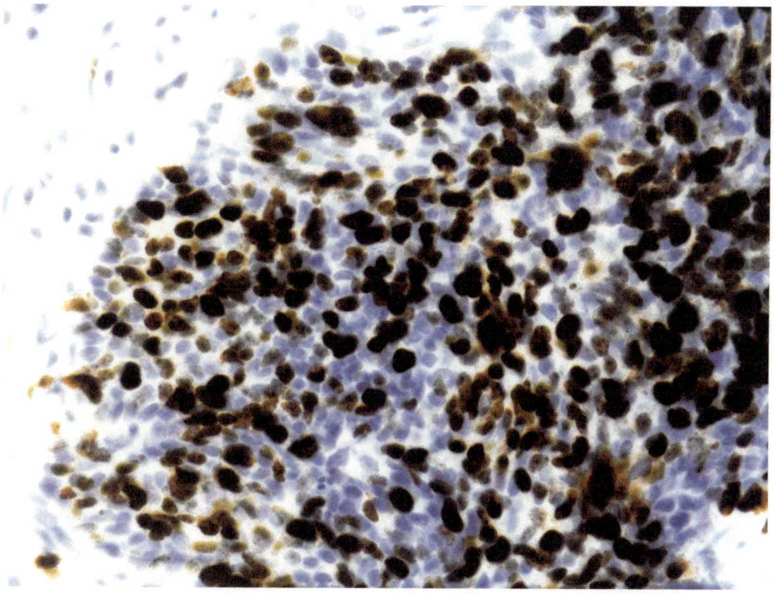

Fig. 5. SCNEC with a ki-67 index of 50%.

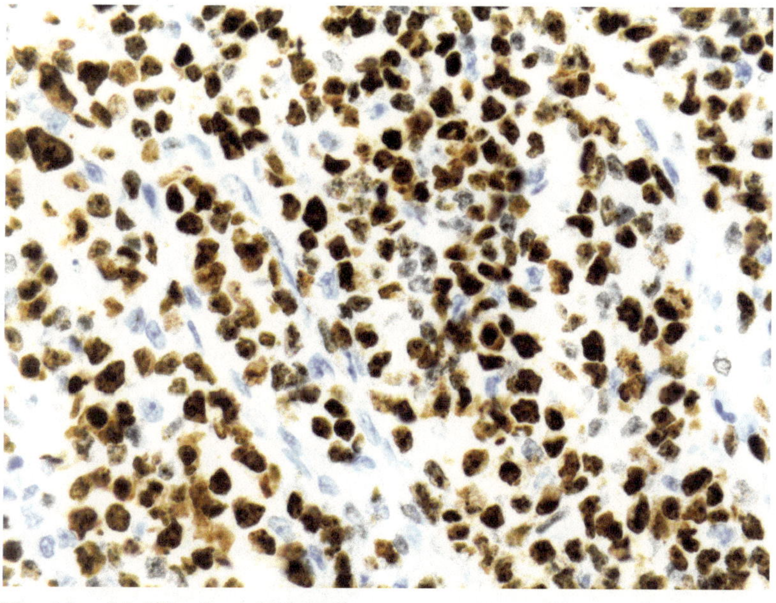

Fig. 6. LCNEC with a ki-67 index of 80-90%

In many patients, metastatic disease is present at time of diagnosis. In some instances the primary can be found, but often the primary will be of uncertain origin but usually considered GI if the metastatic load is dominating in liver and abdomen. Despite rare reports of long-term survivors, surgery alone is inadequate therapy even for apparently localised disease. Many operated patients have a rapid recurrence after surgery. Adjuvant radiotherapy for incompletely resected disease and systemic chemotherapy are widely recommended, although the effectiveness of a combined modality approach has not been firmly established. Despite aggressive multi-modality therapy including surgery and systemic chemotherapy, the median survival in colorectal SCC was six months, with only 15% of patients alive at one-year (Hung 1989). Data from Memorial Sloan Kettering Cancer Centre show a median survival of ten months for patients with colorectal SCC (Bernick et al., 2004). One-year, two-year, and three-year survival was 46%, 26%, and 13%, respectively. There are no significant differences in survival based on pathologic subtypes (Bernick et al., 2004, Shia et al., 2008). In a series of 53 cases of gallbladder SCC, those with disseminated disease had a median survival of eight months after treatment with combination chemotherapy. One and two year survival rates were 28% and 0%, respectively (Fujii et al. 2001). In the SEER database of colorectal NEC, 5-year survival was 21% for all stages, ranging from 73% in localised disease to 6 % in distant disease (Kang et al., 2007).

2.2 Neoadjuvant chemotherapy

Extensive disease (ED) is almost invariably treated by systemic chemotherapy. In contrast, the treatment approach for limited disease (LD), a potentially curable condition, is presently neither consistent nor uniform. While some authors used only local therapies, mostly surgery and occasionally radiotherapy, others advocate the use of chemotherapy, even alone, in these patients. NEC do not respond to treatments usually applied in other neuroendocrine tumours such as somatostatin analogues and interferon (Alhmann et al., 2008, Nilson et al. 2006). For patients with disease localised within an anatomic region (limited disease), initial neoadjuvant therapy with chemotherapy or chemoradiotherapy is an option, followed by surgery if no distant metastases are identified and the locoregional disease is resectable. Usually 2-3 cycles are given before surgery (Figure 7).

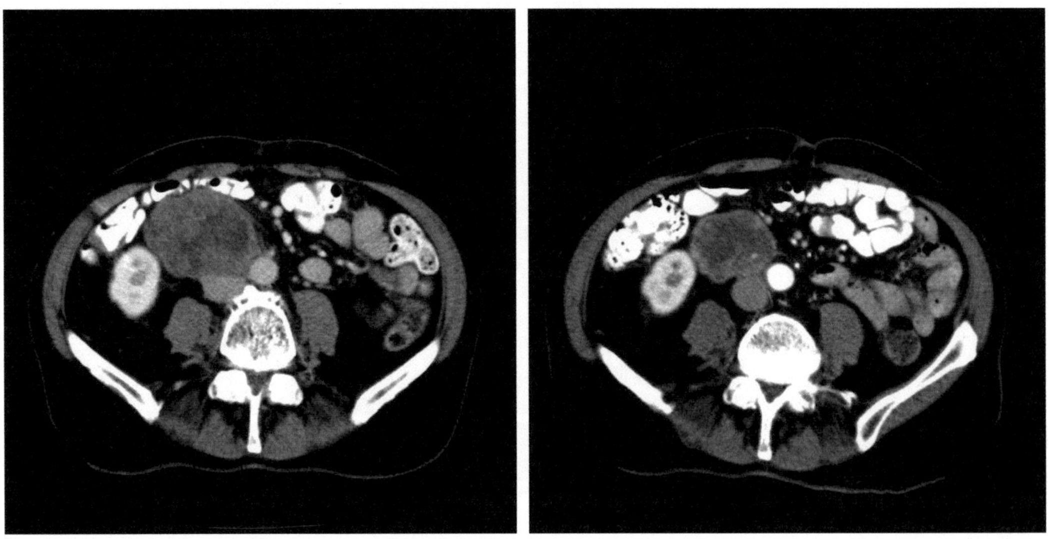

Fig. 7. Partial response after 4 cycles of neoadjuvant cisplatin/etoposide before radical surgery in a patient with unknown primary NEC.

No convincing data exist concerning adjuvant postoperative chemotherapy, but most recommend postoperative chemotherapy with the same drugs for 3-4 months as part of the neoadjuvant approach. Adjuvant or neoadjuvant chemotherapy is based on the effect in a metastatic setting, and is usually given with cisplatin /carboplatin and etoposide with response rates between 41- 67% (Mitry et al., 1999, Moertel et al., 1991). Casas and colleagues highlighted the role of systemic chemotherapy and local treatment in small-cell carcinomas of the oesophagus. In a retrospective series of 199 patients, improved median survival from 5 to 20 months was reported in patients with localised disease who received multi-modal therapy, i.e. surgery, radiation therapy, and systemic treatment (Casas et al., 1997). A prognostic factor analysis found that local therapy only (e.g. surgery alone) was the single most powerful predictor of poor prognosis. In the prognostic factor analysis, chemotherapy was found to be strongly associated with improved survival, both in LD and ED. Recent data from Memorial Sloan Kettering Cancer Centre support the use of induction chemotherapy followed by consolidative chemoradiation for patients with limited disease oesophageal SCNEC (Ku et al., 2008). Median survival was 20 months in this single institute retrospective study of 25 oesophageal SCNEC patients, with two limited disease patients alive and free of disease after five years follow-up. The authors concluded that surgery might not be necessary as part of initial therapy if a clinical complete response is achieved after chemoradiation, and that surgery may be reserved for salvage after documented local failure. In 64 patients with GI NEC seen at Memorial Sloan Kettering Cancer Center between 1980 and 2002,the most common primary tumour locations were in the large bowel and oesophagus (Brenner et al., 2004b). Sixteen patients with LD received chemotherapy, 12 of whom received it in conjunction with either surgery or radiotherapy. Of these, two remained alive with no evidence of disease for at least 64 and 94 months and one expired with no evidence of recurrence after almost 9 years. The authors suggests a potential role for surgery for LD; half of the operated patients retained locoregional control, and four of the six long-term survivors had surgery; two of them with no other treatment. The authors also state that this study supports the effectiveness of chemotherapy on survival in this disease; three of the long-term survivors received chemotherapy and six patients were treated by a combination of surgery and chemotherapy. Two of these had no evidence of disease for over 7 years and locoregional control was preserved in three. At present, in the absence of data derived from prospective clinical trials, they recommend to treat patients with LD with pre- or postoperative chemotherapy.

In contrast to metastatic neuroendocrine tumours with a low ki-67, debulking surgery and surgery for liver metastasis is generally not recommended in NEC patients due to the high ki-67 level. In some patients, however, this may still be an option. In one of our patients, surgery for extensive metastatic disease after neoadjuvant chemotherapy resulted in long time survival (Figure 8) (Sorbye et al., 2007). Similar case reports of neoadjuvant chemotherapy before locoregional treatment of metastatic NEC lesions have been reported (Power et al., 2010).

Altogether, most data support that in patients presenting with limited disease NEC of the gastrointestinal tract, a combination of systemic platinum-based chemotherapy combined with local treatment consisting of radiotherapy, surgery or both offer the best chance for long-term survival. Based on the high rate of micrometastatic disease presentation, several authors suggest that a sequence of neoadjuvant chemotherapy followed by definitive surgery seems appropriate, although the reverse sequence of surgery followed by adjuvant chemotherapy can not be excluded (Brenner et al., 2007).

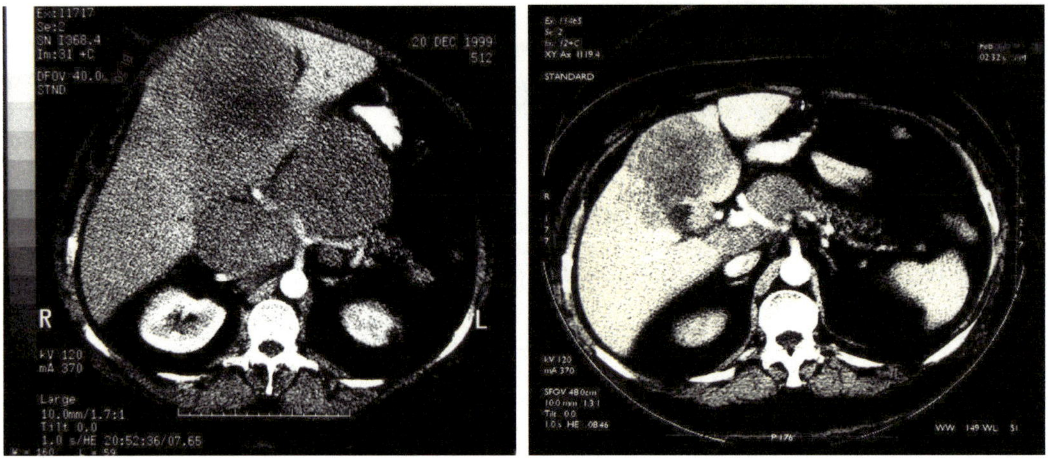

Fig. 8. Partial response of liver metastases and lymph node metastases after 4 cycles of neoadjuvant chemotherapy with cisplatin/etoposide before radical surgery and long-term survival.

3. Neuroendocrine cancer of the uterine cervix

3.1 Background

Neuroendocrine tumours of the uterine cervix represent 1–2% of cervical cancers and are the 2nd most common extra-pulmonary location of the primary tumor for NEC (Crowder et al., 2007). They are classified as typical carcinoid tumours, atypical carcinoid tumours, small-cell neuroendocrine carcinomas (SCNEC) and large-cell neuroendocrine carcinomas (Figure 9). Small-cell neuroendocrine carcinoma is the most common, and is aggressive with a high chance of distant metastasis and poor prognosis, even with combinations of treatments.

The natural history of this disease differs from the more commonly seen squamous cell or adenocarcinoma of the cervix. Patients diagnosed with SCNEC are more likely to have lymph node metastases and lymphovascular space invasion, and their clinical course is frequently marked by local and distant failure. Five-year survival rates vary from 31-36% for early disease and 0-14% for advanced disease (Chen et al., 2008). Long-term survival can be achieved only in patients with limited stage disease. Limited stage disease, which is defined as disease that can be encompassed within a radiation field, is treated with curative intent with combined modality therapy, with approximately 30% of patients achieving a cure (Figure 10). Patients with extensive stage disease - defined as disease outside of these confines - have a dismal prognosis with few surviving beyond two years. Clear treatment recommendations for SCNEC have not been defined. Due to the rarity of this disease it has been difficult to conduct prospective trials. Based on retrospective studies and treatment paradigms established for small-cell lung carcinoma, many clinicians favour the use of combined modality therapy for limited stage disease, definitive chemoradiation therapy for locoregional advanced disease and palliative chemotherapy for metastatic disease. It is not known if these treatment modalities ultimately improve survival. Often, the diagnosis of small-cell is not made until receipt of the final pathology on a radical hysterectomy; once the diagnosis is made, prompt initiation of combined modality therapy should follow post-operatively. The role of surgery for SCNEC is not well studied. It is unclear which patients, if any should undergo radical hysterectomy as opposed to primary combined chemotherapy and radiation therapy. If small cell histology is known, it is probably most appropriate to proceed with chemotherapy followed by surgery and postoperative chemotherapy or postoperative chemoradiation.

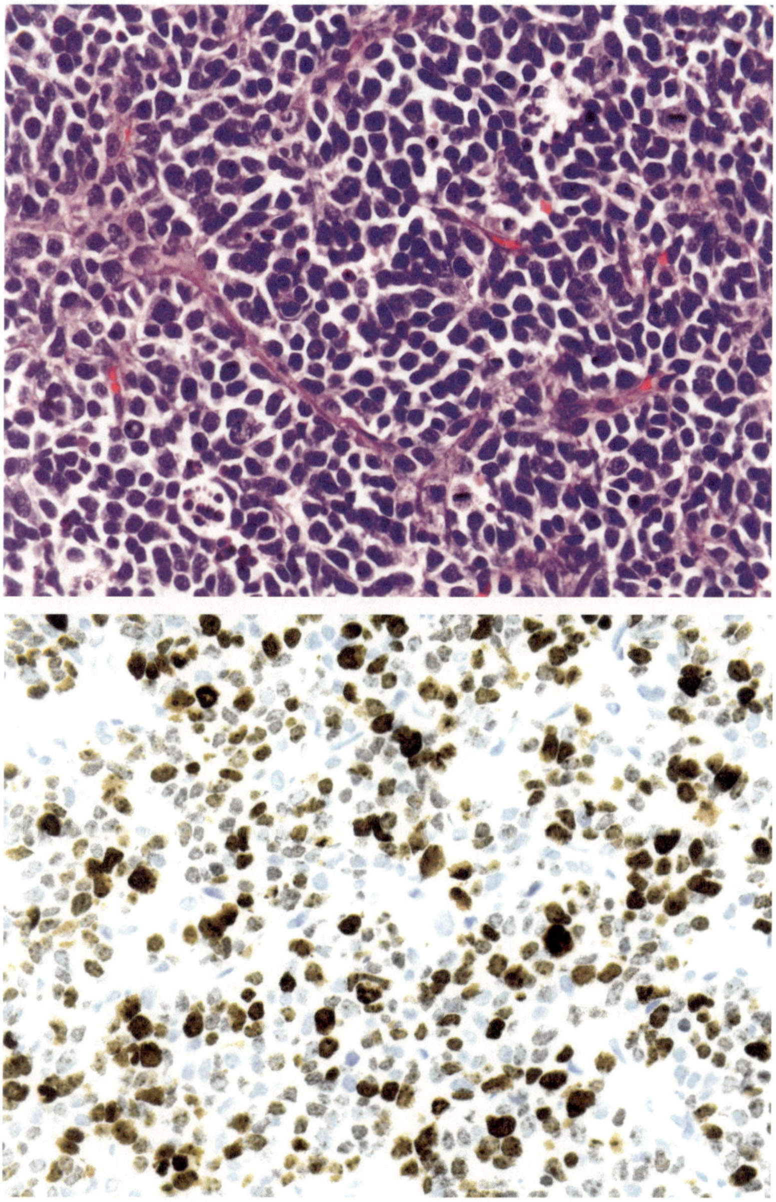

Fig. 9. Small-cell neuroendocrine cancer of uterine cervix, ki-67 about 60%

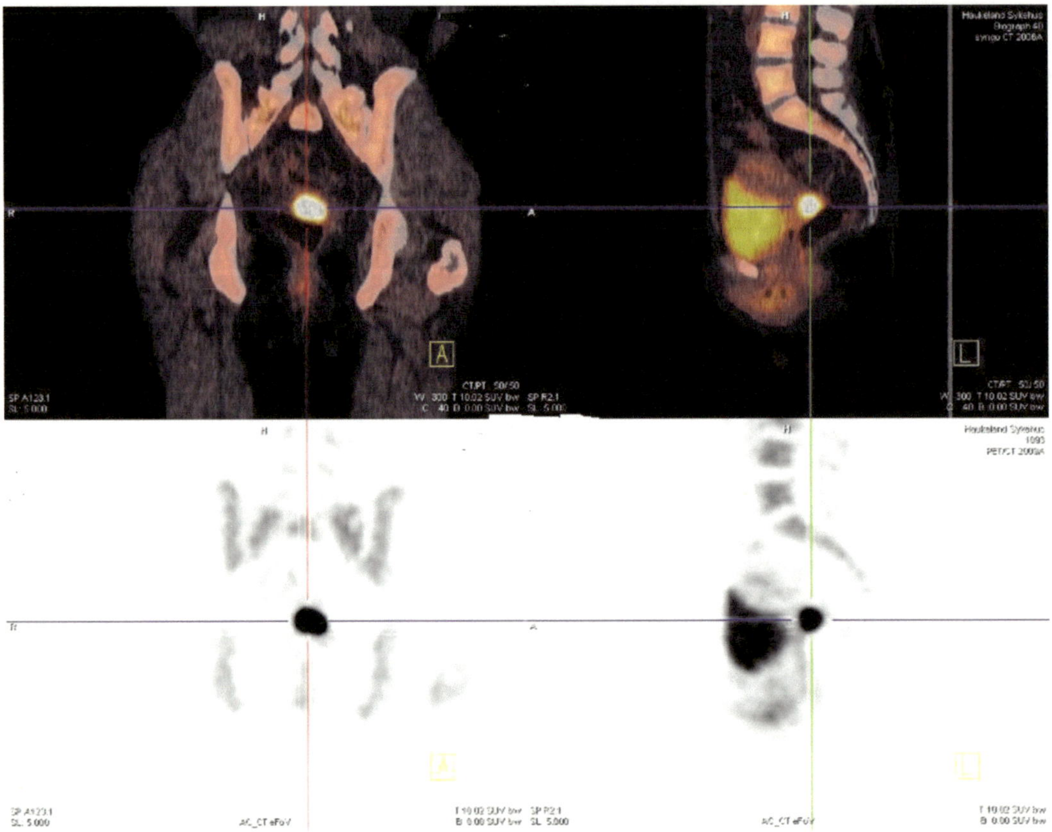

Fig. 10. PET/CT and MRI of a localised uterine cervix NEC before initiation of neoadjuvant chemotherapy.

3.2 Neoadjuvant chemotherapy

In a retrospective review of 188 patients of small-cell carcinoma of the uterine cervix, 135 patients had stages I-IIA, 45 stages IIB-IVA, and 8 stage IVB disease (Cohen et al., 2010). Adjuvant chemotherapy or chemoradiation was associated with improved survival in patients with stages IIB-IVA disease compared with those who did not receive chemotherapy (17.8% vs 6.0%; *P* = .04). On multivariable analysis, early-stage disease and use of chemotherapy or chemoradiation were independent prognostic factors for improved survival. Hoskins et al. reported 31 patients who were treated with protocols using etoposide, cisplatin and radiation therapy with concurrent chemotherapy with or without the addition of carboplatin and paclitaxel (Hoskins et al., 2003). The 3-year failure-free rate of the patients with early stage disease (stage I and II) was 80%. Chang et al. analysed 40 cases of small-cell uterine cervical carcinoma treated with primary hysterectomy followed by adjuvant chemotherapy containing a combination of vincristine, doxorubicin and cyclophosphamide or cisplatin and etoposide (Chang et al., 1998). Median survival was 47 months, signifying the importance of adjuvant chemotherapy for early stage small-cell cervical carcinoma after radical hysterectomy. A recent study from Korea retrospectively reviewed 68 patients (Lee et al., 2008). Seven were treated with radical surgery alone; 11 with neoadjuvant chemotherapy followed by radical surgery; 24 with radical surgery followed by adjuvant chemotherapy; and 26 with radical surgery followed by adjuvant radiation or chemoradiation. After a median follow-up of 44 months, the two-year and five-year survival for all patients was 65% and 47%, respectively. Patients who received neoadjuvant chemotherapy had a worse prognosis than those who did not receive neoadjuvant chemotherapy, but the patients who received neoadjuvant therapy had worse baseline prognostic factors. Adjuvant chemoradiation did not improve survival compared with adjuvant chemotherapy alone. In a study with 17 patients with SCNEC in uterine cervix, all 5 patients with early stage disease without chemotherapy as part of their initial treatment developed distant metastases within 2 years from the diagnosis (Zivanovic et al., 2009). This was in contrast to the 6 patients who were treated with adjuvant platinum- and etoposide-based combination therapy. In this group, only 1 patient developed systemic disease. In a retrospective analyses of 62 patients with large-cell NEC of the uterine cervix, median age was 37 and FIGO stage was: 58% stage I, 16% stage II, 2% stage III and 8% stage IV disease (Embry et al., 2011). Median overall survival for stage I, II, III, and IV cancers was 19, 17, 3, and 1.5 months, respectively. Thirty-seven women (60%) received chemotherapy as part of their initial treatment plan. In a multivariate analysis, earlier stage and the addition of chemotherapy were associated with improved survival. Both platinum agents and platinum and etoposide together were associated with improved survival.

Among 20 patients with neuroendocrine cervical carcinoma, patients with stage Ib_2 or greater received neoadjuvant chemotherapy with vincristine, bleomycin, and platinum (Bermudez et al., 2001). The response was <50% in 2/13 cases (15%), >50% in 9/13 (69%), and complete in 2/13 (15%), and resection was successfully performed in all 13 patients. Patients with initial tumor volume less than 4 cm had no recurrences and 5-year survival was 76%, whereas 75% recurred and 5-year survival was only 18% when initial tumor volume was over 4 cm (Figure 11).

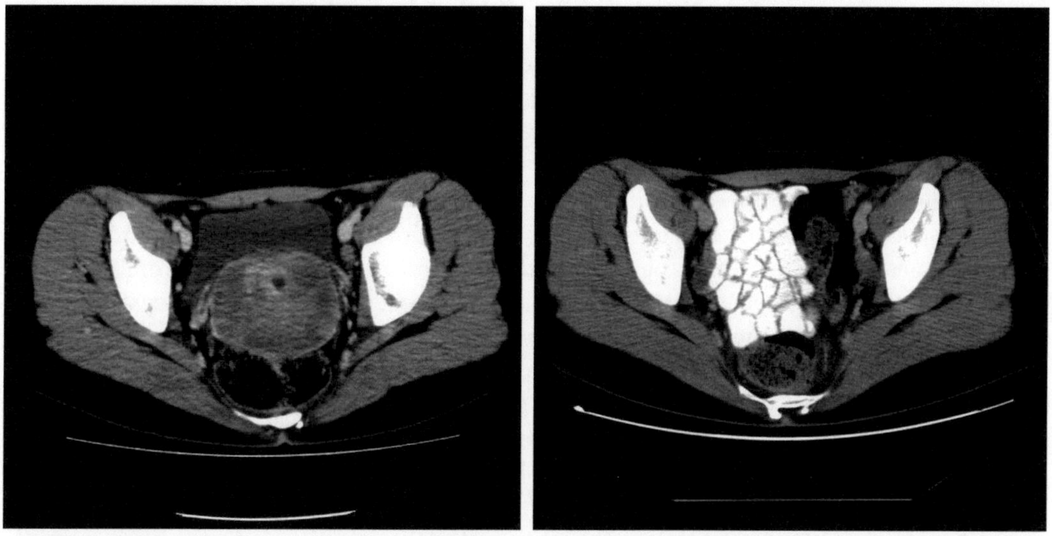

Fig. 11. Complete response of small-cell NEC of uterine cervix after 2 cycles of neoadjuvant chemotherapy with cisplatin and etoposide preceding planned surgery.

Although the comparison between different series is problematic due to selection bias and different treatment strategies, data support that in patients with early stage disease NEC of the uterine cervix, the addition of systemic platinum-based chemotherapy appears to have a protective effect on the development of distant metastases. The association between chemotherapy and local therapy (surgery/radiation) seems to obtain the best results in terms of survival. However, the sequence at which both therapeutic modalities should be used has not been proven yet.

4. Neuroendocrine carcinoma of the bladder

4.1 Background

In the urinary system, the majority of cases have been observed in the bladder and prostate. Small-cell neuroendocrine carcinoma accounts for less than 1% of all bladder tumours, whereas large-cell neuroendocrine carcinoma is even rarer. Like small-cell carcinoma of the lung, small-cell carcinoma of the bladder has a propensity for early metastases. Only about one third (14–44%) of the patients present with limited disease. Given the lack of evidence to the contrary, a radical cystectomy has been considered the "de facto" standard for patients without evidence of metastatic disease. However, the lack of efficacy of this approach is readily apparent; even in recently published series, most patients die within 2 years of cystectomy (Cheng et al., 2004, Quek et al., 2005). Management ranges from cystectomy alone, with or without adjuvant radiation therapy or adjuvant chemotherapy. Recent retrospective reviews suggest better survival with initial chemotherapy followed by local consolidation with cystectomy or radiation (Church & Bahl 2006). The use of preoperative chemotherapy follows from the frequent observation of rapid growth rates and typical upstaging on initial surgery, not uncommonly leading to aborted cystectomy. The benefits of incorporating neoadjuvant chemotherapy can be multifold. Whereas it may take time to schedule an operation or for patients in this age group to complete preoperative clearance, systemic chemotherapy can be initiated quickly, providing timely control of this rapidly growing chemotherapy-sensitive tumor. Tumor can frequently be downstaged, resulting in a surgery that is more likely to achieve negative margins and the pathologic stage after preoperative chemotherapy may provide valuable prognostic information.

4.2 Neoadjuvant chemotherapy

In a retrospective review of 25 patients with neuroendocrine tumor of the bladder, Quek and associates reported significant improvement in recurrence-free and overall survival (OS) in those receiving neoadjuvant or adjuvant chemotherapy with radical cystectomy as compared with radical cystectomy alone (Quek et al., 2005). Walther et al observed that five of seven patients were alive and cancer free at 36 months, most as a result of preoperative chemotherapy (Walther et al., 2002). A study from M.D. Anderson Cancer Centre reported similar results with regard to neoadjuvant chemotherapy but not with adjuvant chemotherapy (Siefker-Radtke et al., 2004). Of the 88 patients 46 underwent cystectomy, including 25 who were treated with initial cystectomy and 21 who received preoperative chemotherapy. For patients treated with initial cystectomy median cancer specific survival (CSS) was 23 months, with 36% disease-free at 5 years. For patients receiving preoperative chemotherapy median CSS had not been reached, although CSS at 5-years was 78% with no cancer related deaths observed beyond 2 years. Notably 7 of 25 patients treated with initial cystectomy received chemotherapy after surgery, but their survival was no better than those treated with cystectomy alone. As others have observed, the pathological stage was higher than clinically appreciated for 56% of patients treated with initial cystectomy. There were no cancer related deaths among patients with disease that was downstaged to pT2 or less. Other studies, however, have shown no survival benefit between cystectomy and multi-modal therapy. Cheng et al. reported no survival benefit in 64 cases of SCC in those undergoing cystectomy alone compared with multi-modal treatment (Cheng et al., 2004). Still, a one-year disease specific survival difference of 66% versus 45% was observed among patients who received combination therapy, compared to those who underwent cystectomy only. A retrospective report from the Mayo Clinic advocates surgery alone in patients with surgically resectable tumours, especially for those with muscle-invasive tumours (pT2N0M0) (Choong et al., 2005). Although it is not clear how many patients were upstaged at surgery, of 12 patients with pT2N0M0 small-cell urothelial cancer, the 3-year OS rate was 63.6%. However, half of these patients experienced relapse. The Mayo Clinic results are also in marked contrast to another retrospective study that suggests an approximately 25% 3-year survival rate in 30 patients with organ-confined disease (≤ pT2N0M0). In a study of 106 cases of SCC bladder cancer, only cisplatin chemotherapy predicted survival on multivariate analysis (Mackay et al., 1998). Initial stage was not independently associated with survival, which strongly suggests that micrometastatic disease is usually present at presentation in clinically localised tumours and systemic metastases are the major cause of mortality. In the most recent study, 4 cycles of neoadjuvant chemotherapy were given to small-cell urothelial cancer in a phase II trial (Sifker-Radtke 2009). 18 patients with surgical resectable cancer received neoadjuvant treatment with a median survival of 58 months, 13 are still cancer free and alive. Pathologic downstaging was quite frequent, with an improved survival in those downstaged to ≤ pT2N0M0. The largest impact on survival seemed to be in patients with muscle-invasive bladder cancer.

In the absence of a large comparative trial, definitive conclusions cannot be drawn regarding the best multi-modality strategy for the treatment of neuroendocrine carcinoma of the bladder. Currently available literature suggests that local therapy with surgery or radiotherapy alone is not optimal, and that integrating chemotherapy can improve long-term disease control. Recent results suggest that neoadjuvant chemotherapy followed by localised therapy to the pelvis may be the optimal strategy. Whether radiation or cystectomy provides optimal local consolidation is not currently known.

5. Neuroendocrine carcinoma of the prostate

5.1 Background

Prostate cancer is one of the most common types of extra-pulmonary small-cell carcinoma, accounting for 10% of all EP-NEC (Asmis et al., 2006). Pure SCC is rare at initial presentation, accounting for less than two percent of all prostate malignancies. Small cell carcinoma prostatic disease has a worse prognosis than SCC bladder disease (Mackey et al., 1998). Three patterns of small-cell carcinoma are known: one third present as pure small-cell carcinoma; one fifth of cases present with combined adenocarcinoma; and approximately half present as recurrence of small-cell carcinoma from conventional adenocarcinoma. Many prostatic adenocarcinomas show areas of focal neuroendocrine differentiation, and many extrapulmonary small-cell carcinomas of the prostate are associated with an adenocarcinoma component. In patients with mixed prostate cancer that has metastasised, it is often unclear whether the metastatic disease is of the adenocarcinoma component, the SCC component or both since biopsies of metastatic lesions are typically not done. Because this type of prostate cancer essentially has two tumor types, it may be beneficial to biopsy any atypical metastatic lesion. Clinically, prostate cancer with SCC component act differently from pure adenocarcinoma. Typical features of a mixed tumor type include; elevated neuroendocrine markers such as serum chromogranin A, low to normal PSA, early disease progression, resistance to androgen deprivation and high-grade disease. Small-cell carcinomas of the prostate do not express androgen receptors. These features warrant aggressive multi-modal therapy. Small-cell neuroendocrine carcinoma of the prostate is a highly aggressive tumor, presenting early metastasis to soft tissues and bone without a commensurate with serum PSA level.

5.2 Neoadjuvant chemotherapy

For patients with mixed adenocarcinoma/SCC prostate cancer, the standard treatment regimen includes hormonal therapy in combination with systemic etoposide/cisplatin chemotherapy. Whether chemotherapy is effective for long term survival for patients with small cell prostate carcinoma is controversial. Vinblastine, doxorubicin, and cyclophosphamide, or platinum (cisplatin or carboplatin) compound-based regimens combined with etoposide, or etoposide and doxorubicin, are recommended for the initial treatment. Therapy usually results in a 60% response rate, median survival is approximately one-year whereas long-term survival is rare (Amato et al., 1992, Palmgren et al., 2007). Immediate chemotherapy with or without hormonal therapy for both pure SCC and mixed adenocarcinoma of the prostate resulted in longer clinical remissions in retrospective study, although none survived (Moore et al., 1992). In a single centre study performed at M.D. Anderson Cancer Centre with 83 patients, 26 had no evidence of metastatic disease at the time of diagnosis (Spiess et al., 2007). The most common form of initial therapy for SCC of the prostate was systemic chemotherapy containing etoposide and/or a platinum compound, given either alone (38 patients), combined with androgen deprivation therapy (ADT) (29 patients), with radiotherapy and ADT (6 patients) or with surgery and ADT (3 patients). The use of systemic chemotherapy was not found to be a predictor of PFS and disease-free survival in this study, because the majority of patients (92%) received it as initial therapy. In a retrospective study of 60 SCC prostate cancer patients, primary surgical therapy was the only parameter that predicted survival on univariate analysis (Mackey et al., 1998). In contrast to bladder SCC, no benefit of chemotherapy was found for prostate primary tumours. Within the framework of the Rare Cancer Network Study, 30 patients suffering from small-cell neuroendocrine prostate cancer were examined, either in an early/localised or an advanced/metastatic stage (Stein et al., 2008). Patients were treated with cisplatin-based chemotherapy, with or without pelvic radiotherapy. Two patients with early disease achieved complete remission for a duration of 19 and 22 months. Twenty-five patients succumbed to massive local and/or distant failure. Despite initial response, the common cisplatin-based chemotherapy plus radiotherapy failed to improve outcome markedly.

In conclusion, for localised non-metastatic small-cell neuroendocrine prostate, initial therapy with platinum-based chemotherapy is usually recommended, but the long term benefit is uncertain.

6. Neuroendocrine carcinoma of the breast

6.1 Background

Neuroendocrine carcinoma of the breast is one of the least common types of breast cancer with data consisting of only case reports in the literature. All the tumours described showed morphological and immunohistochemical similarities to the breast metastases of pulmonary small cell carcinoma, the most distinguishing feature are the absence of primary small-cell cancer elsewhere. In 2003, the World Health Organization (WHO) recommended classification of these tumours into three histologic types: solid, small-cell, and large-cell neuroendocrine carcinoma (Tavassoli et al., 2003). Seventy-four patients with NEC of the breast who were treated at M. D. Anderson Cancer Center were recently analysed. NEC showed a more aggressive course than invasive ductal carcinoma, with a higher propensity for local and distant recurrence and poorer overall survival (Wei et al., 2010). No standard treatment protocol has been defined with certainty due to the small number of cases. Modified radical mastectomy with axillary lymph node dissection seems to be the treatment of choice, with adjuvant radiation, chemotherapy or both, based on the clinical stage and presence of metastasis. Data suggest using different chemotherapy schedules than ordinary used in breast cancer treatment. Most studies show that the SCNEC of breast is a very aggressive neoplasm and has in general a worse prognosis than the usual ductal types, but may have a good prognosis depending on the initial stage of the disease (Wei et al., 2010).

6.2 Neoadjuvant chemotherapy

There are case reports on the use of neoadjuvant chemotherapy for SCC of the breast and one patient with a complete response after cisplatin and etoposide treatment (Mirza & Shahab, 2007). Treatment and outcome information for 60 patients with NEC of the breast at M. D. Anderson Cancer Center show that among 14 patients who received cisplatin-based neoadjuvant chemotherapy only 1 patient had recurrence of disease (Wei et al., 2010). Among the other 46 patients where 38 received postoperative chemotherapy, 18 patients had a recurrence of disease indicating that neoadjuvant chemotherapy might be superior to postoperative treatment.

7. Conclusion

In the absence of large comparative trials, definitive conclusions cannot be drawn regarding the best multi-modality strategy for the treatment of EP-NEC. Currently available literature suggests that local therapy with surgery or radiotherapy alone is not optimal and that integrating platinum-based chemotherapy can improve long-term disease control and survival. Most data support that patients presenting with limited disease EP-NEC of the GI, bladder, breast and uterine cervix should be treated with systemic platinum based chemotherapy combined with local treatment consisting of radiotherapy, surgery or both. The sequence at which both therapeutic modalities should be used has not been proven yet, but recent results for NEC in bladder and breast indicate that neoadjuvant chemotherapy might be superior to postoperative treatment. Secondary surgery can be considered after neoadjuvant chemotherapy in highly selected patients with metastatic disease.

8. Acknowledgements

Dr Lars Helgeland, Dept of Pathology, Haukeland University Hospital, Bergen, Norway, provided histological photos.

9. References

Ahlman H, Nilsson O, McNicol AM, et al. (2008). Poorly-differentiated endocrine carcinomas of midgut and hindgut origin. *Neuroendocrinology*, 87, pp. 40-6.

Amato RJ, Logothetis CJ, Hallinan R, et al. (1992) Chemotherapy for small cell carcinoma of prostatic origin. *J Urol*, 147, pp. 935–937

Asmis TR, Reaume MN, Dahrouge S, et al (2006) Genitourinary small cell carcinoma: a retrospective review of treatment and survival patterns at the Ottawa Hospital Regional Cancer Center. *BJU Int*, 97, pp. 711–715

Bermúdez A, Vighi S, García A & Sardi J. (2001). Neuroendocrine cervical carcinoma: a diagnostic and therapeutic challenge. *Gynecol Oncol*, 82, pp. 32-9.

Bernick PE, Klimstra SD, Shia J *et al.*, (2004), Neuroendocrine carcinomas of the colon and rectum, *Dis Colon Rectum*, 47, pp. 163–169.

Bosman, FT., Carneiro, F., Hruban, RH.& Theise, ND. *WHO Classification of Tumours of the Digestive System*, Fourth Edition. 2010. ISBN 978-92-832-2432-7. WHO Press, Geneva, Switzerland.

Brennan SM, Gregory DL, Stillie A, et al. (2010). Should extrapulmonary small cell cancer be managed like small cell lung cancer? *Cancer*,116, pp. 888–95.

Brenner B, Tang LH, Klimstra DS & Kelsen DP. (2004). Small-cell carcinomas of the gastrointestinal tract: a review. *J Clin Oncol*, 22, pp. 2730-9.

Brenner B, Shah MA, Gonen M, et al. (2004) Small-cell carcinoma of the gastrointestinal tract: a retrospective study of 64 cases. *Br J Cancer*, 90, pp. 1720-6

Brenner B, Tang LH, Shia J, et al. (2007). Small cell carcinomas of the gastrointestinal tract: clinicopathological features and treatment approach. *Semin Oncol*, 34, pp. 43–50.

Casas F, Ferrer F, Farrus B, et al. (1997). Primary small cell carcinoma of the esophagus: a review of the literature with emphasis on therapy and prognosis. *Cancer*, 80, pp. 1366–72.

Chang TC, Lai CH, Tseng CJ et al. (1998). Prognostic factors in surgically treated small cell cervical carcinoma followed by adjuvant chemotherapy, *Cancer* ,83, pp. 712–718

Chen J, Macdonald OK & Gaffney DK. (2008). Incidence, mortality and prognostic factors of small cell carcinoma of the cervix. *Obstet Gynecol*, 111, pp. 1394-402

Cheng L, Pan CX, Yang XJ, et al. (2004). Small cell carcinoma of the urinary bladder: a clinicopathologic analysis of 64 patients. *Cancer*, 101, pp. 957–962.

Choong NW, Quevedo JF & Kaur JS. (2005). Small cell carcinoma of the urinary bladder. The Mayo Clinic experience. *Cancer*, 103, pp.1172–1178.

Church DN & Bahl A. (2006). Clinical review—small cell carcinoma of the bladder. *Cancer Treat Rev*, 32, pp. 588–593.

Cohen JG, Kapp DS, Shin JY et al. (2010) Small cell carcinoma of the cervix: treatment and survival outcomes of 188 patients. *Am J Obstet Gynecol*, 347.e1-6. Epub 2010 Jul 1

Crowder S & Tuller E. (2007). Small cell carcinoma of the female genital tract. *Semin Oncol*, 34, pp. 57–63

Cunningham D, Allum WH, Stenning SP, et al. (2006). Perioperative chemotherapy versus surgery alone for resectable gastroesophageal cancer. *N Engl J Med*, 355, pp. 11–20

Embry JR, Kelly MG, Post MD & Spillman MA.(2011). Large cell neuroendocrine carcinoma of the cervix: prognostic factors and survival advantage with platinum chemotherapy.*Gynecol Oncol*, 120, pp.444-8.

Faggiano A, Sabourin JC, Ducreux M et al. (2007). Pulmonary and extrapulmonary poorly differentiated large cell neuroendocrine carcinomas. *Cancer*, 110, pp. 265-74

Fujii H, Aotake T, Horiuchi T et al., (2001). Small cell carcinoma of the gallbladder: a case report and review of 53 cases in the literature, *Hepatogastroenterology* 48, pp. 1588–1593.

Galanis E, Frytak S & Lloyd RV. (1997). Extrapulmonary small cell carcinoma. *Cancer*, 79, pp. 1729-36.

Garcia-Carbonero R, Capdevila J, Crespo-Herrero G et al. (2010). Incidence, patterns of care and prognostic factors for outcome of gastroenteropancreatic neuroendocrine tumors (GEP-NETs): results from the National Cancer Registry of Spain (RGETNE).*Ann Oncol*, 2, pp. 1794-1803.

Hoskins PJ, Swenerton KD, Pike JA et al. (2003). Small-cell carcinoma of the cervix: fourteen years of experience at a single institution using a combined-modality regimen of involved-field irradiation and platinum-based combination chemotherapy. *J Clin Oncol*,21, pp. 3495-501

Hung SS, Small cell carcinoma of the colon (1989). A case report and literature review, *J Clin Gastroenterol*, 11, pp. 335–339.

Janson ET, Sørbye H, Welin S,et al. (2010). Nordic Guidelines 2010 for diagnosis and treatment of gastroenteropancreatic neuroendocrine tumours. *Acta Oncol*, 49, pp. 740-56.

Kang H, O'Connell JB & Leonardi MJ. (2007). Rare tumors of the colon and rectum: a national review. Int J Colorectal Dis. 22, pp. 183-9.

Kloppel G, Heitz PU, Capella C, et al. (1996). Pathology and nomenclature of human gastrointestinal neuroendocrine (carcinoid) tumors and related lesions. *World J Surg*, 20, pp. 132-141.

Lee JM, Lee KB, Nam JH *et al.*, (2008). Prognostic factors in FIGO stage IB-IIA small cell neuroendocrine carcinoma of the uterine cervix treated surgically: results of a multi-center retrospective Korean study. *Ann Oncol*, 19, pp. 321–326

Lee SS, Lee JL, Ryu MH, et al. (2007). Extrapulmonary small cell carcinoma: single center experience with 61 patients. *Acta Oncol*, 46, pp. 846-51.

Mackey JR, Au HJ, Hugh J, et al: (1998). Genitourinary small cell carcinoma: Determination of clinical and therapeutic factors associated with survival. *J Urol*, 159, 1624-1629.

Mitry E, Baudin E, Ducreux M, et al. (1999). Treatment of poorly differentiated neuroendocrine tumours with etoposide and cisplatin. *Br J Cancer*, 81, pp. 1351-5.

Mirza IA and Shahab N. (2007). Small cell carcinoma of the breast. *Semin Oncol*, 34, pp. 64-66.

Moertel CG, Kvols LK, O'Connell MJ & Rubin J. (1991). Treatment of neuroendocrine carcinomas with combined etoposide and cisplatin. Evidence of major therapeutic activity in the anaplastic variants of these neoplasms. *Cancer*, 68, pp. 227-32.

Moore SR, Reinberg Y & Zhang G (1992) Small cell carcinoma of prostate: effectiveness of hormonal versus chemotherapy. *Urology*, 39, pp. 411–416

NCCN. (2010). *NCCN Clinical practice guidelines in oncology*. National Comprehensive Cancer Network (NCCN); 2010 v10.

Nilsson O, Van Cutsem E, Delle Fave G, et al. (2006). Poorly differentiated carcinomas of the foregut (gastric, duodenal and pancreatic). *Neuroendocrinology*, 84, pp. 212-5.

Nordlinger B, Sorbye H, Glimelius B, et al. (2008). Preoperative chemotherapy with FOLFOX4 and surgery for resectable liver metastases form colorectal cancer. *Lancet*, 371, pp. 1007-1016.

Palmgren S, Karavadia SS & Wakefield MR. (2007). Unusual and underappreciated: small cell carcinoma of the prostate. *Sem Oncol*, 34, pp. 22–29

Power DG, Asmis TR, Tang LH, et al. (2010) High-grade neuroendocrine carcinoma of the colon, long-term survival in advanced disease. *Med Oncol*. 2010 Sep 14. [Epub ahead of print]

Quek ML, Nichols PW, Yamzon J, et al. (2005). Radical cystectomy for primary neuroendocrine tumors of the bladder: the University of Southern California experience. *J Urol*, 174, pp. 93–96.

Shia J, Tang LH, Weiser MR, et al. (2008). Is nonsmall cell type highgrade neuroendocrine carcinoma of the tubular gastrointestinal tract a distinct disease entity? *Am J Surg Pathol*, 32, pp. 719–31.

Siefker-Radtke AO, Dinney CP, Abrahams NA, et al. (2004). Evidence supporting preoperative chemotherapy for small cell carcinoma of the bladder: a retrospective review of the M. D. Anderson cancer experience. *J Urol*, 172, pp. 481–484

Siefker-Radtke AO, Kamat AM, Grossman HB. et al. (2009). Phase II clinical trial of neoadjuvant alternating doublet cehmotherapy with ifosfamide/doxorubicin and etoposide/cisplatin in smallcell urothelial cancer. *J Clin Oncol*, 27, pp. 2592-97.

Spiess PE, Pettaway CA, Vakar-Lopez F *et al.*, (2007). Treatment outcomes of small cell carcinoma of the prostate: a single-center study. *Cancer*, 110, pp. 1729–1737

Solcia E KG, Sobin LH. (2000). *Histological Typing of Endocrine Tumours*. New York: Springer,

Stein ME, Bernstein Z, Abacioglu U et al. Small cell (neuroendocrine) carcinoma of the prostate: etiology, diagnosis, prognosis, and therapeutic implications--a retrospective study of 30 patients from the rare cancer network. Am J Med Sci 2008 336:478-88.

Strosberg J,Coppola D, Klimstra D.S. et al. (2010). The NANETS Consensus Guidelines for the Diagnosis and

Management of Poorly Differentiated (High-Grade) Extrapulmonary Neuroendocrine Carcinomas. *Pancreas*, 39,pp. 799-800.

Sorbye H, Westre B, Horn A. (2007). Curative surgery after neoadjuvant chemotherapy in metastatic poorly differentiated neuroendocrine carcinoma *Eur J Surg Oncol*, 33, pp. 1209-10.

Tavassoli FA & Devilee P. (2003). Pathology and genetics. In: *Tumors of the breat and female genital organs*. WHO classification of tumors series. Lyan, France. IARC Press 2003: pp. 32-34.

Walenkamp AM, Sonke GS & Sleijfer DT. (2009). Clinical and therapeutic aspects of extrapulmonary small cell carcinoma. *Cancer Treat Rev*, 35, pp. 228-236.

Walther PJ (2002). Adjuvant/neoadjuvant etoposide/cisplatin and cystectomy for management of invasive small cell carcinoma of the bladder. *J Urol*, 167, pp. 285.

Wei B, Ding T, Xing Y et al. (2010). Invasive neuroendocrine carcinoma of the breast: a distinctive subtype of aggressive mammary carcinoma. *Cancer*, 116, pp. 4463-73

Welin S, Sorbye H, Sebjornsen S, et al. (2011) Clinical effect of temozolomide-based chemotherapy in poorly differentiated endocrine carcinoma after progression on first-line chemotherapy. *Cancer*. 2011 Mar 31. doi: 10.1002/cncr.26124. (Epub ahead of print)

Zivanovic O, Leitao MM Jr, Park KJ et al. (2009). Small cell neuroendocrine carcinoma of the cervix: Analysis of outcome, recurrence pattern and the impact of platinum-based combination chemotherapy. *Gynecol Oncol*. 112, pp. 590-3.

5

Neoadjuvant Chemotherapy in Gynecologic Cancers

Prapaporn Suprasert
Department of OB&GYN, Faculty of Medicine, Chiang Mai University Chiang Mai Thailand

1. Introduction

Neoadjuvant chemotherapy is introduced in many gynecologic cancers such as cervical and ovarian cancer. The aim of using neoadjuvant chemotherapy is to reduce the tumor size prior to the principle treatment, either radiation or surgery. The benefit of reducing tumor size can increase the operability and decrease the morbidity in many types of gynecologic cancers. Besides this, neoadjuvant chemotherapy might control the micro- metastatic disease to decrease the distant metastasis (Benedetti-Panici et al., 1998; Buda et al., 2005; Chua, 2010). On the other hand, in patients who did not respond to chemotherapy, however, the administration of neoadjuvant chemotherapy risks delaying the principle treatment.
In this chapter, literature pertaining to neoadjuvant chemotherapy for gynecologic cancer will be presented in five parts, categorized by types of cancers; cervical cancer, ovarian cancer, endometrial cancer, vulvar cancer, and vaginal cancer.

2. Cervical cancer

Cervical cancer is the third most common malignancy in women worldwide. The GLOBOCAN project estimates that there will be 530,000 new cases in 2008. The highest incidence is in Africa and Asia. In early stage, the patients may be treated with either surgery or radiation therapy depending on preferences of both patient and physician (Undurraga et al., 2010). Whereas concurrent chemoradiation is the principle treatment in the locally advanced stage, and chemotherapy is the main treatment in advanced stage.
Neoadjuvant chemotherapy has been investigated in cervical cancer with the aim of improving the treatment outcome for over 20 years. This section presents the studies about using neoadjuvant chemotherapy in cervical cancer before radiation and surgery.

2.1 Neoadjuvant chemotherapy before radiation therapy

The rationale of giving neoadjuvant chemotherapy before radiation therapy included reducing tumor volume and radio- sensitizing tumors by decreasing the hypoxic cell fraction in large tumors (Movva et al., 2009). However, several randomized trials of such treatment revealed no survival advantage compared with radiation therapy alone (Chiara et al., 1994; Herod et al., 2000; Lacava et al., 1997; Leborgne et al., 1997; Sundfor et al., 1996; Souhami et al., 1991; Symonds, 2000; Tattersall et al., 1992; Tattersall et al., 1995). Furthermore, the Neoadjuvant Chemotherapy for Locally Advanced Cervical Cancer Meta-Analysis Collaboration Group presented a systematic review and meta-analysis of individual patient data (IPD) from eighteen trials with 2,074 patients. (Neoadjuvant Chemotherapy for Locally Advanced Cervical Cancer Meta-analysis Collaboration,2003). Neoadjuvant chemotherapy before radiation therapy was compared with radiation therapy alone. The result did not show any benefit in overall survival with neoadjuvant chemotherapy. However, when the analyses were re-grouped by the interval and the dose intensity of the chemotherapy, a survival benefit was apparent in patients who received weekly and biweekly cisplatin with a dose of intensity more than 25 mg/m^2/week (Table 1). There was 7% absolute improvement in overall 5-year survival in trials using shorter cycles of neoadjuvant chemotherapy of less than fourteen days. This advantage was also observed in disease-free, locoregional disease-free and matastasis-free survival. In addition, trials that used a dose more than 25 mg/m^2/week showed an improvement of about 3% in 5-year overall survival. Conversely, in trials that administered lower dose of cisplatin (less than 25 kg/m^2/week) demonstrated an 11% reduction in 5-year overall survival. In the meantime, intervals longer than fourteen days trials demonstrated a decrease of 8% in 5-year overall survival. A decrease was also observed in disease-free, locoregional disease-free and matastasis-free survival. The benefit from short cycle and dose intensive cisplatin-based neoadjuvant chemotherapy prior radiation therapy suggested that chemotherapy may effectively control radioresistant cellular clones and decrease the chance of surviving tumor cell regrowth.

Trial grouping	Number of trials	Number of events/patients	HR (95%CI, P value)	Heterogeneity P value	5-year OS (%)
Interval of chemotherapy (days)					
>14	11	639/1214	1.25(1.07-1.46), 0.005	0.238	⇓ 8
≤14	6	417/812	0.76(0.62-0.92), 0.005	0.193	⇑ 7
Neoadjuvant cisplatin dose intensity (mg/m^2)					
<25	7	413/845	1.35(1.11-1.64), 0.002	0.746	⇓ 11%
≥25	11	671/1229	0.91(0.78-1.05), 0.200	0.001	⇑ 3%

Table 1. Overall survival (OS) by frequency of chemotherapy and cisplatin dose intensity in comparison I (Neoadjuvant Chemotherapy for Locally Advanced Cervical Cancer Meta-analysis Collaboration,2003; Gonzalez-Martin et al., 2008)

2.2 Neoadjuvant chemotherapy before concurrent chemoradiation

Studies on neoadjuvant chemotherapy before concurrent chemoradiation is limited. Gonzalez et al. (Duenas-Gonzalez et al., 2002) reported a phase II study that compared neoadjuvant chemotherapy followed by surgery or concurrent chemoradiation with standard concomitant chemoradiation. There were two groups, forty-one patients with cervical carcinoma in stage IB2-IIIB each, in the study. The first group was treated with neoadjuvant chemotherapy. The treatment consisted of cisplatin 100 mg/m^2 given on the first day and gemcitabine 1,000 mg/m^2 given on day 1 and 8, followed by either surgery or concomitant chemoradiation, depending on operability. The second group was treated with six weekly courses of cisplatin 40 mg/m^2 during standard pelvic radiation. Both groups had comparable clinicopathological characteristics. In this study, fourteen cases from the first group underwent chemoradiation after receiving neoadjuvant chemotherapy. Of these patients, thirteen patients had a clinical complete response. Nevertheless, this small number of patients did not conclusively demonstrate a benefit from neoadjuvant chemoradiation prior to concurrent chemoradiation. Further research is required to study this approach.

2.3 Neoadjuvant chemotherapy before surgery

2.3.1 Neoadjuvant chemotherapy before radical surgery versus radical surgery

Several studies revealed that giving neoadjuvant chemotherapy before surgery is effective in reducing tumor size, expediting micrometastasis treatment, improving operability and surgical downstaging (Hwang et al., 2001; Panici et al., 1991; Panici et al., 1991; Sardi et al., 1993). However, the randomized phase III study from the Gynecologic Oncologic Group (GOG) failed to demonstrate a survival benefit when compared to patients who received neoadjuvant chemotherapy followed by radical hysterectomy with patients who underwent surgery alone for bulky stage IB disease (Eddy et al., 2007). In addition, in a recent Cochrane database review, six randomized control trials including 1,072 cervical cancer patients comparing neoadjuvant chemotherapy plus surgery with primary surgery showed only significantly improvements in progression free survival in the neoadjuvant chemotherapy arm. In contrast, overall survival was not improved (Rydzewska et al.,2010).

Cai et al (2006) reported a randomized study of preoperative chemotherapy versus primary radical surgery for stage IB cervical cancer patients. This study was not included in the Cochrane review. In the neoadjuvant chemotherapy arm, patients were given cisplatin 75 mg/m^2 on day 1 plus 5- fluorouracil 24 mg/kg/day on day 1-5 every three weeks, for two courses. The number of studied patients in the neoadjuvant chemotherapy group was fifty-two cases, while the patients in primary surgery group numbered fifty-four cases. The results demonstrated a reduction in pathological risk factors and an improvement in long-term survival in patients who received neoadjuvant chemotherapy.

Another comparative study by Cho et al (2009) compared fifty-one patients who were given neoadjuvant chemotherapy before radical hysterectomy with thirty-five patients who received radical surgery alone in stage IB2-IIA bulky cervical cancer. Both groups were well balanced in age, tumor size, FIGO stage, level of squamous cell cancer antigen, histopathologic type and grade, operating time, estimated blood loss, number of lymph nodes removed and rate of complications. There was a reduction in pathologic tumor size, and there were fewer patients with deep cervical invasion in the neoadjuvant chemotherapy group, and adjuvant radiation was given more frequently in the primary surgical group. However, there was no improvement in 5-year disease free and overall survival. These findings differed slightly from a report from Kim et al (2010). The study expressed the matched - case comparison between neoadjuvant chemotherapy before surgery group and primary surgery group in stage IB1-IIA and found more definitely reduced intermediate and high risk factors in neoadjuvant chemotherapy patients in stage IIA. Although the authors reported no significant difference in progression-free survival and disease recurrence between these two studied groups in stage IB, the patients who received neoadjuvant chemotherapy before surgery showed worse overall survival than the primary surgery group in stage IIA.

The delay in standard treatment is one important issue of concern in patients receiving neoadjuvant chemotherapy. To study this problem, Chen et al (2008) conducted a randomized study in stage IB2-IIB comparing modified preoperative neoadjuvant chemotherapy, (N=72) with primary radical surgery, (N=70). The neoadjuvant chemotherapy regimen consisted of two cycles at fourteen-day intervals of cisplatin 100 mg/m^2 IV given on day 1, mitomicin C 4 mg/m^2 IM given on day 1-5 and 5 - fluorouracil 24 mg/kg/day IV given on day 1-5. A longer tumor-free survival was observed in the neoadjuvant chemotherapy group. When using Cox hazard analysis, however, this did not indicate the therapy modality as a prognostic predictor. The authors further analyzed the survival difference between non-neoadjuvant chemotherapy responders and the patients in the primary surgery group by using Log rank tested. There was no difference in survival between these two groups. Therefore, the modified schedule of neoadjuvant chemotherapy did not adversely delay the treatment in non-neoadjuvant chemotherapy responders.

2.3.2 The type of neoadjuvant chemotherapy before surgery

Many phase II studies have been reported of various neoadjuvant chemotherapy types and schedules (table 2). The response rate was over 80% in the studies using combination

Author (year)	Chemotherapy	Stage	N	outcome
Zanetta et al (1998)	Paclitaxel 175 mg/m^2 D1& cisplatin 50 mg/m^2 D2-3& ifosfamide 5 gm/m2 D2-3 x 3 courses q 3 weeks	IB2-IVA	38	Overall RR 84%,PCR 16%,PPR 18%
Sugiyama et al (1999)	Cisplatin 60 mg/m^2 day 1-3 & Irinothecan 60 mg/m^2 days 1, 8, 15 x 2-3 courses q 4 weeks	IB= IIIB	23	CR 13%,PR 65%
Gonzalez et al (2001)	Cisplatin 100 mg/m^2 & gemcitabine 1000 mg/m^2 D1,8 x 2 courses q 3 weeks	IB2-IIIB	41	Overall RR 95%,PCR 23%
Gonzalez et al (2003)	Carboplatin AUC=6 & paclitaxel 175 mg/m2 x 2 courses q 3 weeks	IB2-IIIB	41	63% received CCRT,CR 95%,PCR=17%, PPR = 20%, 2 years OS=79%
Gonzalez et al (2003)	Oxaliplatin 130 mg/m^2 day 1& Gemcitabine 1250 mg/m^2 days 1, 8 x 3 q 3 weeks	IB-IIB	10	RR 80%, PCR 14%
Termrungru-anglert et al (2005)	Cisplatin 70 mg/m^2 & gemcitabine 1000 mg/m^2 D1,8 x 2 courses q 3 weeks	IB2	28	Overall RR 88.9%, PCR 8.3%,3 year OS = 88.9%
Suprasert et al (2007)	Cisplatin 75 mg/m^2 x 1-2 courses q 3 weeks	IB-IIA	42	PR 4.7%
Bae et al (2008)	cisplatin 60 mg/m^2 D1,2 & etoposide 100 mg/m^2 D1 x 3 courses q 10 days	IB-IIB	99	PRR 69.7%,5-year OS 88.1%,5- year PFS 60.5%
Matsumura et al (2010)	Irinotecan 60 mg/m^2 D1,8,15 & cisplatin 60 mg/m^2 D1 or Irinotecan 60 mg/m^2 D1,8 & nadaplatin 80 mg/m^2 D1 x 1-2 courses q 4 weeks	IB2-IIB	46	Overall RR 80.4%,3- year PFS 86.1%

RR = response rate
CR = complete response
PR = partial response
PCR=pathologic complete response
PPR=pathologic partial response
PRR = pathologic response rate
PFS = Progression-free survival rate
OS = overall survival rate
CCRT = Concurrent chemoradiation

Table 2. Phase II study of neoadjuvant chemotherapy followed by radical surgery neoadjuvant chemotherapy (Duenas-Gonzalez et al., 2001; Duenas-Gonzalez et al., 2003; Duenas-Gonzalez et al., 2003; Matsumura et al., 2010; Termrungruanglert et al., 2005; Sugiyama et al., 1999; Zanetta et al., 1998) but in our study (Suprasert et al., 2007), the response rate of using single cisplatin was very low, 4.5%. The pathologic complete response was in a range of 8.3-23% (Duenas-Gonzalez et al., 2001; Duenas-Gonzalez et al., 2003; Termrungruanglert et al., 2005; Zanetta et al., 1998). Adjuvant radiation was given to patients with intermediate and/or high risk factors in most of the studies, except the study by Matsumura et al (2010). Chemotherapy was administered in patients with high risk factors by using the same regimen as given in the neoadjuvant chemotherapy setting. The authors reported the 3-year progression free survival as 86.1%.

2.4 Neoadjuvant chemotherapy before surgery versus standard radiation therapy

Benedetti-Panici et al. (2002) conducted an Italian multicenter randomized study comparing cisplatin-based neoadjuvant chemotherapy followed by radical surgery versus conventional radiotherapy, in locally advance squamous cell cervical cancer. Two hundreds and ten cases were assigned to the neoadjuvant chemotherapy group and 199 cases were assigned to the conventional radiotherapy group. There was an increase in 5- year overall survival rate for patients who received neoadjuvant chemotherapy. However, when analyzed by FIGO stage, the overall survival rate significantly increased only in stage IB2 to IIB. In more advanced stages, the overall survival rate was not significantly different between the two groups. The result suggested that, the more advanced the stage, the more limited the benefit achievable by neoadjuvant chemotherapy. This could be explained by considering that the large tumor volumes were associated with a large number of hypoxic cells and high proportion of cell population in resting phases. Both events reduced chemosensitivity and probability of developing resistant clones.

Another important study (Neoadjuvant Chemotherapy for Locally Advanced Cervical Cancer Meta-analysis Collaboration, 2003) was a systematic review and meta-analysis of individual patient data from twenty-one randomized trials, which included data from the above study (Benedetti-Panici et al., 2002). Two comparisons were performed in the review. The first one compared neoadjuvant chemotherapy followed by radiotherapy versus the radiotherapy alone as discussed in the previous section (2.1). The other compared neoadjuvant chemotherapy followed by surgery with or without radiation versus radical radiotherapy. Five randomized trials with a total of 872 patients were analyzed. The planned total dose of cisplatin was in a range of 100-300 mg/m^2 in 10-21-day cycles while the radiation dosage was similar in each trial. The results indicated a highly significant effect of neoadjuvant chemotherapy group with overall HR of 0.65 (P=0.00004), which translated into an absolute increase in 5-year overall survival rate from 50% to 64%.

2.5 Neoadjuvant chemotherapy and conservative surgery

Preoperative neoadjuvant chemotherapy could reduce the tumor size and may virtually sterilize micrometastases in the paracervical tissue and pelvic lymph nodes. This effect allows for a less extensive surgery of the cervix instead of radical hysterectomy in stage IB1patients who desire to preserve fertility-sparing. Maneo et al (2008) reported sixteen stage IB1 nulliparous patients treated with three courses of preoperative chemotherapy followed by cold-knife conization and pelvic lymphadenectomy. The chemotherapy regimen for squamous cell carcinoma consisted of cisplatin 75 mg/m^2, paclitaxel 175 mg/m^2 and ifosfamide 5 gm/m^2, for adenocarcinoma, epirubicin 80 mg/m^2 was applied instead of ifosfamide. During a median follow-up of sixty-nine months, no relapse occurred. However, three patients developed carcinoma intraepithelial neoplasia (CIN) after follow- up in long term. Regarding the fertility outcome, ten pregnancies occurred in six patients. The authors concluded that this integrated treatment was feasible.

3. Ovarian cancer

Neoadjuvant chemotherapy was introduced as an alternative management strategy in patients with advanced ovarian cancer approximately two decades ago (Chambers et al. ,1990). Initially, the approach was used only for patients who had significant comorbidities and could not tolerate the cytoreductive surgery. Later on, neoadjuvant chemotherapy has been advocated for the treatment of the patients with multiple sites of metastases ovarian cancer (Ansquer et al., 2001; Schwartz et al., 1999). Other advantages of the neoadjuvant chemotherapy approach include a risk reduction of peri-operative morbidity and a higher rate of optimal resection than primay debulking surgery (Baekelandt, 2003; Huober et al., 2002). The optimal resection outcome is an important factor potentially augmenting survival rate.

To review the above issues, three systematic reviews were published (Bristow & Chi, 2006; Bristow et al., 2007; Kang & Nam, 2009). The first one was presented in 2007 by Bristow et al (Bristow & Chi, 2006). They performed a meta- analysis in twenty-two cohorts studied with 835 patients in stage III-IV ovarian cancer who received neoadjuvant platinum- base that were published in MEDLINE 1989-2005. About 47% of these patients received a taxane. They presented the median overall survival of 24.5 months and found that each incremental increase in pre-operative chemotherapy cycles was associated with a decrease in median survival time of 4.1 months.

In the subsequent year, they presented a second report (Bristow et al., 2007). In that systematic review, they analyzed twenty-six studies published in the English language literature encompassing a total of 1,336 patients treated with neoadjuvant chemotherapy. The common study design was retrospective analysis in twelve reports, followed by retrospective case-control in eight reports, phase I study in four reports, and phase II study in the rest. The authors reported that 10 studies showed inferior survival in patients who received neoadjuvant chemotherapy compared with primary cytoreductive surgery whereas nine studies revealed no significant difference in survival outcome between neoadjuvant chemotherapy and primary cytoreductive surgery. With the heterogenous and predominant retrospective studies in the systematic review, the authors concluded that neoadjuvant chemotherapy should be an alternative management strategy for patients who were felt to be non-optimally resectable by an experienced ovarian cancer surgical team.

The third systematic review was published by Kang et al (2009). Twenty-one studies published between January 1989 and June 2008 met the selection criteria. Due to the heterogeneity in each study, a meta-regression analysis was implemented. The authors found that patients who received neoadjuvant chemotherapy had a lower risk of suboptimal cytoreduction than the patients with primary cytoredutive surgery. Meta-regression analysis revealed that heterogeneity in year of publication, taxane use, and optimal cytoreduction rate influenced median overall survival rate. However, the between- studies variation of the number of neoadjuvant chemotherapy cycles did not influence survival. This finding disagreed with Bristow's report. The authors suggested that the contrary result was due to the difference in statistical models and the study subjects.

In recent years, Vergote et al (2010) presented the large randomized multicenter study of stage IIIC or IV epithelial ovarian cancer, fallopian tube cancer, or primary peritoneal carcinoma patients treated with neoadjuvant platinum-based chemotherapy followed by debulking surgery compared with primary debulking surgery followed by platinum-based chemotherapy. Over 300 patients were included in each arm. The results showed a similar overall survival and progression - free survival in both groups. However, the optimal resection rate was higher in the neoadjuvant chemotherapy arm. On the other hand, the postoperative adverse effects and morbidity tended to be higher after primary debulking than after received neoadjuvant chemotherapy.

With respect to elderly patients, McLean et al (2010) reported the comparative study of the ovarian cancer patients aged over 65 who received neoadjuvant chemotherapy or primary debulking surgery. They found that the overall survival rate did not differ in both treatments. The neoadjuvant group showed a trend toward higher rate of optimal debulking and less surgical complication than primary surgery group.

Although many previous reports suggested the non-inferior outcome of neoadjuvant chemotherapy setting in advanced ovarian cancer patients, the survey results from members of the Society of Gynecologic Oncologists (SGO) revealed that the majority of the respondants did not treat patients with neoadjuvant chemotherapy followed by interval debulking (Dewdney et al., 2010). The result demonstrated that further research would be required to support the role of neoadjuvant chemotherapy in advanced ovarian cancer patients.

4. Endometrial cancer

Most endometrial cancer patients present at an early stage and are cured with hysterectomy and surgical staging alone. The treatment with chemotherapy is predominantly in advanced - stage disease which occurs in only 10-15% of all newly diagnosed cases (Behbakht et al., 1994; Cook et al., 1999). Many studies including a recent meta-analysis demonstrated a survival benefit when a small residual volume could be achieved after cytoreductive surgery in advanced endometrial cancer (Barlin et al.,2010; Bristow et al., 2000; Chi et al., 1997; Goff et al., 1994; Memarzadeh et al., 2002; Numazaki et al., 2009). Neoadjuvant chemotherapy was of proven benefit in advanced ovarian cancer for increase optimal cytoreductive surgery. However, the role of neoadjuvant chemotherapy was still limited in advanced endometrial cancer. Vandenput et al.(2009) investigated the value of neoadjuvant chemotherapy followed by interval debulking in thirty patients with stage IVB endometrial cancer. The most common histology was serous cystadenocarcinoma. Over 80% of these patients received paclitaxel plus carboplatin. The number of cycles before interval debulking was 3-4 cycles. Six patients (13%) were inoperable due to extensive invasion. A total of 22 out of 24 patients (92%) had complete cytoreduction and 8% had optimal cytoreduction (less than 1 cm). The median progression-free survival and overall survival times were 13 and 23 months, respectively. The survival data corresponded to the previous reports which treated stage III-IV uterine papillary serous carcinoma with primary surgery followed by chemotherapy (Memarzadeh et al, 2002; Thomas et al, 2007). The authors suggested that neoadjuvant chemotherapy followed by interval cytoreductive surgery was a reasonable option for endometrial cancer with thansperitoneal spread. Nevertheless, to support this result, further research on the role of neoadjuvant chemotherapy for endometrial cancer is required.

5. Vulvar cancer

Vulvar cancer, an uncommon cancer, represents approximately 4% of all gynecologic cancers. The main treatment consists of vulvectomy plus bilateral groin node dissection in early stage (de Hullu et al., 2004) and more extensive surgery in locally advanced stage (Kehoe, 2006). Although this type of surgery can be curative, it is associated with high morbidity and mortality rates. Neoadjuvant chemotherapy is an alternative approach in locally advanced vulvar cancer patients. The aim of this strategy is to downstage in an effort to avoid the morbidity from such extensive surgery.

Shimizu et al (1990) published the first related case report using a combination of bleomycin, vincristine, mitomicin C and cisplatin for three cycles in an unresectable case with FIGO stage IV squamous cell carcinoma of the vulvar. The patient had a complete response with few toxic effects and successfully underwent a subsequent radical vulvectomy with bilateral groin node dissection. After surgery, the patient was given a further two courses of these chemotherapy regimen. She was still free of disease for 20 months. The next paper was presented by Benedetti-Panici et al (1993). Twenty-one patients with locally advanced squamous cell carcinoma of the vulvar received 2-3 courses of cisplatin , bleomycin and methotrexate followed by radical surgery in operable patients. Of these patients, 10% had a measurable response in the primary tumor and 67% in the groin nodes, without serious morbidity. The operability rate following neoadjuvant chemotherapy was 90% , but only 79% underwent radical surgery. On the other hand, 3- year survival rate was only 24%; 68% of the operated patients recurred 3-17 months after the end of treatment; and 50% had a distant relapse. Furthermore, many previous studies reported overall response rate of 56% and a poor one year survival rate of 32% with the different chemotherapeutic regimen of bleomycin, methotrexate and lomustine (van Doorn et al., 2006; de Hullu et al., 2004; de Hullu & van der Zee, 2006). In contrast, Geisler et al. (2006) reported the very impressive outcome of cisplatin 50 mg/m^2 day 1 plus 5-fluorouracil 1,000 mg/m^2 day 1-5 using as neoadjuvant chemotherapy setting in ten patients with advanced vulvar cancer involving the anal sphincter and/or urethra. All studied patients underwent surgery except one who had a synchronous renal cell carcinoma and died prior to surgery. They demonstrated a response rate approaching 100%.

More recently, to identify the best regimen for this neoadjuvant setting, Domingues et al. (2010) analyzed three various neoadjuvant chemotherapy regimens consisting of 20 mg/m^2 continuous perfusion on day 1-10 of bleomycin, 100 mg/m^2 of paclitaxel (weekly), and 60-80 mg/m^2 of cisplatin on day 1 plus 750 mg/m^2 of 5- fluorouracil on day 1-4 utilized in locally advanced vulvar cancer in a 12-year period, to find the best regimen. The best response and overall survival rate was associated with using bleomycin. The authors hypothesized the contrary results from Geisler's report that might be from the different of the number of studied patients and dosage of chemotherapy.

To identify the real value of any regimen of neoadjuvant chemotherapy in patients with locally advanced vulvar cancer, a large multicenter, and prospective study will ultimately be required.

6. Vaginal cancer

The data on neoadjuvant chemotherapy in vaginal cancer is limited, due to the rarity of the disease. Benedetti Panici et al (2008) reported on eleven patients with stage II vaginal cancer who received paclitaxel 175 mg/m^2 and cisplatin 75 mg/m^2 every three weeks for three

courses followed by radical hysterectomy and vaginectomy. Three patients (27%) had a complete response and seven patients (64%) experienced a partial clinical response without serious toxicity. With a median follow-up time of 75 months, two patients (18%) had disease recurrence and one of them died of disease. The authors concluded that neoadjuvant chemotherapy followed by radical surgery is a feasible therapeutic strategy with good short and long-term results.
In recent years, case reports of two vaginal cancer patients using different neoadjuvant chemotherapy were published. The first one was presented by Takemoto et al (2009). They described a 69-year-old woman with stage III primary vaginal adenocarcinoma at recto-vaginal space. She received neoadjuvant chemotherapy consisting of paclitaxel and carboplatin following by pelvic and vaginal radiotherapy. She experienced a complete remission and remained free from recurrence one year after treatment. The other case report was released by LV et al. (2010). They presented a 41-year-old vaginal cancer patient who had a large lesion occupying the entire length of the left latero- posterior vaginal walls with left paravaginal tissue involvement. A biopsy showed a poorly differentiated squamous cell carcinoma. She was given two courses of bleomycin 15 mg/m^2 on day 1-2 and cisplatin 70 mg/m^2 on day1 every fourteen days followed by radical hysterectomy, radical vaginectomy and bilateral extraperitoneal pelvic lymphadenectomy. After the resection margins and all lymph nodes were confirmed negative by frozen section, vaginal reconstruction with bilateral pudendal thigh fasciocutaneous flaps were performed. She received four courses of bleomycin and cisplatin chemotherapy postoperatively. At 30 months, the patient was clinically free of disease and had a good sexual life.

7. Conclusion

In many gynecologic cancers, especially in cervical cancer and ovarian cancer, neoadjuvant chemotherapy has been explored to improve the operability and decrease the morbidity of radical surgery, without adversely affecting survival. However, research to discover the best regimen is still necessary. In some cancers such as in endometrium, vulvar and vagina, there are few publications, and further studies are required in the future.

8. References

(2003). Neoadjuvant chemotherapy for locally advanced cervical cancer: a systematic review and meta-analysis of individual patient data from 21 randomised trials. Neoadjuvant Chemotherapy for Locally Advanced Cervical Cancer Meta-analysis Collaboration. *Eur J Cancer*, Vol 39, No.17, pp.2470-86.

Ansquer, Y., Leblanc, E.K, Morice, P., Dauplat, J., Mathevet, P., Lhommé, C., Scherer, C., Tigaud, J.D., Benchaib, M., Fourme, E., Castaigne, D., Querleu, D. & Dargent, D. (2001). Neoadjuvant chemotherapy for unresectable ovarian carcinoma: a French multicenter study. *Cancer*, Vol 91,No.12,pp.2329-2334.

Bae, J.H., Lee, S.J., Lee, A., Park, Y.G., Bae, S.N., Park, J.S. & Namkoong, S.E. (2008). Neoadjuvant cisplatin and etoposide followed by radical hysterectomy for stage 1B-2B cervical cancer. *Gynecol Oncol*, Vol 111,No.3,pp.444-448.

Baekelandt, M. (2003). The potential role of neoadjuvant chemotherapy in advanced ovarian cancer. *Int J Gynecol Cancer*,Vol 13,Suppl. 2,pp.163-168.

Barlin, J.N., Puri, I. & Bristow, R.E. (2010). Cytoreductive surgery for advanced or recurrent endometrial cancer: a meta-analysis. *Gynecol Oncol*, Vol. 118,No.1,pp.14-18.

Behbakht, K., Yordan, E.L., Casey, C., DeGeest, K., Massad, L.S., Kirschner, C.V. & Wilbanks, G.D. (1994). Prognostic indicators of survival in advanced endometrial cancer. *Gynecol Oncol* , Vol 55, No. 3 Pt 1,pp.363-367.

Benedetti-Panici, P., Greggi, S., Scambia, G., Salerno, G. & Mancuso, S. (1993). Cisplatin (P), bleomycin (B), and methotrexate (M) preoperative chemotherapy in locally advanced vulvar carcinoma. *Gynecol Oncol,* Vol 50, No.1,pp. 49-53.

Benedetti-Panici, P., Greggi, S., Scambia, G., Amoroso, M., Salerno. M.G., Maneschi. F., Cutillo, G., Paratore. M.P., Scorpiglione. N. & Mancuso, S. (1998). Long-term survival following neoadjuvant chemotherapy and radical surgery in locally advanced cervical cancer. *Eur J Cancer* , Vol 34, No.3,pp. 341-346.

Benedetti-Panici, P., Greggi, S., Colombo, A., Amoroso, M., Smaniotto, D., Giannarelli, D., Amunni, G., Raspagliesi, F., Zola, P., Mangioni, C. & Landoni ,F. (2002). Neoadjuvant chemotherapy and radical surgery versus exclusive radiotherapy in locally advanced squamous cell cervical cancer: results from the Italian multicenter randomized study. *J Clin Oncol* ,Vol 20, No.1,pp. 179-188.

Benedetti Panici, P., Bellati, F., Plotti, F., Di Donato, V., Antonilli, M., Perniola, G., Manci, N., Muzii, L. & Angioli, R. (2008). Neoadjuvant chemotherapy followed by radical surgery in patients affected by vaginal carcinoma. *Gynecol Oncol,* Vol 111, No.2,pp. 307-311.

Bristow, R.E., Zerbe, M.J., Rosenshein, N.B., Grumbine, F.C. & Montz, F.J. (2000). Stage IVB endometrial carcinoma: the role of cytoreductive surgery and determinants of survival. *Gynecol Oncol,* Vol 78, No.2,pp. 85-91.

Bristow, R. E. & Chi, D.S. (2006). Platinum-based neoadjuvant chemotherapy and interval surgical cytoreduction for advanced ovarian cancer: a meta-analysis. *Gynecol Oncol,* Vol 103, No.3,pp. 1070-1076.

Bristow, R.E., Eisenhauer, E.L., Santillan, A. & Chi, D.S. (2007). Delaying the primary surgical effort for advanced ovarian cancer: a systematic review of neoadjuvant chemotherapy and interval cytoreduction. *Gynecol Oncol,*Vol 104,No2,pp. 480-90.

Buda, A., Fossati, R., Colombo, N., Fei, F., Floriani, I., Gueli Alletti, D., Katsaros, D., Landoni, F., Lissoni, A., Malzoni, C., Sartori, E., Scollo, P., Torri, V., Zola, P. & Mangioni, C. (2005). Randomized trial of neoadjuvant chemotherapy comparing paclitaxel, ifosfamide, and cisplatin with ifosfamide and cisplatin followed by radical surgery in patients with locally advanced squamous cell cervical carcinoma: the SNAP01 (Studio Neo-Adjuvante Portio) Italian Collaborative Study. *J Clin Oncol,*Vol 23,No.18,pp 4137-4145.

Cai, H.B., Chen, H.Z. & Yin, H.H. (2006). Randomized study of preoperative chemotherapy versus primary surgery for stage IB cervical cancer. *J Obstet Gynaecol Res,* Vol 32, No.3,pp. 315-323.

Chambers, J.T., Chambers, S.K., Voynick, I.M. & Schwartz, P.E. (1990). Neoadjuvant chemotherapy in stage X ovarian carcinoma. *Gynecol Oncol,* Vol 37, No.3, pp. 327-331.

Chen, H., Liang, C., Zhang, L., Huang, S. & Wu, X. (2008). Clinical efficacy of modified preoperative neoadjuvant chemotherapy in the treatment of locally advanced (stage IB2 to IIB) cervical cancer: randomized study. *Gynecol Oncol,* Vol 110, No.3,pp 308-315.

Chi, D.S., Welshinger, M., Venkatraman, E.S. & Barakat, R.R.(1997). The role of surgical cytoreduction in Stage IV endometrial carcinoma. *Gynecol Oncol* , Vol 67, No.1,pp 56-60.

Chiara, S., Bruzzone, M., Merlini, L., Bruzzi, P., Rosso, R., Franzone, P., Orsatti, M., Vitale, V., Foglia, G., Odicino, F., et al. (1994). Randomized study comparing chemotherapy plus radiotherapy versus radiotherapy alone in FIGO stage IIB-III cervical carcinoma. GONO (North-West Oncologic Cooperative Group). *Am J Clin Oncol*, Vol 17, No.4, pp. 294-297.

Cho, Y.H., Kim, D.Y., Kim, J.H., Kim, Y.M., Kim, Y.T. & Nam, J.H. (2009). Comparative study of neoadjuvant chemotherapy before radical hysterectomy and radical surgery alone in stage IB2-IIA bulky cervical cancer. *J Gynecol Oncol*, Vol 20, No.1,pp. 22-27.

Chua, T. C.(2010). Neoadjuvant chemotherapy or primary surgery in advanced ovarian cancer. *N Engl J Med* , Vol 363, No.24,pp. 2371.

Cook, A.M., Lodge, N. & Blake, P. (1999). Stage IV endometrial carcinoma: a 10 year review of patients.*Br J Radiol* , Vol 72, No.857, pp. 485-488.

de Hullu, J.A., Oonk, M.H. & van der Zee, A.G. (2004). Modern management of vulvar cancer. *Curr Opin Obstet Gynecol*, Vol 16, No.1,pp. 65-72.

de Hullu, J.A.&van der Zee, A.G. (2006). Surgery and radiotherapy in vulvar cancer. *Crit Rev Oncol Hematol*, Vol 60, No.1,pp. 38-58.

Dewdney, S.B., Rimel, B.J., Reinhart, A.J., Kizer, N.T., Brooks, R.A., Massad, L.S. & Zighelboim. I. (2010). The role of neoadjuvant chemotherapy in the management of patients with advanced stage ovarian cancer: survey results from members of the Society of Gynecologic Oncologists. *Gynecol Oncol* ,Vol 119, No.1,pp. 18-21.

Domingues, A.P., Mota, F., Durão, M., Frutuoso, C., Amaral, N. & de Oliveira, C.F. (2010). Neoadjuvant chemotherapy in advanced vulvar cancer. *Int J Gynecol Cancer*, Vol 20, No.2,pp. 294-298.

Dueñas-Gonzalez, A., Lopez-Graniel, C., Gonzalez, A., Reyes, M., Mota, A., Muñoz, D., Solorza, G., Hinojosa, L.M., Guadarrama, R., Florentino, R., Mohar, A., Meléndez, J., Maldonado, V., Chanona, J., Robles, E.& De la Garza, J. (2001). A phase II study of gemcitabine and cisplatin combination as induction chemotherapy for untreated locally advanced cervical carcinoma. *Ann Oncol* , Vol 12, No.4,pp .541-547.

Dueñas-González, A., Rivera, L., Mota, A., López-Graniel, C., Guadarrama, A., González, A., Chanona, G., Cabrera, P. & de la Garza, J. (2002). The advantages of concurrent chemoradiation after neoadjuvant chemotherapy for locally advanced cervical carcinoma. *Arch Med Res*, Vol 33, No.2,pp .201-202.

Dueñas-Gonzalez, A., López-Graniel, C., González-Enciso. A., Cetina. L., Rivera. L., Mariscal. I., Montalvo. G., Gómez. E., de la Garza. J., Chanona. G. & Mohar, A. (2003). A phase II study of multimodality treatment for locally advanced cervical cancer: neoadjuvant carboplatin and paclitaxel followed by radical hysterectomy and adjuvant cisplatin chemoradiation. *Ann Oncol*, Vol 14, No.8, pp. 1278-1284.

Dueñas-González, A., López-Graniel, C., González ,A., Gomez, E., Rivera, L., Mohar ,A., Chanona ,G., Trejo-Becerril, C.& de la Garza ,J. (2003). Induction chemotherapy with gemcitabine and oxaliplatin for locally advanced cervical carcinoma. *Am J Clin Oncol*, Vol 26, No.1,pp. 22-25.

Eddy, G.L., Bundy, B.N., Creasman, W.T., Spirtos, N.M., Mannel, R.S., Hannigan, E. & O'Connor, D. (2007). Treatment of ("bulky") stage IB cervical cancer with or without neoadjuvant vincristine and cisplatin prior to radical hysterectomy and pelvic/para-aortic lymphadenectomy: a phase III trial of the gynecologic oncology group. *Gynecol Oncol* , Vol 106, No.2, pp. 362-369.

Geisler, J.P., Manahan, K.J. & Buller, R.E. (2006). Neoadjuvant chemotherapy in vulvar cancer: avoiding primary exenteration. *Gynecol Oncol*, Vol 100, No.1, pp. 53-57.

Goff, B.A., Goodman, A., Muntz. H.G., Fuller, A.F. Jr, Nikrui, N. & Rice, L.W.(1994). Surgical stage IV endometrial carcinoma: a study of 47 cases. *Gynecol Oncol* , Vol 52, No.2, pp. 237-240.

González-Martín, A., González-Cortijo. L., Carballo. N., Garcia. J.F., Lapuente. F., Rojo. A. & Chiva, L.M. (2008). The current role of neoadjuvant chemotherapy in the management of cervical carcinoma. *Gynecol Oncol*, Vol 110, No.3 Suppl 2,pp. S36-40.

Herod, J., Burton, A., Buxton, J., Tobias, J., Luesley, D., Jordan ,S., Dunn, J. & Poole, C.J. (2000). A randomised, prospective, phase III clinical trial of primary bleomycin, ifosfamide and cisplatin (BIP) chemotherapy followed by radiotherapy versus radiotherapy alone in inoperable cancer of the cervix. *Ann Oncol*, Vol 11, No.9, pp. 1175-1181.

Huober, J., Meyer, A., Wagner, U. & Wallwiener, D. (2002). The role of neoadjuvant chemotherapy and interval laparotomy in advanced ovarian cancer. *J Cancer Res Clin Oncol*, Vol 128, No.3, pp. 153-160.

Hwang, Y.Y., Moon, H., Cho, S.H., Kim, K.T., Moon, Y.J., Kim, S.R. & Kim, D.S. (2001). Ten-year survival of patients with locally advanced, stage ib-iib cervical cancer after neoadjuvant chemotherapy and radical hysterectomy. *Gynecol Oncol*, Vol 82, No.1, pp. 88-93.

Kang, S. & Nam, B.H. (2009). Does neoadjuvant chemotherapy increase optimal cytoreduction rate in advanced ovarian cancer? Meta-analysis of 21 studies. *Ann Surg Oncol*, Vol 16, No.8, pp. 2315-2320.

Kehoe, S. (2006). Treatments for gynaecological cancers. *Best Pract Res Clin Obstet Gynaecol* , Vol 20, No.6,pp. 985-1000.

Kim, H.S., Kim, J.Y., Park, N.H., Kim, K., Chung, H.H., Kim, Y.B., Kim, J.W., Kim, H.J., Song, Y.S. & Kang, S.B. (2010). Matched-case comparison for the efficacy of neoadjuvant chemotherapy before surgery in FIGO stage IB1-IIA cervical cancer. *Gynecol Oncol*, Vol 119, No.2,pp. 217-224.

Lacava, J.A., Leone, B.A., Machiavelli, M., Romero, A.O., Perez, J.E., Elem, Y.L., Ferreyra, R., Focaccia, G., Suttora, G., Salvadori, M.A., Cuevas, M.A., Acuña, L.R., Acuña, J.R., Langhi, M., Amato, S., Castaldi, J., Arroyo, A. & Vallejo, C.T. (1997). Vinorelbine as neoadjuvant chemotherapy in advanced cervical carcinoma. *J Clin Oncol*, Vol 15, No.2, pp. 604-9.

Leborgne, F., Leborgne, J.H., Doldán, R., Zubizarreta, E., Ortega, B., Maisonneuve, J., Musetti, E., Hekimian, L. & Mezzera, J. (1997). Induction chemotherapy and radiotherapy of advanced cancer of the cervix: a pilot study and phase III randomized trial. *Int J Radiat Oncol Biol Phys*, Vol 37, No.2, pp. 343-350.

Lv, L., Sun, Y., Liu, H., Lou, J. & Peng, Z. (2010). Neoadjuvant chemotherapy followed by radical surgery and reconstruction of the vagina in a patient with stage II primary vaginal squamous carcinoma. *J Obstet Gynaecol Res*, Vol 36, No.6, pp. 1245-1248.

Maneo, A., Chiari, S., Bonazzi, C. & Mangioni, C. (2008). Neoadjuvant chemotherapy and conservative surgery for stage IB1 cervical cancer. *Gynecol Oncol*, Vol 111, No.3,pp. 438-443.

Matsumura, M., Takeshima, N., Ota, T., Omatsu, K., Sakamoto. K., Kawamata. Y., Umayahara, K., Tanaka, H., Akiyama, F.& Takizawa ,K. (2010) .Neoadjuvant chemotherapy followed by radical hysterectomy plus postoperative chemotherapy but no radiotherapy for Stage IB2-IIB cervical cancer-irinotecan and platinum chemotherapy. *Gynecol Oncol* , Vol 119, No.2,pp. 212-216.

McLean, K.A., Shah, C.A., Thompson, S.A., Gray, H.J., Swensen, R.E. & Goff, B.A. (2010). Ovarian cancer in the elderly: outcomes with neoadjuvant chemotherapy or primary cytoreduction. *Gynecol Oncol*, Vol 118, No.1,pp. 43-46.

Memarzadeh, S., Holschneider, C.H., Bristow, R.E., Jones, N.L., Fu, Y.S., Karlan, B.Y., Berek, J.S. & Farias-Eisner, R. (2002). FIGO stage III and IV uterine papillary serous carcinoma: impact of residual disease on survival. *Int J Gynecol Cancer* , Vol 12, No.5,pp. 454-458.

Movva, S., Rodriguez, L., Arias-Pulido, H. & Verschraegen, C. (2009). Novel chemotherapy approaches for cervical cancer. *Cancer*, Vol 115, No.14, pp. 3166-3180.

Numazaki, R., Miyagi, E., Konnai, K., Ikeda, M., Yamamoto, A., Onose, R., Kato, H., Okamoto, N., Hirahara, F. & Nakayama, H. (2009). Analysis of stage IVB endometrial carcinoma patients with distant metastasis: a review of prognoses in 55 patients. *Int J Clin Oncol* , Vol 14, No.4, pp. 344-350.

Panici, P.B., Greggi, S., Scambia, G., Ragusa, G., Baiocchi, G., Battaglia, F., Coronetta, F. & Mancuso, S. (1991). High-dose cisplatin and bleomycin neoadjuvant chemotherapy plus radical surgery in locally advanced cervical carcinoma: a preliminary report. *Gynecol Oncol* , Vol 41, No.3, pp. 212-216.

Panici, P.B., Scambia, G., Baiocchi, G., Greggi, S., Ragusa, G., Gallo, A., Conte, M., Battaglia, F., Laurelli, G., Rabitti, C., et al. (1991). Neoadjuvant chemotherapy and radical surgery in locally advanced cervical cancer. Prognostic factors for response and survival. *Cancer*, Vol 67, No.2, pp. 372-379.

Rydzewska, L., Tierney, J., Vale, C.L. & Symonds, P.R. (2010). Neoadjuvant chemotherapy plus surgery versus surgery for cervical cancer. *Cochrane Database Syst Rev*, No1: CD007406.

Sardi, J., Sananes, C., Giaroli, A., Bayo, J., Rueda, N.G., Vighi, S., Guardado, N., Paniceres, G., Snaidas, L., Vico, C., et al. (1993). Results of a prospective randomized trial with neoadjuvant chemotherapy in stage IB, bulky, squamous carcinoma of the cervix. *Gynecol Oncol* , Vol 49, No.2, pp. 156-165.

Schwartz, P.E., Rutherford, T.J., Chambers, J.T., Kohorn, E.I. & Thiel, R.P. (1999). Neoadjuvant chemotherapy for advanced ovarian cancer: long-term survival. *Gynecol Oncol* , Vol 72, No.1, pp. 93-99.

Shimizu, Y., Hasumi, K. & Masubuchi, K. (1990). Effective chemotherapy consisting of bleomycin, vincristine, mitomycin C, and cisplatin (BOMP) for a patient with inoperable vulvar cancer. *Gynecol Oncol* , Vol 36, No.3, pp. 423-427.

Souhami, L., Gil, R.A., Allan, S.E., Canary, P.C., Araújo, C.M., Pinto, L.H. & Silveira, T.R. (1991). A randomized trial of chemotherapy followed by pelvic radiation therapy in stage IIIB carcinoma of the cervix. *J Clin Oncol*, Vol 9, No.6, pp. 970-977.

Sugiyama, T., Nishida, T., Kumagai, S., Nishio, S., Fujiyoshi, K., Okura, N., Yakushiji, M., Hiura, M. & Umesaki, N. (1999). Combination therapy with irinotecan and cisplatin as neoadjuvant chemotherapy in locally advanced cervical cancer. *Br J Cancer*, Vol 81, No.1, pp. 95-98.

Sundfør, K., Tropé, C.G., Högberg, T., Onsrud, M., Koern, J., Simonsen, E., Bertelsen, K. & Westberg, R. (1996). Radiotherapy and neoadjuvant chemotherapy for cervical carcinoma. A randomized multicenter study of sequential cisplatin and 5-fluorouracil and radiotherapy in advanced cervical carcinoma stage 3B and 4A. *Cancer*, Vol 77, No.11, pp. 2371-2378.

Suprasert, P., Thongsong, T., Srisomboon, J. & Chailert, C. (2007). Efficacy of cisplatin in early stage cervical cancer with a long waiting period for surgery. *Asian Pac J Cancer Prev*, Vol 8, No.1, pp. 51-54.

Symonds, R. P. (2000). Audit of treatment by radiotherapy of carcinoma of the cervix in the UK in 1993: worse than expected results. *Clin Oncol (R Coll Radiol)*, Vol 12, No.6, pp. 343-344.

Takemoto, S., Ushijima, K., Nakaso, K., Fujiyoshi, N. & Kamura, T. (2009). Primary adenocarcinoma of the vagina successfully treated with neoadjuvant chemotherapy consisting of paclitaxel and carboplatin. *J Obstet Gynaecol Res*, Vol 35, No.3, pp. 579-583.

Tattersall, M.H., Ramirez, C. & Coppleson, M. (1992). A randomized trial comparing platinum-based chemotherapy followed by radiotherapy vs. radiotherapy alone in patients with locally advanced cervical cancer. Int J *Gynecol Cancer*, Vol 2, No.5, pp. 244-251.

Tattersall, M.H., Lorvidhaya, V., Vootiprux, V., Cheirsilpa, A., Wong, F., Azhar, T., Lee, H.P., Kang, S.B., Manalo, A., Yen, M.S., et al. (1995). Randomized trial of epirubicin and cisplatin chemotherapy followed by pelvic radiation in locally advanced cervical cancer. Cervical Cancer Study Group of the Asian Oceanian Clinical Oncology Association. *J Clin Oncol*, Vol 13, No.2, pp. 444-451.

Termrungruanglert, W., Tresukosol, D., Vasuratna, A., Sittisomwong, T., Lertkhachonsuk, R. & Sirisabya, N. (2005).Neoadjuvant gemcitabine and cisplatin followed by radical surgery in (bulky) squamous cell carcinoma of cervix stage IB2. *Gynecol Oncol*, Vol 97, No.2,pp. 576-581.

Thomas, M.B., Mariani, A., Cliby, W.A., Keeney, G.L., Podratz, K.C. & Dowdy, S.C. (2007). Role of cytoreduction in stage III and IV uterine papillary serous carcinoma. *Gynecol Oncol*, Vol 107, No.2, pp. 190-193.

Undurraga, M., Loubeyre, P., Dubuisson, J.B., Schneider, D. & Petignat, P. (2010). Early-stage cervical cancer: is surgery better than radiotherapy? *Expert Rev Anticancer Ther*, Vol 10, No.3,pp. 451-460.

van Doorn, H.C., Ansink, A., Verhaar-Langereis, M. & Stalpers, L. (2006). Neoadjuvant chemoradiation for advanced primary vulvar cancer. *Cochrane Database Syst Rev*, No. 3: CD003752.

Vandenput, I., Van Calster, B., Capoen, A., Leunen, K., Berteloot, P., Neven, P., Moerman, P., Vergote, I. & Amant, F. (2009). Neoadjuvant chemotherapy followed by interval debulking surgery in patients with serous endometrial cancer with transperitoneal spread (stage IV): a new preferred treatment?. *Br J Cancer*, Vol 101, No.2,pp. 244-249.

Vergote, I., Tropé, C.G., Amant, F., Kristensen, G.B., Ehlen, T., Johnson, N., Verheijen, R.H., van der Burg, M.E., Lacave, A.J., Panici, P.B., Kenter, G.G., Casado, A., Mendiola, C., Coens, C., Verleye, L., Stuart, G.C., Pecorelli, S., Reed, N.S, & European Organization for Research and Treatment of Cancer-Gynaecological Cancer Group; NCIC Clinical Trials Group. (2010). Neoadjuvant chemotherapy or primary surgery in stage IIIC or IV ovarian cancer. *N Engl J Med*, Vol 363, No.10,pp. 943-953.

Zanetta, G., Lissoni, A., Pellegrino, A., Sessa, C., Colombo, N., Gueli-Alletti, D. & Mangioni, C. (1998). Neoadjuvant chemotherapy with cisplatin, ifosfamide and paclitaxel for locally advanced squamous-cell cervical cancer. Ann Oncol, Vol 9, No.9,pp. 977-980.

6

Neoadjuvant Chemotherapy in Ovarian Cancer

Jasmeet Chadha Singh and Amy Tiersten
New York University Medical Center
USA

1. Introduction

Ovarian cancer is the second most common gynecological malignancy occurring in about 200,000 women worldwide out of which close to 125,000 die from the disease. In the United States, ovarian cancer is detected in about 21,000 women resulting in about 14,000 deaths (Parkin, Bray et al. 2005; Sankaranarayanan and Ferlay 2006; Jemal, Siegel et al. 2009). The majority of women diagnosed with ovarian cancer, are usually diagnosed in the advanced stage of the disease (Yancik 1993). This chapter highlights major developments that have led to emergence of neoadjuvant chemotherapy (NAC) as a useful strategy for managing advanced ovarian carcinoma.

For many years, primary cytoreductive surgery (PCS) followed by adjuvant chemotherapy with a platinum based agent has been the standard of care for management of advanced ovarian cancer (Griffiths 1975; 1994; Hoskins, McGuire et al. 1994; Curtin, Malik et al. 1997; Berek, Trope et al. 1999; Bristow, Tomacruz et al. 2002; Kyrgiou, Salanti et al. 2006). The Gynecologic Oncology Group (GOG) defines optimal cytoreduction as leaving residual disease less than one centimeter in maximum tumor diameter. Residual disease after cytoreduction is a known risk factor for disease recurrence and poor survival. In a GOG study, compared to patients with microscopic residual disease, patients with 0.1 to 1.0 cm and >1.0 cm residual disease had an increased risk of recurrence (HR = 1.96; 95% CI, 1.70 to 2.26; and HR = 2.36; 95% CI, 2.04 to 2.73, respectively) and death (HR = 2.11; 95% CI, 1.78 to 2.49; P<.001; and HR = 2.47; 95% CI, 2.09 to 2.92, respectively) (Winter, Maxwell et al. 2007).

However, there are recent studies challenging this GOG definition of optimal cytoreduction. These studies have shown even better survival rates when post surgical tumor size is reduced to no visible disease. A retrospective study divided the cohort of 465 patients undergoing surgery into no visible residual disease, residual tumor size <0.5 centimeter, 0.6-1 centimeter, 1-2 centimeter or greater than 2 centimeter. The survival outcomes of the above five cohorts were 106 months, 66 months, 48 months, 33 months and 34 months respectively. The overall survival rate was significantly better in the group cytoreduced to no visible disease. The group with residual tumor size <1 cm had better survival outcomes compared to group of patients with >1cm residual disease (Chi, Eisenhauer et al. 2006).

Another study comparing patients that had been cytoreduced to no visible disease to patients cytoreduced to less than 1 cm versus more than 1 cm concluded that the former group had better overall (OS) and progression free survival (PFS) as well as lesser platinum resistance (Eisenhauer, Abu-Rustum et al. 2008).

Debate exists as to whether the observed survival benefits for cytoreducted patients are a function of tumor biology or surgical effort. Hientz et al observed that cytoreduction is easier to obtain in young patients with low grade tumor, smaller sized metastases and no ascites (Heintz, Van Oosterom et al. 1988). One study also showed that women who could not be optimally debulked had higher frequency of pelvic and paraortic lymph node metastases (Burghardt, Girardi et al. 1991). Hacker et al reported that presence of extensive metastatic disease was by itself a poor prognostic marker despite optimal cytoreduction (Hacker, Berek et al. 1983). Friedlander reported that the size of largest residual tumor was not an independent prognostic factor when newer variables such as DNA ploidy were included in multivariate analysis. (Friedlander, Hedley et al. 1988)

2. Neoadjuvant chemotherapy: Role in ovarian cancer

Neoadjuvant chemotherapy is defined as chemical cytoreduction occurring prior to any significant attempt at surgical reduction of the tumor. On the other hand, interval debulking surgery (IDS) refers to secondary surgical cytoreduction in patients who could not be optimally cytoreducted in the first surgical attempt. This involves administrating chemotherapy after primary surgery and then repeating the surgical procedure in hopes of achieving optimal cytoreduction. An EORTC study that randomized 319 patients who had residual disease of more than 1 centimeter after primary surgery and received three cycles of cyclophosphamide and Cisplatin to undergo either debulking surgery or no surgery. Progression free survival and overall survival were both significantly higher in the group that underwent interval debulking surgery. However, a large prospective GOG trial showed that this approach did not improve progression free survival or overall survival when compared to post operative chemotherapy alone (Rose, Nerenstone et al. 2004).

Neoadjuvant chemotherapy has been proposed for patients with advanced ovarian cancer where the disease extent would deem optimal cytoreduction extremely difficult or impossible (Ledermann 2010). Studies have shown that neoadjuvant chemotherapy can improve quality of life in patients over an extended period of time. One study analyzing quality of life of patients receiving neoadjuvant chemotherapy using EORTC quality of life questionnaire as a tool assessing global health, symptom improvement and functional status reported that life overall quality of life improved after neoadjuvant chemotherapy and continues to improve up to a period of 12 months. (Chan, Ng et al. 2003).

2.1 Patient selection

Several studies have tried to define the group of patients in whom, due to the advanced and unresectable nature of their disease, primary surgery would be difficult or have a suboptimal result. These patients could potentially benefit from neoadjuvant chemotherapy (Markman 2010; Weinberg, Rodriguez et al. 2010). Nelson et al. were the first to study CT imaging criteria to define cytoreducibility by primary surgery. Forty two patients with epithelial ovarian carcinoma underwent preoperative CT scan. Primary tumor was scored as non cytoreducible if the following characteristics were present: attachment of omentum to spleen, >2 centimeter of disease in mesentery, liver, gallbladder fossa, diaphragm, paraaortic suprarenal lymph nodes, and pericardial nodes, pulmonary or pleural involvement. This study concluded that CT scan was a sensitive tool to predict optimal cytoreduciblity (sensitivity= 92.3 percent) with specificity being 79.3 percent. Addition of Ca-125 to upper limits of 36 units/ml, 65 units/ml or 100 units/ml did not enhance CT prediction of accuracy (Chi, Franklin et al. 2004).

Preliminary studies indicate that higher Ca-125 levels (>2000 U/ml) may be a risk factor for suboptimal cytoreduction and hence may prompt initial cytoreduction before proceeding with primary surgery. In a retrospective review of 314 patients, 94 patients who received neoadjuvant chemotherapy had more advanced disease ($p<0.001$) and had higher CA-125 levels (p<0.001). Optimal cytoreduction rate was significantly higher in the neoadjuvant chemotherapy group (81.9% vs. 50%, p<0.001) but progression free survival was similar in both groups. However, in patients with CA-125 levels >2000 U/ml, progression free survival was significantly higher in neoadjuvant chemotherapy group. (HR= 0.62, 95% CI = 0.24-0.96, P=0.037)(Kang, Kim et al. 2011).

Recently, RNA microarray analysis has been used to identify gene expression associated with optimal debulking. After looking at more than 22,000 genes in forty four study patients by the means of RNA microarray analysis, Berchuck et al were able to identify a set of 32 genes which are potentially strong predictors of optimal or suboptimal debulking (Berchuck, Iversen et al. 2004).

2.2 Outcomes

Neoadjuvant chemotherapy followed by surgery has shown to improve perioperative outcomes such optimal cytoreduction, decrease blood loss, and reduce length of hospitalization. (Fanfani, Ferrandina et al. 2003; Milam, Tao et al. 2011)

Several small studies of patients with advanced ovarian cancer have demonstrated that neoadjuvant chemotherapy is associated with same progression free survival and overall survival as the patients treated conventionally.(Giannopoulos, Butler-Manuel et al. 2006) (Chambers, Chambers et al. 1990; Schwartz, Chambers et al. 1994) However, there are also some studies which show significantly improved survival with neoadjuvant chemotherapy.(Hou, Kelly et al. 2007) (Kuhn, Rutke et al. 2001)

The cost of caring for patients who have had an extensive but suboptimal surgery may be greater than those treated with neoadjuvant chemotherapy. (Schwartz, Chambers et al. 1994) These studies also demonstrate that neoadjuvant chemotherapy is associated with lesser surgical morbidity such as blood loss, shorter operative times and shorter length of hospital and ICU stay.(Lawton, Redman et al. 1989; Chambers, Chambers et al. 1990; Jacob, Gershenson et al. 1991; Lim and Green 1993; Schwartz, Chambers et al. 1994; Vergote, De Wever et al. 1998; Schwartz, Rutherford et al. 1999) One retrospective study of 116 patients showed worse outcomes with neoadjuvant chemotherapy with greater survival in primary surgery group (53% vs. 30%, p=0.03). However, in this study, patients in the neoadjuvant chemotherapy group were significantly older (p<0.001), had higher grade of disease (p<0.005) and when adjusted for age and grade, patients there was no difference in overall survival (p=0.95) (Steed, Oza et al. 2006).

The largest randomized control trial to analyze the role of neoadjuvant chemotherapy in advanced stage ovarian carcinoma was performed by Vergote et al. In this study, 718 patients with stage IIIc or IV ovarian carcinoma were randomized to primary debulking surgery or neoadjuvant chemotherapy. Primary debulking surgery group had attempt at cytoreduction in the beginning followed by 3 cycles of platinum based chemotherapy, followed by interval debulking if needed, followed by 3 additional cycles of chemotherapy. 704 patients were required in order to show noninferiority with respect to survival between primary debulking surgery and neoadjuvant chemotherapy, with a one-sided type I error of 0.05 and a power of 80%. The expected median survival in the primary debulking surgery arm was 31 months. The expected optimal debulking rate (≤ 1 centimeter) was 50% in the primary debulking surgery. It was found that percentage of patients with large size metastases (>10 centimeter and >2 centimeter) was fewer in the group that received neoadjuvant chemotherapy. 53 percent of patients in neoadjuvant chemotherapy group had no residual disease after interval debulking while the corresponding number in primary debulking surgery group was 21 percent only. Optimal cytoreduction defined as residual tumor <1 centimeter could be obtained in 82 percent of patients in neoadjuvant chemotherapy group and 46 percent patients in primary debulking surgery group. There was lower incidence of post operative mortality and morbidity (hemorrhage, fever, fistula formation) in neoadjuvant chemotherapy group. Both the groups had similar progression free (12 months) and overall survival (29 months for primary debulking surgery vs. 30 months for neoadjuvant chemotherapy, HR 0.98 (95% C.I. 0.85-1.14)). There did not seem to be a subgroup based on stage III or IV, age, WHO performance, histological type, countries with high or low optimal debulking rate for which primary debulking surgery or neoadjuvant chemotherapy followed by interval debulking surgery result in better survival. In multivariate analysis, optimal debulking was the strongest independent prognostic factor for overall survival ($p<0.0001$). Hence, it can be concluded from this study that optimal debulking should remain the goal of every surgical effort but the timing of this procedure (primary debulking surgery or interval debulking surgery) does not seem to affect outcomes. Due to the lower morbidity of interval debulking surgery compared with primary debulking surgery and the similar survival, neoadjuvant chemotherapy can be considered a preferred treatment in these patients with stage IIIC/IV ovarian cancer. Interval cytoreductive surgery is also currently a subject of the Chemotherapy or Upfront surgery in Ovarian Cancer Patients (CHORUS) study in Canada and the United Kingdom.

One possible arguement against neoadjuvant chemotherapy is that it deprives potential candidates of intraperitoneal chemotherapy. Studies (Smith, Moon et al. 2009), *Barnett abs. SGO 2007)* have shown that intraperitoneal therapy can be successfully incorporated post-operatively in patients that are able to be optimally debulked following neoadjuvant chemotherapy. Intraperitoneal therapy was well tolerated in these studies.(Tiersten, Liu et al. 2009)

Though there are no standard predictors of response to neoadjuvant chemotherapy, reduction in volume of ascites and decreasing Ca-125 values are the most studied parameters. A randomized phase 2 multicenter trial evaluated early response criteria and surgical outcomes in patients with advanced stage (stage IIIC or IV) ovarian carcinoma with large volume ascites treated with neoadjuvant chemotherapy. Patient were randomized into receiving 2/6 vs. 3/6 cycles of carboplatin and docetaxel preoperatively and response was measured by assessing residual ascites volume and CA-125 levels. It was found that reduction in ascites volume to <500ml and CA-125 to <50% of initial value, were predictors of good response (Polcher, Mahner et al. 2009).

Neoadjuvant chemotherapy followed by cytoreductive surgery has shown to yield better results in advanced ovarian cancer then compared to chemotherapy only approach. Another retrospective study of 129 patients with stage IV ovarian cancer showed that patients who were treated with neoadjuvant chemotherapy followed by cytoreductive surgery had a median survival of 45.5 months, which was significantly better than patients who did not have cytoreductive surgical procedure (15.1 months) ($p<0.01$)(Rafii, Deval et al. 2007).

A phase two study to assess the safety and efficacy of neoadjuvant chemotherapy (four cycles of carboplatin and paclitaxel) followed by debulking surgery followed by four more cycles of chemotherapy for mullerian carcinoma was done in Japan. Out of the fifty-three patients who received neoadjuvant chemotherapy, 47 underwent interval debulking surgery (89%). Twenty two (42%) patients achieved complete clinical remission which was also the primary endpoint. Complete resection of tumor could be performed in 55% (29/53) patients. Median overall and progression free survival was 45 and 14 months respectively. Main toxicity of chemotherapy regimen was neutropenia (grade 4 in 70% patients) and anemia (Onda, Kobayashi et al. 2009).

Although, ability of neoadjuvant chemotherapy to help achieve optimal cytoreduction is an important end point in most of the above trials, it is important to note that significance of achieving optimal surgical cytoreduction is still unclear. Some studies define it to be one of the most important indicators of prognosis (Eisenkop, Spirtos et al. 2003; Aletti, Dowdy et al. 2006; Chi, Eisenhauer et al. 2006), others have demonstrated less benefit. A meta-analysis of fifty eight studies analyzing about 6900 patients demonstrated that maximal cytoreduction in advanced ovarian cancer led to only a modest improvement in outcomes, however, it was the use of platinum based chemotherapy which had the most pronounced effect (Hunter, Alexander et al. 1992).
The results of various studies analyzing the outcomes of neoadjuvant chemotherapy in advanced ovarian cancer are summarized in table 1.

Study type	Author	# Patients	Stage	Optimal cytoreduction (NAC VS. PDS)	OS (NAC VS. PDS)
Randomized control trial	Vergote et al (Vergote, Trope et al. 2010)	670	IIIc-IV	82% vs. 46% (p= NS)	30m vs. 29m (p=0.98)
Randomized control trial	Kumar et al	128	IIIc- IV	83% vs. 13% (p<0.001)	41m vs. 42 m (p=ns)
Prospective non randomized	Kuhn et al (Kuhn, Rutke et al. 2001)	63	IIIc	More in NAC group (p=0.004)	42m vs. 23m (0.007)
Retrospective	Steed et al (Steed, Oza et al. 2006)	116	IIIb-IV	48% vs. 14% (p<0.01)	P=0.95 when adjusted for age and grade
Retrospective	Hou et al (Hou, Kelly et al. 2007)	172	IV	95% vs. 71% (p<0.001)	31m vs. 20m (p<0.01)
Retrospective	Ansquer et al (Ansquer, Leblanc et al. 2001)	54	IIIc- IV	91% vs. 82%	Higher in NAC group (p<0.01)
Non randomized prospective trial	Giannopoulos et al (Giannopoulos, Butler-Manuel et al. 2006)	64	IIIc-IV	82.9% vs. 62.1% (p=0.061)	Not calculated
Retrospective	Schwartz, chambers	29	IIIc-IV	Not calculated	P= 0.26
Retrospective	Schwartz, Rutherford	265	IIIc-IV	Not calculated	1.09y vs. 2.18y (P=0.1578)

Table 1. Studies comparing primary debulking surgery (PDS) to interval debulking after neoadjuvant chemotherapy (NAC), OS. overall survival

2.3 Number of cycles of NAC

In an analysis of patients treated with neoadjuvant chemotherapy, 18 patients were operated after three cycles of neoadjuvant chemotherapy and 32 patients received six cycles of neoadjuvant chemotherapy. There was no significant difference in survival after three and six cycles of chemotherapy (20 vs. 15 months, p = 0.27). The main factors influencing treatment results were optimal cytoreduction and tumor grade. The side effect frequency and profile was also similar in the two groups (Bidzinski, Danska-Bidzinska et al. 2005).

3. Conclusion

There is reasonable evidence to suggest that neoadjuvant chemotherapy has a role in carefully selected group of patients with advanced ovarian cancer, in whom primary surgery will be impossible or suboptimal due to existing comorbidities or extent of the disease. It has also been documented that patients undergoing neoadjuvant chemotherapy followed by surgery have a much better quality of life and require a shorter time to return to baseline. Moreover, neoadjuvant chemotherapy demonstrates clear benefit in terms of shorter hospital stays and lesser post-operative morbidity. Although, the landmark trial investigating the role on neoadjuvant chemotherapy in advanced ovarian cancer did not show a survival advantage, it does demonstrate that neoadjuvant chemotherapy increases chances of optimal cytoreduction. In such patients, primary chemotherapy followed by surgical resection is an acceptable management option.

4. References

(1994). "National Institutes of Health Consensus Development Conference Statement. Ovarian cancer: screening, treatment, and follow-up." Gynecol Oncol 55(3 Pt 2): S4-14.

Aletti, G. D., S. C. Dowdy, et al. (2006). "Aggressive surgical effort and improved survival in advanced-stage ovarian cancer." Obstet Gynecol 107(1): 77-85.

Ansquer, Y., E. Leblanc, et al. (2001). "Neoadjuvant chemotherapy for unresectable ovarian carcinoma: a French multicenter study." Cancer 91(12): 2329-2334.

Berchuck, A., E. S. Iversen, et al. (2004). "Prediction of optimal versus suboptimal cytoreduction of advanced-stage serous ovarian cancer with the use of microarrays." Am J Obstet Gynecol 190(4): 910-925.

Berek, J. S., C. Trope, et al. (1999). "Surgery during chemotherapy and at relapse of ovarian cancer." Ann Oncol 10 Suppl 1: 3-7.

Bidzinski, M., A. Danska-Bidzinska, et al. (2005). "Analysis of the treatment of ovarian cancer patients with neo-adjuvant chemotherapy--preliminary results." Eur J Gynaecol Oncol 26(4): 423-426.

Bristow, R. E., R. S. Tomacruz, et al. (2002). "Survival effect of maximal cytoreductive surgery for advanced ovarian carcinoma during the platinum era: a meta-analysis." J Clin Oncol 20(5): 1248-1259.

Burghardt, E., F. Girardi, et al. (1991). "Patterns of pelvic and paraaortic lymph node involvement in ovarian cancer." Gynecologic oncology 40(2): 103-106.

Chambers, J. T., S. K. Chambers, et al. (1990). "Neoadjuvant chemotherapy in stage X ovarian carcinoma." Gynecologic oncology 37(3): 327-331.

Chan, Y. M., T. Y. Ng, et al. (2003). "Quality of life in women treated with neoadjuvant chemotherapy for advanced ovarian cancer: a prospective longitudinal study." Gynecol Oncol 88(1): 9-16.

Chi, D. S., E. L. Eisenhauer, et al. (2006). "What is the optimal goal of primary cytoreductive surgery for bulky stage IIIC epithelial ovarian carcinoma (EOC)?" Gynecol Oncol 103(2): 559-564.

Chi, D. S., C. C. Franklin, et al. (2004). "Improved optimal cytoreduction rates for stages IIIC and IV epithelial ovarian, fallopian tube, and primary peritoneal cancer: a change in surgical approach." Gynecol Oncol 94(3): 650-654.

Curtin, J. P., R. Malik, et al. (1997). "Stage IV ovarian cancer: impact of surgical debulking." Gynecol Oncol 64(1): 9-12.

Eisenhauer, E. L., N. R. Abu-Rustum, et al. (2008). "The effect of maximal surgical cytoreduction on sensitivity to platinum-taxane chemotherapy and subsequent survival in patients with advanced ovarian cancer." Gynecol Oncol 108(2): 276-281.

Eisenkop, S. M., N. M. Spirtos, et al. (2003). "Relative influences of tumor volume before surgery and the cytoreductive outcome on survival for patients with advanced ovarian cancer: a prospective study." Gynecol Oncol 90(2): 390-396.

Fanfani, F., G. Ferrandina, et al. (2003). "Impact of interval debulking surgery on clinical outcome in primary unresectable FIGO stage IIIc ovarian cancer patients." Oncology 65(4): 316-322.

Friedlander, M. L., D. W. Hedley, et al. (1988). "Prediction of long-term survival by flow cytometric analysis of cellular DNA content in patients with advanced ovarian cancer." Journal of clinical oncology : official journal of the American Society of Clinical Oncology 6(2): 282-290.

Giannopoulos, T., S. Butler-Manuel, et al. (2006). "Clinical outcomes of neoadjuvant chemotherapy and primary debulking surgery in advanced ovarian carcinoma." European journal of gynaecological oncology 27(1): 25-28.

Giannopoulos, T., S. Butler-Manuel, et al. (2006). "Clinical outcomes of neoadjuvant chemotherapy and primary debulking surgery in advanced ovarian carcinoma." Eur J Gynaecol Oncol 27(1): 25-28.

Griffiths, C. T. (1975). "Surgical resection of tumor bulk in the primary treatment of ovarian carcinoma." Natl Cancer Inst Monogr 42: 101-104.

Hacker, N. F., J. S. Berek, et al. (1983). "Primary cytoreductive surgery for epithelial ovarian cancer." Obstetrics and gynecology 61(4): 413-420.

Heintz, A. P., A. T. Van Oosterom, et al. (1988). "The treatment of advanced ovarian carcinoma (I): clinical variables associated with prognosis." Gynecologic oncology 30(3): 347-358.

Hoskins, W. J., W. P. McGuire, et al. (1994). "The effect of diameter of largest residual disease on survival after primary cytoreductive surgery in patients with suboptimal residual epithelial ovarian carcinoma." Am J Obstet Gynecol 170(4): 974-979; discussion 979-980.

Hou, J. Y., M. G. Kelly, et al. (2007). "Neoadjuvant chemotherapy lessens surgical morbidity in advanced ovarian cancer and leads to improved survival in stage IV disease." Gynecologic oncology 105(1): 211-217.

Hou, J. Y., M. G. Kelly, et al. (2007). "Neoadjuvant chemotherapy lessens surgical morbidity in advanced ovarian cancer and leads to improved survival in stage IV disease." Gynecol Oncol 105(1): 211-217.

Hunter, R. W., N. D. Alexander, et al. (1992). "Meta-analysis of surgery in advanced ovarian carcinoma: is maximum cytoreductive surgery an independent determinant of prognosis?" Am J Obstet Gynecol 166(2): 504-511.

Jacob, J. H., D. M. Gershenson, et al. (1991). "Neoadjuvant chemotherapy and interval debulking for advanced epithelial ovarian cancer." Gynecologic oncology 42(2): 146-150.

Jemal, A., R. Siegel, et al. (2009). "Cancer statistics, 2009." CA Cancer J Clin 59(4): 225-249.

Kang, S., T. J. Kim, et al. (2011). "Interaction between preoperative CA-125 level and survival benefit of neoadjuvant chemotherapy in advanced epithelial ovarian cancer." Gynecol Oncol 120(1): 18-22.

Kuhn, W., S. Rutke, et al. (2001). "Neoadjuvant chemotherapy followed by tumor debulking prolongs survival for patients with poor prognosis in International Federation of Gynecology and Obstetrics Stage IIIC ovarian carcinoma." Cancer 92(10): 2585-2591.

Kyrgiou, M., G. Salanti, et al. (2006). "Survival benefits with diverse chemotherapy regimens for ovarian cancer: meta-analysis of multiple treatments." J Natl Cancer Inst 98(22): 1655-1663.

Lawton, F. G., C. W. Redman, et al. (1989). "Neoadjuvant (cytoreductive) chemotherapy combined with intervention debulking surgery in advanced, unresected epithelial ovarian cancer." Obstetrics and gynecology 73(1): 61-65.

Ledermann, J. A. (2010). "Primary chemotherapy: the future for the management of advanced ovarian cancer?" Int J Gynecol Cancer 20(11 Suppl 2): S17-19.
Lim, J. T. and J. A. Green (1993). "Neoadjuvant carboplatin and ifosfamide chemotherapy for inoperable FIGO stage III and IV ovarian carcinoma." Clinical oncology 5(4): 198-202.
Markman, M. (2010). "Recent studies that influence the chemotherapeutic paradigm in the management of advanced ovarian cancer." F1000 Med Rep 2.
Milam, M. R., X. Tao, et al. (2011). "Neoadjuvant chemotherapy is associated with prolonged primary treatment intervals in patients with advanced epithelial ovarian cancer." Int J Gynecol Cancer 21(1): 66-71.
Onda, T., H. Kobayashi, et al. (2009). "Feasibility study of neoadjuvant chemotherapy followed by interval debulking surgery for stage III/IV ovarian, tubal, and peritoneal cancers: Japan Clinical Oncology Group Study JCOG0206." Gynecol Oncol 113(1): 57-62.
Parkin, D. M., F. Bray, et al. (2005). "Global cancer statistics, 2002." CA Cancer J Clin 55(2): 74-108.
Polcher, M., S. Mahner, et al. (2009). "Neoadjuvant chemotherapy with carboplatin and docetaxel in advanced ovarian cancer--a prospective multicenter phase II trial (PRIMOVAR)." Oncol Rep 22(3): 605-613.
Rafii, A., B. Deval, et al. (2007). "Treatment of FIGO stage IV ovarian carcinoma: results of primary surgery or interval surgery after neoadjuvant chemotherapy: a retrospective study." Int J Gynecol Cancer 17(4): 777-783.
Rose, P. G., S. Nerenstone, et al. (2004). "Secondary surgical cytoreduction for advanced ovarian carcinoma." N Engl J Med 351(24): 2489-2497.
Sankaranarayanan, R. and J. Ferlay (2006). "Worldwide burden of gynaecological cancer: the size of the problem." Best Pract Res Clin Obstet Gynaecol 20(2): 207-225.
Schwartz, P. E., J. T. Chambers, et al. (1994). "Neoadjuvant chemotherapy for advanced ovarian cancer." Gynecologic oncology 53(1): 33-37.
Schwartz, P. E., T. J. Rutherford, et al. (1999). "Neoadjuvant chemotherapy for advanced ovarian cancer: long-term survival." Gynecologic oncology 72(1): 93-99.
Smith, H. O., J. Moon, et al. (2009). "Southwest Oncology Group Trial S9912: intraperitoneal cisplatin and paclitaxel plus intravenous paclitaxel and pegylated liposomal doxorubicin as primary chemotherapy of small-volume residual stage III ovarian cancer." Gynecologic oncology 114(2): 206-209.
Steed, H., A. M. Oza, et al. (2006). "A retrospective analysis of neoadjuvant platinum-based chemotherapy versus up-front surgery in advanced ovarian cancer." Int J Gynecol Cancer 16 Suppl 1: 47-53.
Tiersten, A. D., P. Y. Liu, et al. (2009). "Phase II evaluation of neoadjuvant chemotherapy and debulking followed by intraperitoneal chemotherapy in women with stage III and IV epithelial ovarian, fallopian tube or primary peritoneal cancer: Southwest Oncology Group Study S0009." Gynecol Oncol 112(3): 444-449.
Vergote, I., I. De Wever, et al. (1998). "Neoadjuvant chemotherapy or primary debulking surgery in advanced ovarian carcinoma: a retrospective analysis of 285 patients." Gynecologic oncology 71(3): 431-436.
Vergote, I., C. G. Trope, et al. (2010). "Neoadjuvant chemotherapy or primary surgery in stage IIIC or IV ovarian cancer." N Engl J Med 363(10): 943-953.
Weinberg, L. E., G. Rodriguez, et al. (2010). "The role of neoadjuvant chemotherapy in treating advanced epithelial ovarian cancer." J Surg Oncol 101(4): 334-343.
Winter, W. E., 3rd, G. L. Maxwell, et al. (2007). "Prognostic factors for stage III epithelial ovarian cancer: a Gynecologic Oncology Group Study." J Clin Oncol 25(24): 3621-3627.
Yancik, R. (1993). "Ovarian cancer. Age contrasts in incidence, histology, disease stage at diagnosis, and mortality." Cancer 71(2 Suppl): 517-523.

7

Neoadjuvant Chemotherapy in the Treatment of Cervical Cancer

Lua Eiriksson, Gennady Miroshnichenko and Allan Covens
Division of Gynecologic Oncology, University of Toronto
Canada

1. Introduction

The treatment of cervical cancer has seen great advances since the first radical hysterectomy was performed by Ernst Wertheim in 1898. Breakthroughs in surgical techniques, including total laparoscopic approaches, sentinel lymph node mapping, and fertility-sparing procedures have dramatically reduced the morbidity of definitive treatment, while preserving oncologic outcomes. Increasingly conservative approaches are being proposed, based on individual patient and tumour characteristics.

Cervical cancer was previously thought to be chemo-resistant, and therefore chemotherapy was used only for recurrent or metastatic disease. However, after responses were noted to platinum-based regimens (Friedlander et al., 1983, 1984), interest in the use of chemotherapy was reignited, particularly in the neoadjuvant setting. Whether prior to surgery or radiotherapy, the use of neoadjuvant chemotherapy in cervical cancer has been actively studied, in multiple settings and diverse patient populations, showing promise with acceptable toxicity profiles.

In this chapter, the use of neoadjuvant chemotherapy in the treatment of cervical cancer will be reviewed. The rationale will be explored followed by the evidence for its effectiveness prior to surgery, radiotherapy, and fertility-sparing procedures. An approach to patient selection will be provided, and chemotherapeutic regimens will be compared, concluding with areas of ongoing and future research.

2. Rationale for neoadjuvant chemotherapy in cervical cancer

One of the motivations behind neoadjuvant chemotherapy in the treatment of cervical cancer was to reduce tumour size in order to facilitate surgical resection. This was an objective, primarily in low resource countries, where cervical cancer is one of the most common causes of female cancer mortality (World Health Organization, 2011) and access to radiotherapy for patients with locally advanced tumours is limited. Tumour size reduction would not only simplify surgical procedures, but also potentially transform inoperable tumours to resectable. In conjunction with the reduction of lymph node metastases, neoadjuvant chemotherapy prior to surgery may decrease the need for postoperative radiotherapy or chemo-radiotherapy, minimizing long-term treatment-related complications, particularly in sexually active women. Prior to surgery, the blood supply to the tumour is uncompromised, allowing improved drug delivery and distribution. Local control might also be improved with early control of micrometastases.

In the setting of pelvic recurrence, the anticipated morbidity of salvage surgery after neoadjuvant chemotherapy followed by surgery would seemingly be less than that following failed radiotherapy, introducing an additional benefit to the avoidance of primary radiotherapy.

Applications prior to radiotherapy have also been envisioned, including the reduction in tumour size and distortion of pelvic anatomy to facilitate radiotherapy. The effectiveness of radiotherapy might also be improved through decreased tumour cell hypoxia and subsequently improved radiosensitivity with platinum-based agents. The administration of chemotherapy prior to radiotherapy, rather than concurrently, could decrease the radiotherapy-induced toxicity. Although attractive in theory, the benefit of chemotherapy prior to radiotherapy has not been established, particularly in the era of concurrent chemo-radiotherapy (National Cancer Institute, 1999).

Some studies have shown that the response to neoadjuvant chemotherapy may serve as an important prognostic factor, guiding the direction of subsequent therapy. Whether the response to neoadjuvant chemotherapy simply identifies a subset of patients who are destined to fare better than non-responders has been questioned. However, as a group, those receiving neoadjuvant chemotherapy have in some studies demonstrated improved progression-free and overall survival. These studies will be reviewed, highlighting study designs, treatment protocols, statistical analyses, author conclusions, and unanswered questions.

Finally, neoadjuvant chemotherapy may optimize a patient's pathologic risk factors, introducing the option of fertility-sparing treatment to a patient who would otherwise not be a candidate. In this setting, neoadjuvant chemotherapy offers benefits other than an equivalent oncologic outcome.

3. Neoadjuvant chemotherapy prior to surgery versus surgery alone

3.1 Rationale

While radical surgery or radiotherapy have been shown to be equally effective in the treatment of early stage cervical cancer (stage IB1), with equivalent disease-free and overall survival (Landoni et al., 1997), patients with locally advanced disease (FIGO IB2 - IVA) are typically treated with radical radiotherapy, including external beam and intracavitary treatments. However, neoadjuvant chemotherapy may transform previously inoperable tumours to those that are resectable. This may be desirable in patients who wish to avoid radiotherapy, or for whom radiotherapy is not available. The former patients may include young women seeking to maintain ovarian and sexual function, patients having previously received pelvic radiotherapy for other diagnoses, or patients needing to avoid the toxicities of radiotherapy due to comorbid diseases such as inflammatory bowel disease or connective tissue disorders with significant vasculitis.

Neoadjuvant chemotherapy may also be administered prior to radical surgery to improve progression-free or overall survival. By minimizing pathologic factors that contribute to poor prognosis and disease recurrence, chemotherapy prior to surgery may not only render previously inoperable tumours operable, but also decrease the risk of recurrence for patients having operable tumours with high risk features. If survival benefit is associated with improved pathological response, and improved pathological response is possible with neoadjuvant chemotherapy prior to surgery, it is possible that with optimized chemotherapy regimens, neoadjuvant chemotherapy could lead to a survival advantage in select patients with high risk features.

3.2 Tumour size reduction

The first question to be addressed is whether there is evidence to support the use of neoadjuvant chemotherapy in the reduction of tumour size. Sardi *et al.* (Sardi et al., 1986) first described a cohort of 8 patients treated with vincristine, bleomycin, and cisplatin (VBP) every 21 days, similar to the conventional protocol of Friedlander (Friedlander et al., 1984), with the substitution of vincristine for vinblastine. While reduction in tumour volumes overall was 48%, only 62.5% of patients displayed a central response, and only 28.5% responded in the parametria. A modified protocol was therefore administered to a cohort of 25 patients. This "Quick VBP" protocol was intensified, given every 10 days, which yielded a 92% central response rate, and 94.6% parametrial response, with an average regression in tumour volume of 73.5% overall. While the conventional cohort had a larger average pre-treatment tumour volume (78.4 cm^3 versus 55.7 cm^3), when stratified by stage, the "Quick VBP" protocol produced an 82% reduction in stage IIIB disease, compared to 50.1% using the conventional protocol.

Sardi *et al.* (Sardi et al., 1993) later conducted a randomized trial of radical surgery plus adjuvant radiotherapy with or without neoadjuvant chemotherapy in patients with bulky stage IB2 disease. Of the 74 patients randomized to receive neoadjuvant chemotherapy, delivered via the "Quick VBP" protocol (vincristine, bleomycin and cisplatin every 10 days for 3 cycles), 92% of patients responded (40.5% complete response, 51.4% partial response). The average change in tumour size was from 63 cm^3 to 31 cm^3. Significant reductions in tumour size to less than 25% of original volume were noted in those receiving VBP (55% in the VBP arm versus 7% in the control arm, $p < 0.00001$). Similarly, the number of patients with final tumour size less than 2 cm was significantly greater in those receiving VBP (62% versus 4% in the control arm, $p < 0.0001$), despite similar mean tumour volume between groups at randomization. This cisplatin-containing protocol of neoadjuvant chemotherapy showed efficacy in reducing tumour volume to <25% in roughly half of patients with bulky stage IB2 disease.

Given these results, it seemed promising that neoadjuvant chemotherapy may be used to reduce tumour size in order to facilitate primary surgery.

3.3 Reduction in poor prognostic factors

As suggested by Benedetti-Panici *et al.*, (Benedetti-Panici et al., 2002) one category of patients who may derive the greatest benefit from neoadjuvant chemotherapy are those with bulky stage IB2 disease. These patients are at risk for subclinical parametrial infiltration, lymph node metastases, and vascular space invasion, all of which are poor prognostic factors and for which adjuvant radiotherapy is commonly offered. Sardi *et al.* (Sardi et al., 1993) randomized 146 patients to receive radical surgery followed by adjuvant radiotherapy plus or minus neoadjuvant chemotherapy using the "Quick VBP" protocol (every 10 days for 3 cycles). All but three patients randomized to neoadjuvant chemotherapy and all but six patients randomized to control underwent radical hysterectomy. A significant reduction in tumour volume ($p < 0.0001$), incidence of vascular space invasion (15% vs. 57%, $p<0.00001$), parametrial infiltration (3% vs. 22%, $p<0.00001$), and lymph node metastases (7% vs. 31%, $p < 0.0005$) was found in patients having received neoadjuvant chemotherapy versus control, respectively. In 9% (7/74) of "Quick VBP" patients there was no evidence of residual disease on surgical specimen.

3.4 Improvement in progression-free and overall survival

While surrogate markers of treatment effectiveness might suggest neoadjuvant chemotherapy is of benefit, what is of greatest interest to patients and clinicians is whether neoadjuvant chemotherapy confers a survival advantage. The following studies, presented individually and later analyzed collectively, sought to compare patients receiving neoadjuvant chemotherapy prior to surgery versus surgery alone.

3.4.1 Neoadjuvant chemotherapy, surgery and radiotherapy in stage IB squamous carcinoma of the cervix

Sardi *et al.* (Sardi et al., 1997) performed a randomized controlled trial of patients with stage IB disease (>2 cm), comparing radical hysterectomy and whole pelvis adjuvant radiotherapy with or without neoadjuvant chemotherapy (cisplatin, vincristine, and bleomycin) (Table 1). All patients underwent a staging laparotomy. If the tumour was found to be resectable, a radical hysterectomy, with para-aortic lymphadenectomy, was performed, followed by whole pelvis radiotherapy (50 Gy). Conversely, if the cancer was found to be unresectable, patients received 50-60 Gy to the whole pelvis followed by 25-35 Gy of intracavitary treatment.
Two hundred and five patients were randomized, 102 to neoadjuvant chemotherapy and 103 to the control arm. For all patients, improved overall survival was noted in those receiving neoadjuvant chemotherapy compared to controls (81% vs. 66% at 8 years, $p = 0.05$).
While pathologic risk factors such as lymph node metastases (19% vs. 2%, $p = 0.04$) and vascular space invasion (38% vs. 2%, $p = 0.007$) were significantly improved in patients with stage IB1 disease receiving neoadjuvant chemotherapy, there was no difference in overall survival at 8 years in this subgroup (82% with neoadjuvant chemotherapy versus 77% control).
Patients with stage IB2 disease, however, demonstrated improved overall survival following neoadjuvant chemotherapy (80% versus 61% at 9 years, $p < 0.01$). This benefit was driven by an increased rate of operability (100% (61/61) versus 86% (48/56), $p < 0.01$) and possibly an improvement in pathologic risk factors in those receiving neoadjuvant chemotherapy compared to controls. Of all patients with resectable tumours, greater survival was noted in those who had received neoadjuvant chemotherapy (81% vs. 69% at 7 years, $p = 0.05$).
The incidence of high-risk pathologic features was similar between controls and patients who did not respond to neoadjuvant chemotherapy. In those who responded, however, there were significantly fewer with lymph node metastases (6% vs. 40%, $p < 0.0001$), vascular space invasion (10% vs. 60%, $p = 0.009$) and parametrial involvement (2% vs. 34%, $p = 0.001$). Neoadjuvant chemotherapy appeared beneficial in decreasing the incidence of pelvic recurrences for those patients with stage IB2 disease (23% vs. 6%, $p < 0.01$). However, rates of distant metastases were the same for stage IB patients overall.
The authors concluded that in patients with stage IB1 disease there was no difference in operability or survival, and minimal difference in pathologic features, suggesting limited benefit of neoadjuvant chemotherapy in this patient population. However, patients with stage IB2 disease had a significant increase in operability, and survival.
While offering an alternative to radical radiotherapy in patients with stage IB2 disease, all patients in this study underwent adjuvant radiotherapy. Therefore, those receiving neoadjuvant chemotherapy underwent triple modality treatment in order to derive benefit. How their survival would compare to the current standard treatment of chemo-radiotherapy is also unclear. There were methodological issues in this study; violation of intention-to-treat analysis took place, with the exclusion of 3 control and 2 neoadjuvant

chemotherapy patients who did not complete treatment. Multiple interim analyses were performed, ultimately leading to early closure of the study, and finally there was no pre-stated sample-size calculation.

3.4.2 Neoadjuvant chemotherapy and surgery in bulky stage IB carcinoma of the cervix

Protocol GOG #141 (Eddy et al., 2007) was a multicentre randomized trial of radical hysterectomy and pelvic/para-aortic lymphadenectomy with or without neoadjuvant chemotherapy (vincristine and cisplatin) for patients with "bulky" stage IB2 disease (Table 1). Primary endpoints were overall and progression-free survival as well as tumour operability. Patients received adjuvant radiotherapy in the presence of surgical or pathological risk factors. Unfortunately, due to slow accrual, this study was closed prematurely after randomizing 288 patients (145 to neoadjuvant chemotherapy, 143 to control), only 70% of the calculated sample size. There was no difference between treatment groups in recurrence rates, death rates, operability, and proportion receiving adjuvant radiotherapy. The authors concluded that neoadjuvant chemotherapy did not offer any additional objective benefit to patients undergoing neoadjuvant chemotherapy prior to surgical management of stage IB cervical cancer. However, the study was underpowered to make any definitive conclusions.

3.4.3 Neoadjuvant chemotherapy and surgery in stage IB2 – IIB carcinoma of the cervix

One proposed explanation for the lack of survival benefit from neoadjuvant chemotherapy prior to definitive treatment of locally advanced cervical cancer is the delay in treatment for chemotherapy non-responders, resulting in the development of chemo-resistant cell populations or cross-resistance to radiotherapy. Chen *et al.* (Chen et al., 2008) attempted to evaluate whether high-dose, short-term neoadjuvant chemotherapy prior to surgery (Table 1) could improve response and survival rates. Patients with stage IB2 - IIB disease were randomized to undergo surgical management with or without neoadjuvant chemotherapy (cisplatin, mitomycin C, and 5-fluorouracil). Post-operative pelvic radiotherapy was used for patients with lymph node metastases, parametrial or vaginal involvement, lymph vascular space invasion, and/or ovarian metastases.

Overall, almost 70% of patients had either a complete or partial response to chemotherapy. Pathologic findings were significantly reduced, with decreased pelvic lymph node metastases (25.0% vs. 42.9%, $p = 0.02$) and parametrial involvement (25.0% vs. 41.4%, $p = 0.04$). In chemotherapy "responders" versus "non-responders", significant reductions were noted in pelvic lymph node metastases (16.0% vs. 45.5%, $p = 0.008$) and parametrial involvement (16.0% vs. 45.5%, p = 0.008). Four of the 6 patients with a complete response had no residual tumour in the final pathologic specimen.

There was no difference in recurrence between treatment arms. However, those who responded to chemotherapy had fewer recurrences compared to non-responders (16.3% vs. 47.4%, $p = 0.01$). Using the method of Kaplan and Meier, there was a significant difference in the 4-year overall survival between treatment arms (71.0% with neoadjuvant chemotherapy versus 58.0% with control, $p = 0.04$). To control for confounders, Cox proportional hazards regression modeling was used. In this analysis, tumour size, lymph node metastases, and FIGO stage were significant independent predictors of prognosis, while treatment type was not.

Study	Eligibility	Intervention Arms	Resectability	Overall Survival	Follow-up
Sardi 1997 (Argentina) N = 205	SCC 1B1 (>2 cm) 1B2	n = 103 1B1 (n = 47); 1B2 (n = 56) Staging Laparotomy or Radical Hysterectomy + PALND + Whole Pelvis Radiotherapy (50 Gy)	1B1 100% 1B2 86%	1B1: 77% (8 y) 1B2: 61% (9 y)	67 months
		n = 102 1B1 (n = 41); 1B2 (n = 61) Cisplatin 50 mg/m2 Vincristine 1mg/m2 Bleomycin 25 mg/m2 (D 1-3) Every 10 days x 3 cycles	1B1 100% 1B2 100%	1B1: 82% (8 y) 1B2: 80% (9 y)	
Benedetti-Panici 2002 (Italy) N = 409	SCC IB2- III	n = 210 Cisplatin ≥240 mg/m2 (total dose) (± Bleomycin, Vincristine, Ifosfamide) Over 6 – 8 weeks Radical Hysterectomy	78%	5 y OS: 56.5% IB2-IIB 64.7%	79 months
		n = 199 EBRT 45-50 Gy + Intracavitary 20-30 Gy.		5 y OS: 44.4% IB2-IIB: 46.4%	
Napolitano 2003 (Italy) N = 192	SCC IB- IIIB	n = 106 Cisplatin 50 mg/m2 Vincristine 1mg/m2 Bleomycin 25 mg/m2 (D 1,3) 3 cycles every 3 weeks Radical Hysterectomy, PLND	100%	5 y OS IB-IIA: 78.6% IIB: 68.7%	--
		n = 86 Radical Hysterectomy, PLND (Stage I-IIB) EBRT 50-60 Gy, Intracavitary 30 Gy (Stage IIIA-B)	81%	5 y OS IB-IIA: 73.2% IIB: 64.3%	
Cai 2006 (China) N = 106	SCC Stage IB	n = 52 Cisplatin 75 mg/m2 5-FU 24 mg/kg/d (D 1-5) 2 cycles every 3 weeks Radical Hysterectomy + PLND	100%	5 y OS: 84.6% 1B1: 85.7% 1B2: 84.2%	62 months
		n = 54 Radical Hysterectomy + PLND		5 y OS: 75.9% 1B1: 75% 1B2: 76.7%	

Study	Eligibility	Intervention Arms	Resectability	Overall Survival	Follow-up
Eddy 2007 (USA) N = 288	Stage 1B2	n = 145 Cisplatin 50 mg/m^2 Vincristine 1 mg/m^2 3 cycles every 10 days Radical Hysterectomy, P+PALND	78%	3 y OS: 67.7% 5 y OS: 63.3%	62 months
		n = 143 Radical Hysterectomy, P+PALND	79%	3 y OS: 69.3% 5 y OS: 60.7%	
Chen 2008 (China) N = 142	Stage IB2-IIB	n =72 Cisplatin 100 mg/m^2 Mitomicin C 4 mg/m^2 IM (D1-5) 5-Fluorouracil 24 mg/kg/day (D1-5) 2-3 cycles every 2 weeks Radical Hysterectomy + PLND	100%	4 y OS: 71%	48 months
		n = 70 Radical Hysterectomy + PLND	100%	4 y OS: 58%	

N - number of patients enrolled; SCC- squamous cell carcinoma; n - number of patients in treatment arm; P+PALND - pelvic and para-aortic lymph node dissection; D - cycle day; OS - overall survival

Table 1. Randomized Controlled Trials of Neoadjuvant Chemotherapy Prior to Surgery versus Surgery Alone

When regression modeling stratified the neoadjuvant treatment group into responders and non-responders, response to chemotherapy became an independent prognostic factor for survival ($p = 0.005$), and chemotherapy-responders had significantly improved tumour-free survival compared to non-responders ($p < 0.0001$).

The authors concluded that response to treatment was significantly associated with tumour-free survival, recurrence, and served as an independent prognostic factor, suggesting that in this research protocol, neoadjuvant chemotherapy did not translate into a recurrence or disease-free survival benefit overall, but rather, identified a subgroup of patients with improved prognosis. Those with poor response would have had minimal delay to definitive treatment, given the high-dose and abbreviated treatment in the trial protocol.

This study did not report results of overall survival, and no difference could be found in disease-free survival in the unstratified analysis. Whether this was due to insufficient sample-size or a lack of true effect cannot be determined. Intention-to-treat analysis was violated with the exclusion of two post-surgical patients who underwent no further treatment, and 1 patient was excluded from the survival analysis due to death from other causes. With 1/3 of patients requiring adjuvant radiotherapy, and a lack of overall survival benefit, the merits of neoadjuvant chemotherapy, despite surrogate markers of effect, such as decreased lymph node metastases and parametrial involvement, is questionable.

3.4.4 Neoadjuvant chemotherapy and surgery in stage IB – IIIB cervical carcinoma

A randomized study of neoadjuvant chemotherapy using cisplatin, vincristine and bleomycin (Table 1) reported by Napolitano *et al.* (Napolitano et al., 2003) looked at patients with stage IB - IIIB squamous cell carcinoma. All patients in the neoadjuvant chemotherapy arm underwent radical surgery, while control patients with stage IB - IIB disease underwent radical surgery, and patients with stage IIIA - IIIB disease underwent radiotherapy. Adjuvant radiotherapy was administered to all resectable patients with parametrial infiltration, lymph node metastases or positive surgical margins. Random allocation was planned such that 55% of patients received neoadjuvant chemotherapy.

While a difference in 5-year disease-free survival for those with stage IB - IIA disease was found (77% vs. 64%, $p = 0.05$), there was no difference in overall survival for either stage IB - IIA or stage IIB - IIIB patients. Not only was a sample size calculation lacking, but intention-to-treat analysis of progression-free survival was violated when 20 patients were excluded from the analysis (4 patients with stage III disease unresponsive to chemotherapy and 16 control patients).

3.4.5 Neoadjuvant chemotherapy and surgery in stage IB cervical carcinoma

Cai *et al.* (Cai et al., 2006) presented a randomized controlled trial of patients with stage IB squamous cell and adenocarcinoma of the cervix, receiving neoadjuvant chemotherapy (cisplatin/5-fluorouracil) followed by surgery versus surgery alone. Patients received adjuvant radiotherapy for high-risk features such as deep cervical invasion, parametrial invasion, or lymph node metastases. Primary outcomes were 5-year overall survival, and secondary outcomes included progression-free survival and disease recurrence. Patients receiving neoadjuvant chemotherapy had an improved 5-year disease-free survival (83% vs. 74%, $p = 0.04$) and overall survival (85% vs. 76%, $p = 0.01$).

Although these results might suggest a survival advantage with neoadjuvant chemotherapy, 62% of patients receiving neoadjuvant chemotherapy (vs. 54% of controls) also received adjuvant radiotherapy. Whether the survival advantage seen was related to the chemotherapy, or the combined modality treatment of chemotherapy followed by radiotherapy, is not clear.

As in many similar studies, a sample size calculation was not explicitly stated, and intention-to-treat analysis was violated (1 patient with protocol violation was excluded from the analysis), the latter compromising the validity of the study results.

3.4.6 Neoadjuvant chemotherapy and surgery in patients with locally advanced squamous cell carcinoma of the cervix

If a consistent benefit were to exist with the use of neoadjuvant chemotherapy in select patients with locally advanced cervical cancer, the choice of chemotherapeutic protocol would be challenging, given the variety and number of protocols used.

Buda *et al.* (Buda et al., 2005) sought to determine whether a 3 drug regimen (paclitaxel/ ifosfamide/cisplatin [TIP]) conferred benefit over a 2 drug protocol (ifosfamide/cisplatin [IP]) and whether pathologic response to treatment was associated with survival. This randomized, phase II trial of patients with FIGO stage IB2 - IVA disease, examined neoadjuvant chemotherapy prior to radical surgery. Patients who achieved an optimal response (either complete resolution of tumour, or tumour less than 3 mm on final specimen) received 2 additional courses of chemotherapy after surgery with the same agents used in the neoadjuvant treatment. Those found to be inoperable due to progression of disease despite chemotherapy were offered radical radiotherapy, and those with lymph node metastases, parametrial involvement, tumour "cut-through" or suboptimal response underwent adjuvant radiotherapy or chemo-radiotherapy.

Cisplatin and ifosfamide were chosen due to their proven benefit in the neoadjuvant and salvage settings. Paclitaxel was added to the experimental arm as favourable results had also been noted with its use. The purpose of the study was to determine the optimal chemotherapeutic regimen for a future planned randomized clinical trial of neoadjuvant chemotherapy prior to surgery, versus chemo-radiotherapy.

While optimal pathologic response rates were greater in patients receiving TIP (48% vs. 23%, $p = 0.0004$), there was no significant difference in treatment failure rate or hazard of death. Rates of grade 3 and 4 neutropenia, anemia and thrombocytopenia were greater with TIP treatment ($p = 0.02$). Treatment delays and dose reductions were necessary in 35% of patients receiving TIP versus 18% receiving IP. There were 4 treatment related deaths, 1 receiving TIP and 3 receiving IP, the majority of which were in women greater than 70 years with pre-existing renal disease, suggesting the need for careful patient selection. Response to chemotherapy predicted prognosis, with average death rates higher in the group not achieving optimal response (HR 5.88, 95% CI 2.5 – 13.84, $p < 0.0001$).

The authors concluded that the TIP regiment was associated with a greater response than the IP regimen. This did not translate into a survival benefit. However the study was only powered for treatment response, not overall and disease-free survival.

To determine the incremental benefit of ifosfamide to the TIP protocol, the same Italian Collaborative Group performed a randomized phase II study comparing TIP to paclitaxel/cisplatin (TP) prior to radical surgery (Lissoni et al., 2009). Women with inoperable tumours underwent radical radiotherapy, while women with lymph node metastases, parametrial invasion, positive margins, or suboptimal response underwent either external beam radiotherapy or chemo-radiotherapy. Those with either a complete or partial response underwent 2 additional courses of chemotherapy after surgery with the same chemotherapeutic agents as their neoadjuvant treatment.

An optimal pathologic response was achieved in 25% of patients receiving TP compared to 43% receiving TIP ($p = 0.03$). This was driven primarily by the response of patients with stage IB2 disease (53% vs. 24% responding to TIP vs. TP, respectively). The authors felt that the TP regimen demonstrated less efficacy than expected, while the TIP regimen, showing superior response rates, was associated with considerable toxicity. Grade 3-4 leukopenia and neutropenia were significantly more frequent in those receiving ifosfamide (78% vs. 29%, $p < 0.0001$). However only 2 of 49 patients who achieved an optimal response to chemotherapy required adjuvant radiotherapy.

There was no difference in progression-free or overall survival, although this study was not powered to address these outcomes.

While the authors present the option of neoadjuvant chemotherapy as a valid alternative to chemo-radiotherapy, the toxicity of treatment must be considered. Furthermore, while adequate sample size was achieved, the study population in this trial was much younger than the general population with cervical cancer, with better performance status, limiting the external validity and generalizability of these results. Lastly, until such time as a randomized comparison of neoadjuvant chemotherapy followed by surgery versus concomitant chemo-radiotherapy is performed, conclusions regarding the use of neoadjuvant chemotherapy and surgery as a legitimate alternative to radiotherapy cannot be justified.

3.5 Criticisms of data

The majority of published trials comparing neoadjuvant chemotherapy prior to surgery versus surgery alone are small studies, most of which are inconclusive. Conflicting results have been found, with some studies showing significant improvement in survival (Sardi et al., 1997) and others showing significant detriment (Tattersall et al., 1995). Tierney *et al.* (Tierney et al., 1999) therefore sought to compile the results of published reports in a systematic review and meta-analysis, in order to increase the statistical power to detect a difference in survival should one exist. Using published summary data from trial reports, this meta-analysis was found to be of limited benefit, since only a subset of trials had yet been published, and some failed to include sufficient survival data to be used in the analysis. Therefore, no firm conclusions could be made.

3.6 Systematic review and meta-analysis

A decade passed and the question was revisited. Does neoadjuvant chemotherapy prior to surgery in women with operable tumours confer a survival advantage over surgery alone? A systematic review and meta-analysis, performed by Rydzewska *et al.* (Rydzewska et al., 2010) was published in the Cochrane library, examining the role of neoadjuvant chemotherapy in women with early or locally advanced cervical cancer. The primary outcome was overall survival. Secondary outcomes were progression-free survival, local and distant recurrence rates, rates of resection, and surgical morbidity. Six trials were included, with a total of 1072 women with FIGO stage IB – IIIB disease, using trial report data (Table 1). All trials used cisplatin-based chemotherapy. While data on overall survival, progression-free survival, resection rates, pathologic response, and recurrence were not available for all trial participants, the authors found that neoadjuvant chemotherapy prior to surgery resulted in an improved progression-free survival (HR = 0.76, 95% CI 0.62 - 0.94, p = 0.01). These results were similar when random effects modeling was applied (to control for study heterogeneity) (HR = 0.73, 95% CI 0.56 - 0.96, p = 0.03). However, there was no difference in overall survival (HR = 0.85, 95% CI 0.67 - 1.07, p = 0.17) (with minimal heterogeneity).

Studies showed great variation in local and distant recurrences, and rates of tumour resectability. Significantly increased rates of radical resection following neoadjuvant chemotherapy were seen in two trials (Napolitano et al., 2003; Sardi et al., 1997), while no difference was seen in three others (Cai et al., 2006; Chen et al., 2008; Eddy et al., 2007). However, statistical modeling to combine study results showed no overall benefit to neoadjuvant chemotherapy in radical resection rates, local or distant recurrences.

Meanwhile, measures of pathologic response demonstrated a significant decrease in adverse pathologic findings in patients undergoing neoadjuvant chemotherapy. There were fewer patients with lymph node metastases (OR = 0.54, 95% CI 0.39 - 0.73, p < 0.0001) and parametrial invasion (OR = 0.58, 95% CI 0.41 - 0.82, p = 0.002). Significant heterogeneity between studies was again noted, making pooled comparisons of studies inappropriate. However, when statistical adjustment was performed, using random effects modeling, the differences in pathologic response remained significant. While in some trials the improvement in pathologic response was associated with improved local and distant control and overall and progression-free survival, this was not a uniform observation across studies. Survival according to neoadjuvant chemotherapy was unaffected by total cisplatin dose, chemotherapy cycle length, or cervical cancer stage (FIGO IB versus FIGO II – IIIB). Surgical morbidity was not increased in patients undergoing neoadjuvant chemotherapy.

In 1 of the studies included in this meta-analysis (Sardi et al., 1997), all patients received post-operative adjuvant radiotherapy, regardless of risk factors. In 4 others, (Cai et al., 2006; Chen et al., 2008; Eddy et al., 2007; Napolitano et al., 2003), between 36% and 61% of patients received adjuvant radiotherapy due to risk factors identified at the time of surgery. If the objective of neoadjuvant chemotherapy prior to surgery is to decrease the need for adjuvant radiotherapy, this goal has not been achieved.

Rydzewska *et al.* highlight the discrepancy between overall survival and progression-free survival, indicating that overall survival and progression-free survival would be expected to be similar, given that most recurrences and deaths from cervical cancer take place within the first 3 years. However, bias may have been introduced, as 1 study did not present results for overall survival (Chen et al., 2008) and 1 study excluded patients with unfavourable prognoses (those not responding to chemotherapy) from the analysis of progression-free survival, but not overall survival (Napolitano et al., 2003). Therefore, given the available evidence, there is no survival benefit to neoadjuvant chemotherapy prior to surgery in patients with operable tumours, and the noted benefit in progression-free survival should be interpreted with caution.

3.7 Conclusions

Following review of the available evidence, there does not appear to be a consistent benefit in overall survival to neoadjuvant chemotherapy prior to surgery versus surgery alone. Studies suggesting an improvement in survival utilized adjuvant radiotherapy in the majority of patients, obscuring the impact of neoadjuvant chemotherapy. While different rates of pathologic response may be noted, these do not translate into a survival advantage.

4. Neoadjuvant chemotherapy prior to radiotherapy versus radiotherapy alone

4.1 Rationale

The use of neoadjuvant chemotherapy prior to radiotherapy was introduced in order to attempt improved survival in patients with locally advanced cervical cancer. While treatment consisted mainly of radical radiotherapy, cure rates were still low due to local and distant recurrences. The objective of neoadjuvant chemotherapy, therefore, was to eradicate subclinical or clinical distant metastases and to improve the local disease control by achieving a reduction in tumour size. Large tumour masses often cause anatomic distortion, affecting the placement of vaginal and cervical radiation sources. Therefore, a decrease in tumour size prior to radiotherapy might also facilitate the accurate delivery of radiation.

Theoretical benefits to neoadjuvant chemotherapy prior to radiotherapy include increased radiosensitivity and decreased hypoxic cell fractions with tumour size reduction (Eddy, 1996; Souhami et al., 1991), improved drug delivery and distribution to the tissues prior to radiation vasculitis (Eddy, 1996; Tokuhashi et al., 1997), and possible radiation potentiation using platinum-based regimens.

4.2 Objectives

The objective of this review is to determine whether neoadjuvant chemotherapy prior to radiotherapy improves response rates, disease-free and overall survival with acceptable toxicity profiles. The following collection of studies (Table 2) addresses the impact of neoadjuvant chemotherapy followed by radical radiotherapy versus radiotherapy alone.

Author	Stage	Neoadjuvant Chemotherapy	Radiation	Comparison	Response	Overall Survival	Median Follow-up
Souhami 1991 N = 91	SCC IIIB	Bleomycin 15U q12h (D1-4) Vincristine 1mg/m^2 Mitomycin 10mg/m^2 Cisplatin 50mg/m^2 Every 3 weeks x 3 cycles	EBRT 50 Gy Intra-cavitary 40 Gy	CT + RT	CR 47% PR 25%	23%	>34 months
				RT	CR 32% PR 27% (p = NS)	39% (p = 0.02)	
Tattersall 1992 N = 71	IIB – IVA	Cisplatin 50mg/m^2 Vinblastine 4mg/m^2 Bleomycin 15mg (D1,8,15) Every 3 weeks x 3 cycles	EBRT 40-55 Gy	CT + RT	CR 65% PR 29%	141 weeks[1]	37 months
				RT	CR 73% PR 16%	167 weeks	
Chiara 1994 N = 61	SCC + ASQ IIB – III	Cisplatin 60mg/m^2 Every 15 days 2 cycles before RT 4 cycles after RT	EBRT 60 Gy Intra-cavitary 40 Gy	CT + RT + CT	CR 42% PR 36%	72%	36 months
				RT	CR 41% PR 41%	83% (p = NS)	
Kumar 1994 N = 184	SCC IIB – IVA	Bleomycin 15mg Ifosfamide 1g/m^2 (D1-5) Cisplatin 50mg/m^2 Every 3 weeks x 2 cycles	EBRT 50 Gy Intraca-vitary 30 Gy	CT + RT	CR 4% PR 68%	38%	30 months
				RT	CR 69%	43% (p = NS)	22 months
Tattersall 1995 N = 260	IIB – IVA	Cisplatin 60mg/m^2 Epirubicin 110mg/m^2 Every 3 weeks x 3 cycles	EBRT 30-35 Gy Intra-cavitary 30-35 Gy	CT + RT	CR 43% PR 29%	--	16 months
				RT	CR 65% PR 27%	-- (p = 0.02)	
Sundfor 1996 N = 94	SCC IIIB – IVA	Cisplatin 100mg/m^2 5-FU 1000mg/m^2 (D 1-5) Every 3 weeks x 3 cycles	EBRT 65 Gy	CT + RT	CR 56% PR 24%	26 months	46 months
				RT	CR 61% PR 20%	22 months (p = NS)	45 months
Leborgne 1997 N = 96	IB – IVA	Cisplatin 50mg/m^2 Bleomycin 25mg/m^2 (D1-3) Vincristine 1mg/m^2 Every 10 days x 3 cycles	EBRT 20-60 Gy Intra-cavitary 30 Gy	CT + RT	CR12% PR 50%[2]	--	43 months
				RT	--	--	
Sardi 1998 N = 144	SCC IIB	Vincristine 1mg/m^2 Bleomycin 25mg/m^2 (D1-3) Cisplatin 50mg/m^2 Every 10 days x 3 cycles	EBRT 50 Gy Intra-cavitary 35-40 Gy	CT + RT	72%[2]	54%	84 months
				RT	--	48% (p = NS)	

Author	Stage	Neoadjuvant Chemotherapy	Radiation	Comparison	Response	Overall Survival	Median Follow-up
Herod 2000 N = 172	IB – IVA	Bleomycin 30mg Ifosfamide 5g/m[2] Cisplatin 50mg/m[2] Every 4 weeks x 2-3 cycles	According to Institution Policy	CT + RT	CR 53% PR 16%	3 years[1]	108 months
				RT	CR 37% PR 22%	2 years	
Tabata 2003 N = 61	SCC IIIB – IVA	Bleomycin 5mg/body (D1-7) Vincristine 0.7mg/m[2] (D7) Mitomycin 7mg/m[2] (D7) Cisplatin 10mg/m[2] (D1-7) Every 4 weeks x 3 cycles	EBRT 50 Gy Intra-cavitary 40 Gy	CT+RT	CR 53% PR 31%	43%	--
				RT	CR 35% PR 41%	52% (p = NS)	

[1]Median Survival; [2]Response to Chemotherapy; SCC - Squamous Cell Carcinoma; ASQ - Adenosquamous; EBRT - External Beam Radiotherapy; CT – Chemotherapy; RT – Radiotherapy; CR - Complete Response; PR - Partial Response

Table 2. Neoadjuvant Chemotherapy Prior to Radiotherapy versus Radiotherapy Alone

4.3 Data

There are over 20 randomized clinical trials exploring the role of neoadjuvant chemotherapy prior to radical radiotherapy. The trials differ in chemotherapeutic regimens, dosing schedules, inclusion criteria and control arms. However, while generally underpowered, all studies fail to detect a benefit of neoadjuvant chemotherapy prior to radiotherapy versus radiotherapy alone. In the era of concurrent chemo-radiotherapy, the concept of neoadjuvant chemotherapy prior to radiotherapy has seen reduced momentum. Some might argue that the correct dose, drug, or indication has yet to be identified or defined. Perhaps the approach of neoadjuvant chemotherapy prior to radiotherapy may warrant revisiting if new chemotherapeutic agents are introduced. In the meantime, the literature suggests no benefit, and indeed, perhaps harm, when chemotherapy precedes primary radiotherapy.

Souhami *et al.* (Souhami et al., 1991) was one of the first to publish a randomized, controlled trial, comparing patients receiving radiotherapy with or without neoadjuvant bleomycin, vincristine, mitomycin and cisplatin (BOMP). A complete response was seen following chemotherapy in 25% of patients. Following the completion of radiotherapy, there was no difference in response between treatment groups. Of the 91 patients with Stage IIIB disease, the 5-year survival was significantly superior in those receiving radiotherapy alone (39% versus 23%, p = 0.02). The mortality was driven predominantly by excess toxicity to chemotherapy, as there was no difference in locoregional or distant failures. The mortality due to chemotherapy was 10%. This trial was closed early due to the identified survival advantage in the control group.

Tattersall *et al.* (Tattersall et al., 1992) randomized 71 patients with stage IIB – IVA disease to radiation with or without neoadjuvant chemotherapy delivered as 3 cycles of cisplatin, vinblastine, and bleomycin. At a median follow-up of 3.1 years there was no significant difference in overall survival. There were no excess complications of pelvic radiotherapy following neoadjuvant chemotherapy, suggesting that neoadjuvant chemotherapy prior to radiotherapy can be tolerated, however 7 of 34 patients randomized to neoadjuvant chemotherapy did not receive all 3 cycles. In both treatment arms the complete or partial response rate to radiotherapy was 89 - 94%, suggesting that the delay to receiving radiotherapy due to chemotherapy did not reduce the prospects of local disease control from pelvic radiotherapy. This study was underpowered, with a calculated sample size of 180 participants per arm. The trial was terminated early due to poor patient accrual and included 32 stage IIB, 3 stage IIIA, 29 stage IIIB, and 7 stage IVA patients, limiting the generalizability of results to patients with more advanced stage disease.

Kumar *et al.* (Kumar et al., 1994) randomized 184 patients with squamous cell carcinoma of the cervix, Stage IIB - IVA, to receive 2 cycles of bleomycin, ifosfamide, and cisplatin followed by radiotherapy (n = 94), versus radiotherapy alone (n = 90). At a median follow-up of 30 months and 22 months, respectively, there was no difference in overall or disease-free survival. When stratified by stage, there remained no difference in disease-free survival. This study was limited by sample size, with no pre-specified sample size calculation. Furthermore, the dose of cisplatin, at 50 mg/m^2 every 3 weeks, for 2 rather than 3 cycles, may have been insufficient to effect a response, as only 4.5% had a complete response to chemotherapy.

Chiara *et al.* (Chiara et al., 1994) randomized 61 patients with stage IIB - III disease to neoadjuvant and adjuvant cisplatin chemotherapy plus radiotherapy versus radiotherapy alone. The former group received 2 cycles of cisplatin prior to radiotherapy, followed by 4 cycles following radiotherapy. While chemotherapy did not worsen the morbidity of radiotherapy, follow-up at 3 years revealed no difference in recurrence, overall or progression-free survival. The study was limited by sub-therapeutic radiotherapy, with maximum total doses between 55 and 60 Gy, as well as a lack of pre-specified sample-size.

Tattersall *et al.* (Tattersall et al., 1995) then randomized 260 patients with stage IIB - IVA disease to neoadjuvant chemotherapy with 3 cycles of cisplatin and epirubicin plus radiation, versus radiation alone. While tolerance to the combined treatment was acceptable, and 63% of patients responded to chemotherapy alone, there was a significantly higher pelvic failure rate ($p < 0.003$) and lower disease-free survival ($p = 0.02$) at 3 years in those who received neoadjuvant chemotherapy.

Sundfor *et al.* (Sundfor et al., 1996) randomized 94 patients with Stage IIIB - IVA disease to 3 cycles of cisplatin and fluorouracil plus radiotherapy versus radiotherapy alone. At a median follow-up of 44 months there was no difference in survival, time to recurrence, local control, and metastases. There was suggestion of cross-resistance between chemotherapy and radiotherapy, as those who did not respond to chemotherapy were less likely to be cured by radiotherapy. This study planned for 150 patients per treatment arm, and was therefore underpowered.

Leborgne *et al.* (Leborgne et al., 1997) randomized 97 patients with bulky Stage IB - IVA disease to radiotherapy with or without 3 cycles of vincristine, bleomycin and cisplatin ("Quick VBP"). At 43 months follow-up there was no difference in locoregional control or disease-free survival. This study was also underpowered, planning for 75 patients per arm. Dose intensity was suboptimal in both groups. Compliance with chemotherapy was only 85%, and patients on chemotherapy received a lower dose of radiotherapy to the parametria compared to controls. Lesion downsizing and clinical down-staging did not translate into a prolongation of disease-free survival. The study was stopped prematurely due to unequal response between the two arms, although no interim analysis was planned in the original protocol.

Sardi *et al.* (Sardi et al., 1998) performed a randomized trial of 295 stage IIB patients, divided between four arms. Patients either received radiotherapy alone (n = 73), surgery plus adjuvant radiotherapy (n = 75), neoadjuvant chemotherapy ("Quick VBP") plus radiotherapy (n = 71), neoadjuvant chemotherapy plus surgery and adjuvant radiotherapy (n = 76). At 7 years there was no difference in survival between treatment arms with the exception of tumours larger than 5 cm, where survival was improved with chemotherapy (66% vs. 36%, $p < 0.05$). Response to chemotherapy predicted survival.

Herod *et al.* (Herod et al., 2000) looked at the use of neoadjuvant chemotherapy followed by radiotherapy versus radiotherapy alone using bleomycin, ifosfamide, and cisplatin (BIP) in patients with stage IIB - IVA disease. This randomized multicentre trial of patients with inoperable cervical cancer found no difference in complete or partial response (59% with radiotherapy versus 69% with neoadjuvant chemotherapy followed by radiotherapy) or overall survival. In this study individual centres were permitted to choose their radiation protocol, approved by the Radiotherapy Steering Group prior to patient study entry. This trial was closed early due to poor patient accrual as media interest resulted in the demand, by patients and clinicians, for the new treatment off study. Despite the relatively well-tolerated BIP protocol, which contributed to rapid symptom relief in many patients (pain, bleeding and discharge), the power to detect a clinically significant difference of 15% in overall survival was only 50% given the study size.

Finally, one of the most recent studies comparing neoadjuvant chemotherapy prior to radiotherapy versus radiotherapy alone is that of Tabata *et al.* (Tabata et al., 2003). The choice of chemotherapeutic agents was based on reports of clinical efficacy of bleomycin, vincristine, mitomycin and cisplatin (BOMP). The overall response rate was 84% in those receiving neoadjuvant chemotherapy and radiotherapy compared to a 76% response to radiotherapy alone. Again, there was no difference in 5-year survival.

4.4 Systematic review and meta-analysis

Given the importance of the persistent question, whether neoadjuvant chemotherapy prior to surgery or radiotherapy has the potential to increase overall and disease-free survival, an updated systematic review and meta-analysis, using individual patient data, was performed to re-analyze the available trial data. The advantages of individual patient data over the use of published reports in a meta-analysis include: more sensitive time-to-event data, the ability to include non-published trials, the examination of different effects between treatment subgroups, and the use of updated follow-up. This was initiated and coordinated by the Medical Research Council (UK) Clinical Trials Unit and carried out by the Neoadjuvant Chemotherapy for Cervical Cancer Meta-analysis Collaboration (Tierney, et al., 2009) and published in 2009 in the Cochrane library. Trials opening after January 1975 and closing before September 2000 were included, examining the effects of neoadjuvant chemotherapy for patients with locally advanced cervical cancer (FIGO stage IB - IVA). Two outcomes were explored: 1) the effects of neoadjuvant chemotherapy prior to local treatment versus local treatment alone, and 2) neoadjuvant chemotherapy followed by surgery (with or without adjuvant radiotherapy) versus radiotherapy alone.

Trials comparing neoadjuvant chemotherapy prior to local treatment versus local treatment alone (the majority of which examined radiotherapy as the local treatment of choice), were included. Individual data on 2074 patients, from 18 trials, was obtained. This represented 92% of patients eligible from randomized trials performed between 1975 and 2000.

The majority of patients receiving neoadjuvant chemotherapy were administered cisplatin-containing regimens, with varying doses, dosing schedules, and drug combinations. Radiation treatments also varied by external beam and intracavitary dosing, and total dose received (55 - 80 Gy).

The median age of patients in this analysis was 48 years (range of median age across trials was 40-59 years) with good performance status. Patients were included with moderate or poorly differentiated stage II - III tumours of squamous cell histology, the greatest proportion made up of stage III disease (44%). The median follow-up overall was 5.7 years (range of median follow-up across trials was 1.5 - 9.0 years).

A major limitation of this meta-analysis was the significant level of heterogeneity between studies for all outcomes measured. The authors acknowledge that to combine the outcomes, given the significant differences noted between studies, would be inappropriate. However, when studies were grouped according to chemotherapy cycle length (greater or less than 14 days) or dose intensity (greater or less than 25 mg/m^2 per week), a large proportion of the heterogeneity was explained.

The authors found that cycles lasting longer than 14 days had a pooled Hazard Ratio of 1.25 (p = 0.005), suggesting a 25% increase in the risk of death in those receiving neoadjuvant chemotherapy, and an absolute reduction in 5-year survival of 8% (from 45% to 37%). Those with cycles lasting less than 14 days had a pooled Hazard Ratio of 0.83 (p = 0.05), suggesting a 17% decrease in the risk of death, and an absolute improvement in 5-year overall survival of 7% (from 45% to 52%). Heterogeneity was still present between studies with cycle length less than 14 days. When a small trial with an extreme Hazard Ratio (3.37) was excluded, the pooled Hazard Ratio became 0.76 (p = 0.005) with minimal heterogeneity.

When grouped according to cisplatin dose intensity, some of the heterogeneity between study results was explained. Those trials using cisplatin doses less than 25 mg/m^2 per week had a pooled Hazard Ratio of 1.35 (p = 0.002), suggesting a 35% increase in the risk of death and an 11% absolute reduction in 5-year survival (from 45% to 34%). Those trials using cisplatin doses greater than 25 mg/m^2 per week had a pooled Hazard Ratio of 0.91 (p = 0.2), suggesting a potential decrease of 9% in the risk of death, and a 3% absolute improvement in 5-year overall survival (from 45% to 48%). This analysis, however, was limited by the considerable heterogeneity, particularly amoung the trials with high dose intensity, making pooled analyses somewhat inappropriate.

These results are of interest, however, as they suggest that neoadjuvant chemotherapy may be beneficial if applied with adequate chemotherapy dose at optimal treatment intervals.

4.5 Criticisms of data

While some studies display improvement in disease-free or overall survival, other studies have shown detriment. The majority of trials are compromised by inadequate sample sizes as well as suboptimal use of both chemotherapy as well as radiotherapy. Given the variety of treatment protocols, interpretation of the data is difficult, as the most efficient and least toxic regimen of neoadjuvant chemotherapy is difficult to identify. The greatest limitation, however, is the lack of clinical trials comparing neoadjuvant chemotherapy to radiation protocols that incorporate concurrent chemo-radiotherapy. Until a benefit can be demonstrated, above and beyond the survival advantage of chemo-radiotherapy, the use of neoadjuvant chemotherapy prior to radiotherapy cannot be considered an alternative.

4.6 Conclusions

As studied thus far, there is no convincing evidence that neoadjuvant chemotherapy improves survival. The randomized studies are limited by inadequate numbers to allow definitive conclusions, and many employ sub-optimal chemotherapy or radiation protocols. While surrogate markers, such as pathologic response and decreased tumour size may be promising, neoadjuvant chemotherapy prior to radiotherapy is not supported in the literature, and at present should only be considered in the setting of clinical trials where comparisons are made with the current standard treatment using concurrent chemo-radiation protocols.

5. Neoadjuvant chemotherapy prior to surgery versus radical radiotherapy

5.1 Rationale

The current standard of care in the treatment of bulky and locally advanced cervical cancer (stage IB2 - IIIB) is concurrent chemo-radiotherapy (Keys et al., 1999; Morris et al., 1999; Peters et al., 2000; Rose et al., 1999; Whitney et al., 1999). In the midst of ongoing trials investigating neoadjuvant chemotherapy prior to surgery or radiotherapy in the treatment of locally advanced cervical cancer, a National Cancer Institute Alert stated that "strong consideration should be given to the incorporation of chemotherapy with radiotherapy in women who require radiotherapy for the treatment of cervical cancer (National Cancer Institute, 1999). In a systematic review and meta-analysis of clinical trials, a 29% reduction in the risk of death, and overall survival benefit of 12% at 5-years was suggested by the results. Randomized studies of neoadjuvant chemotherapy prior to radiotherapy versus radiotherapy alone, and neoadjuvant chemotherapy prior to surgery versus surgery alone were not able to reveal a consistent survival advantage. Whether neoadjuvant chemotherapy would allow patients to avoid radical radiotherapy is addressed in the following studies comparing neoadjuvant chemotherapy prior to surgery versus radiotherapy alone.

5.2 Data

Benedetti-Panici *et al.* (Benedetti-Panici et al., 2002) randomized 409 patients with stage IB2 - III squamous cell carcinoma to receive either neoadjuvant cisplatin-containing chemotherapy plus radical hysterectomy (with pelvic lymph node dissection) or standard radiotherapy. Of the 210 patients randomized to receive neoadjuvant chemotherapy and surgery, 164 underwent surgery, and 109 had negative lymph nodes and surgical resection margins. Therefore, 52% (109/210) of patients, who would otherwise have received radical radiotherapy, were treated with neoadjuvant chemotherapy and radical surgery only. Interestingly, there were 22 patients who demonstrated no residual tumour on final pathology, suggesting that in some patients, sufficient treatment may be with neoadjuvant chemotherapy alone.

Although 78% (164/210) of patients were made operable with neoadjuvant chemotherapy, the remaining 22% (46/210) received primary radiotherapy, and 34% (55/164) of those undergoing surgery required adjuvant treatment. Neoadjuvant chemotherapy therefore did not avoid radiotherapy in 48% (101/210) of patients. Not included in this figure are those patients who, despite negative lymph nodes and surgical margins, might be considered for adjuvant radiotherapy based on other high-risk features. The added morbidity of treatment with combined chemotherapy, radical surgery, and adjuvant radiotherapy may outweigh the perceived benefits to a select subset of patients.

When compared to primary radiotherapy, however, Benedetti-Panici *et al.* found a survival benefit to neoadjuvant chemotherapy followed by surgery (Benedetti-Panici et al., 2002). When analyzed according to intention-to-treat principles, overall survival and progression-free survival were superior in those receiving neoadjuvant chemotherapy (overall survival 56.5% vs. 44.4%, respectively, $p = 0.01$; progression-free survival 55.4% vs. 41.3%, respectively, $p = 0.02$). While encouraging, this survival advantage was not uniformly distributed. When analyzed by stage, the significant benefit was seen mainly in patients with stage IB2 - IIB disease, and on subgroup analysis, in those with stage IB2 - IIA disease only. There was no significant survival advantage in patients treated for stage III disease. Radical surgery was possible in 85.5% of stage IB2 – IIB patients, compared to 55% with stage III disease ($p = 0.0001$) and there was a higher incidence of persistent disease in the lymph nodes and parametria in patients with stage III disease compared to stage IB2 – IIB (50% vs. 37%).

The median dose of radiotherapy received by control patients was only 70 Gy, and intracavitary treatment was not possible in 28% of patients. The generally accepted dose of radiotherapy is 85-90 Gy to Point A. Whether a difference in survival would persist if neoadjuvant chemotherapy plus surgery were compared to controls receiving a standard dose of primary radiotherapy or primary chemo-radiotherapy is unclear.

5.3 Systematic review and meta-analysis

Five randomized trials, including the work of Benedetti-Panici *et al* (Benedetti-Panici et al. 2002) were included in the systematic review and meta-analysis performed by the Neoadjuvant Chemotherapy for Cervical Cancer Meta-Analysis Collaboration. In this portion of the analysis, neoadjuvant chemotherapy prior to surgery versus radiotherapy alone was examined, and individual patient data was used (Tierney et al., 2009). A total of 872 patients, representing 97% of patients from known randomized trials were included. Patients received either cisplatin-containing neoadjuvant chemotherapy followed by surgery, or external beam radiotherapy (45-60 Gy) with subsequent intracavitary treatments (25-40 Gy).

The median age of study participants was 49 years (range 42 - 58 between trials), with good performance status. The majority had moderate to poorly differentiated tumours, stage IB - III, with squamous cell histology. Median follow-up was 5 years (range 3.9 to 9 years). The primary endpoint of the analysis was survival.

In 3 trials (Sardi et al., 1996; Sardi et al., 1998; Benedetti-Panici et al., 2002) patients receiving neoadjuvant chemotherapy followed by surgery demonstrated improved survival compared to those receiving radiotherapy alone. When all 5 trials were combined together, the direction of effect remained significant, with a Hazard Ratio of 0.65 ($p = 0.0004$) suggesting a 35% reduction in the risk of death and a 14% absolute improvement in survival at 5 years (from 50% to 64%). There was some heterogeneity between trial results.

In 2 of the trials included in the meta-analysis, greater than 90% of patients randomized to neoadjuvant chemotherapy also received adjuvant radiotherapy, and in 2 trials, 28% and

32% of neoadjuvant chemotherapy patients received adjuvant radiotherapy. The comparison being made, therefore, can be considered as triple modality treatment versus radiotherapy alone for many patients studied.

5.4 Conclusions

In the handful of studies exploring neoadjuvant chemotherapy prior to surgery versus radiotherapy alone, it is suggested that some patients may benefit from neoadjuvant chemotherapy followed by surgical resection. However, if the objective is to avoid primary or adjuvant radiotherapy, this goal is not easily achieved, and many patients may be subjected to triple modality treatment with the associated toxicity. Furthermore, since control arms were administered suboptimal doses of radiation, the survival advantage seen with neoadjuvant chemotherapy may not be replicated if compared to standard doses of radiation or radiation with concurrent chemotherapy.

6. Neoadjuvant chemotherapy prior to fertility-sparing surgery

6.1 Background

Radical hysterectomy with pelvic lymphadenectomy is currently considered the standard of care in the treatment of young women with stage 1B1 cervical cancer.

However, recently, greater emphasis is being placed on quality of life as well as minimization of long-term morbidity for those who survive cancer treatment. Cancer-related infertility has significant psychosocial impact on those who undergo treatment for gynecologic malignancies, including increasing rates of depression, stress and sexual dysfunction (Carter et al., 2005). Where possible, it is of foremost importance for gynecologic oncologists to minimize such effects, improving not only oncologic outcomes, but also the emotional well-being of their patients. A prominent concern of young women undergoing treatment for cervical cancer is the preservation of childbearing function in the post-treatment period.

The possibility of maintaining high cure rates while preserving the reproductive organs has been an area of active research over the past 10 years. Due to improvements in cervical screening, more women have been identified with early stage disease for whom fertility-sparing treatments can be considered. These advances also come at a time when greater proportions of newly diagnosed cases of cervical cancer are in nulliparous women (as many have postponed childbearing). The option of preservation of fertility is of great concern to a majority of such patients.

Options for the surgical management of early-stage cervical cancer include cervical conization or radical trachelectomy, the latter of which may be performed via a trans-abdominal or trans-vaginal approach.

Radical vaginal trachelectomy, first described by Dargent in 1994, involves removal of the cervix, the parametria, and part of the vaginal cuff, while preserving the uterine fundus, ovaries and fallopian tubes. This procedure, in combination with a laparoscopic pelvic lymphadenectomy, is the most common and accepted fertility- sparing procedure for early-stage cervical cancer. When compared to historic cohorts, this procedure has a comparably recurrence (4% - 5%) and mortality (2.5% - 3%) (Dursun et al., 2007; Plante et al., 2004; Plante, 2008). However, the removal of the cervix and paracervical tissue has been associated with cervical insufficiency, with a two-fold increase in second-trimester losses compared to the general population, and a 30% incidence of preterm delivery (Beiner & Covens, 2007; Boss et al., 2005; Plante, 2008). Due to the placement of a permanent cervical cerclage at the time of trachelectomy, cesarean section is required to achieve delivery.

An alternative to radical vaginal trachelectomy is the radical abdominal trachelectomy, performed either open or laparoscopically (Abu-Rustum et al., 2008; Cibula et al., 2005; Geisler et al., 2008). While oncologic outcomes have yet to be compared, the abdominal approach may extend the inclusion criteria for patients interested in fertility sparing to those with larger primary cervical lesions (up to 4 cm in diameter). Patient selection is still restricted to those without evidence of metastatic disease (Del Priore et al., 2004; Ungar et al., 2005).

The most recent consideration is whether a radical trachelectomy is required for all invasive cervical cancers, or whether more conservative treatments might be offered, such as cone biopsy or simple trachelectomy. Recent publications have shown promising results, suggesting that such an approach may be acceptable for individually selected "low-risk" patients (Covens et al., 2002; Rob et al., 2008; Smith et al., 2010)..

6.2 Rationale

The eligibility criteria for fertility-sparing surgery typically requires lesions less than 2 cm in diameter, and less than 2/3rsd cervical stromal invasion, based on clinico-pathologic studies among patients with stage IA1- 1B1 disease (Covens et al., 2002). As such, it is not uncommon for women to be denied the option of fertility-preserving surgery in preference for radical radiotherapy.

The objective of neoadjuvant chemotherapy in patients seeking fertility preservation is primarily a reduction in the tumour size in order to facilitate resection. With complete or partial response to chemotherapy, tumours measuring 3 - 4 cm in diameter may become operable. Cure rates would be expected to be similar to those receiving primary radiotherapy, as the use of adjuvant radiotherapy for high risk pathologic findings would tend to negate any difference.

6.3 Neoadjuvant chemotherapy prior to fertility-preserving surgery

The use of neoadjuvant chemotherapy to reduce tumour size and potentially "sterilize" micrometastases in the paracervical tissues and pelvic lymph nodes has been investigated in several randomized controlled trials. If successful, a woman with a previously inoperable tumour may become a surgical candidate. Unfortunately studies were inconclusive, either due to methodological flaws or limitations in patient accrual and sample size (Benedetti-Panici et al., 2002; Cai et al., 2006; Chen et al., 2008; Eddy et al., 2007; Napolitano et al., 2003; Sardi et al., 2007).

A review of the literature describing neoadjuvant chemotherapy prior to fertility-preserving surgery reveals only a handful of publications, all of which are case-series. The largest series, by Maneo *et al.* (Maneo et al., 2008), explored the role of neoadjuvant chemotherapy followed by cold knife conization and pelvic lymphadenectomy. The single-centre study enrolled 51 nulliparous patients with Stage IB1 cervical cancer. Patients were deemed eligible if they were younger than 40 years of age, with tumor size less than 3 cm and had no lymphovascular space involvement. Neoadjuvant chemotherapy consisted of three cycles of cisplatin 75 mg/m^2, paclitaxel 175 mg/m^2 and ifosfamide 5 g/m^2 (substituted by epirubicin 80 mg/m^2 in cases of adenocarcinoma) every 3 weeks. Thirty patients (59%) decided against the planned conservative therapy and 1 patient refused conservative surgery following completion of chemotherapy. Among 20 patients receiving the treatment protocol, all but 4 showed a clinical response to chemotherapy and eventually underwent a cold knife conization. The 4 women who were ineligible for conservative surgical treatment underwent radical hysterectomy, and 2 received adjuvant radiotherapy due to positive lymph node metastases. After the completion of neoadjuvant chemotherapy all 16 remaining patients demonstrated a complete clinical remission or minimal persistence of disease. There were no severe chemotherapy-associated toxicities, and only 1 patient was unable to tolerate all 3 cycles due to the development of hepatic toxicity. There were no perioperative complications, and only 1 patient developed cervical stenosis. Among patients who completed the planned protocol there were no recurrences after a median follow-up of 69 months. There were 10 pregnancies among 6 of 9 patients attempting to conceive, resulting in one spontaneous miscarriage and 9 term deliveries.

The authors concluded that neoadjuvant chemotherapy followed by cold knife conization and pelvic lymphadenectomy should be used with caution, with careful patient selection and inclusion only of motivated women with a strong desire for future childbearing, recognizing the limitations of a small sample size in the assessment of oncologic outcomes.

Plante *et al.*, from Canada, reported a single-institution's experience using neoadjuvant chemotherapy followed by vaginal radical trachelectomy (Plante et al., 2006). Three patients had stage IB1 cervical lesions with tumour size ranging from 3 to 4 cm. Neoadjuvant chemotherapy consisted of 3 cycles every 3 weeks of paclitaxel 175 mg/m^2 on day 1, cisplatin 75 mg/m^2 on day 2 and ifosfamide 5 g/m^2 over 24 hours with mesna 5 g/m^2 on day 2 and 3 g/m^2 on day 3 with continuous hydration. One patient developed febrile neutropenia following the first cycle of chemotherapy. Reduction of tumor size was reported in 2 patients. Over a period of 2 months all patients underwent successful laparoscopic sentinel lymph node dissection followed by pelvic lymphadenectomy and vaginal radical trachelectomy with no perioperative complications. Postsurgical pathological examination revealed no residual disease and focal carcinoma in-situ in 2 and 1 patient, respectively. None of the patients had parametrial or lymph node involvement. At the time of report, all patients were alive without evidence of disease.

A single case report from China (Liu et al., 2008) described a 24 year old nulliparous woman with a 2 cm cervical lesion encroaching the left vaginal fornix. It was a poorly differentiated squamous cell carcinoma without evidence of lympho vascular space invasion. She was treated with one cycle of bleomycin 15 mg/m^2 on day 1 and 2, and cisplatin 70 mg/m^2 on day 1. She underwent a trans-peritoneal lymphadenectomy 10 days later followed by radical abdominal trachelectomy. The final pathology demonstrated only focal residual disease (5.5 mm by 3 mm). The patient recovered well and 2 years later delivered at 35 weeks gestation via cesarean section.

Robova *et al.*, from the Czech Republic, described their group's experience with 5 patients under the age of 40 with Stage IB1 cervical cancers greater than 2 cm in diameter with less than 2/3rsd stromal invasion (Robova et al., 2008). All patients received 3 cycles of neoadjuvant chemotherapy every 10 days consisting of cisplatin 75 mg/m^2 and ifosfamide 2 g/m^2 (substituted by doxorubicin 35 mg/m^2 in cases of adenocarcinoma). Patients underwent laparoscopic sentinel lymph node dissection followed by simple trachelectomy. Tumours ranged in size from 20 by 15 mm to 44 by 36 mm. There were 3 cases of squamous cell carcinoma, and 2 cases of adenocarcinoma. All cases had lympho-vascular space involvement. Final pathology revealed no residual tumor in 2 patients, microscopic residual tumor in 2 patients, and a 13 by 6 mm residual tumor in 1 patient. At the time of publication, all patients were reported alive with 2 full term pregnancies achieved in 2 patients, conceived 5 and 8 months following completion of treatment.

6.4 Conclusions

Fertility preservation with successful obstetrical outcomes is possible following neoadjuvant chemotherapy and fertility-sparing surgery. At present, however, the management of locally advanced cervical cancer in women wishing to preserve fertility is supported by only 25 published cases.

The most commonly used chemotherapeutic regimens are combinations of platinum, paclitaxel and ifosfamide given in 3 cycles. This combination has been the most widely studied in the neoadjuvant setting for patients with cervical cancer undergoing further radical surgery (Benedetti-Panici et al., 2002; Cai et al., 2006; Chen et al., 2008; Eddy et al., 2007; Napolitano et al., 2003; Sardi et al., 2007). However, alkylating agents such as ifosfamide and cisplatin can be detrimental to ovarian follicles, and less gonadotoxic regimens should be evaluated in the future (Plante et al., 2006).

In the absence of long-term follow-up and greater patient numbers, conclusions regarding safety, efficacy and reproductive outcomes are only speculative. This approach should therefore be considered to be experimental, performed only in carefully selected patients, in centers with high levels of expertise.

7. Ongoing research

While neoadjuvant chemotherapy in the treatment of cervical cancer has shown limited benefit in the majority of patients for whom radical surgery or chemo-radiotherapy is available, there are questions regarding its utility that remain unanswered. Neoadjuvant chemotherapy followed by surgery has not been compared to chemo-radiotherapy, for instance, nor has neoadjuvant chemotherapy prior to chemo-radiotherapy been examined.

There are currently two ongoing randomized phase III trials exploring neoadjuvant chemotherapy followed by surgery versus chemo-radiotherapy. These include EORTC Protocol 55994 and NCT00193739. Eligibility for the former study includes FIGO stage IB2, IIA > 4 cm and IIB disease. Activated in March of 2002, this study is currently open, with a targeted sample size of 686 patients. While limited by unstandardized neoadjuvant chemotherapy protocols, these results may help to determine whether neoadjuvant chemotherapy prior to surgery is a useful alternative to chemo-radiotherapy. Given the different levels of response seen with varying chemotherapeutic regimens (Buda et al., 2005; Lissoni et al., 2009), the use of a generic platinum-based protocol, and allowing centres to select their protocol, may again lead to inconclusive results. The latter study, activated in September 2003, with a targeted sample size of 730 patients, was scheduled to close in September 2010. Eligibility includes FIGO stage IB2 - IIB squamous cell carcinoma, and the study will compare 3 cycles of paclitaxel-carboplatin neoadjuvant chemotherapy followed by surgery versus concomitant chemo-radiotherapy.

Phase II studies include the NCRI Gynaecological Cancer Clinical Studies Group investigation "CxII" of weekly neoadjuvant carboplatin/paclitaxel followed by radical chemo-radiotherapy. Including patients with FIGO stage IB2 - IVA disease, this study was closed in November of 2008 and is currently in follow-up. As carboplatin-based regimens are expected to display similar effectiveness to cisplatin, but with easier administration and less toxicity, results of response rate and feasibility are intended to identify a regimen to be used in a subsequent phase III trial. Results presented at ASCO 2009 (McCormack et al., 2009) suggested high response rates with limited grade 3 and 4 toxicity.

8. Conclusions

The primary objectives of neoadjuvant chemotherapy in the treatment of cervical cancer include improvement in tumour characteristics to allow avoidance of radiotherapy, prolonged disease-free and overall survival, and facilitation of fertility-sparing surgery.

While some evidence supports the use of neoadjuvant chemotherapy in patients with early stage disease to permit surgical resection, improving pathologic risk factors and operability, a large proportion of patients ultimately require adjuvant radiotherapy, negating the benefit of neoadjuvant chemotherapy, and subjecting patients to triple modality treatments. Control patients received suboptimal doses of radiotherapy, however, making any comparison of treatment invalid and uninterpretable. How neoadjuvant chemotherapy followed by surgery in early stage disease compares to radiotherapy with concurrent chemotherapy has not been studied, and therefore, given the demonstrated survival advantage of primary chemo-radiotherapy, the use of neoadjuvant chemotherapy followed by surgery cannot be recommended as a superior or even equivalent option at this time.

Upon review of the available evidence, there has been no consistently proven benefit in overall survival to neoadjuvant chemotherapy prior to surgery (versus surgery alone) or radiotherapy (versus radiotherapy alone). Most randomized studies include inadequate patient numbers to support conclusions. The effect of neoadjuvant chemotherapy is then obscured by the addition of adjuvant radiotherapy.

Fertility preservation with successful obstetrical outcomes following neoadjuvant chemotherapy and fertility-sparing surgery has been possible. Women who would otherwise be treated with radiotherapy may be made operable. While promising, this approach is supported only by case series, and should therefore still be considered experimental.

In summary, neoadjuvant chemotherapy in the treatment of cervical cancer has limited applicability. Any use of such therapy should be in the setting of appropriately powered clinical trials, with comparisons made to the current standard of treatment using optimal chemo-radiation protocols.

9. References

Abu-Rustum, NR, et al. (2008). Surgical and pathologic outcomes of fertility-sparing radical abdominal trachelectomy for

FIGO stage Ib1 cervical cancer. *Gynecologic Oncology,* Vol.111, No. 2, (November 2008), pp. 261–264, ISSN 0090-8258

Beiner ME,Covens A. (2007). Surgery insight: radical vaginal trachelectomy as a method of fertility preservation for cervical cancer. *Nature Clinical Practice Oncology,* Vol.4, No. 6, (June 2007), pp. 353–361, ISSN 1743-4254

Benedetti-Panici, P, et al. (2002). Neoadjuvant chemotherapy and radical surgery versus exclusively radiotherapy in locally advanced squamous cell cervical cancer: results from the Italian multi-centre randomised study. *Journal of Clinical Oncology*, Vol.20, No.1, (January 2002), pp. 179–188, ISSN 1527-7755

Boss, EA, et al. (2005). Pregnancy after radical trachelectomy: a real option? *Gynecologic Oncology*, Vol.99, No.3, Supp.1, (December 2005), pp. 152–156, ISSN 0090-8258

Buda, A, et al. (2005). Randomized trial of neoadjuvant chemotherapy comparing paclitaxel, ifosfamide, and cisplatin with ifosfamide and cisplatin followed by radical surgery in patients with locally advanced squamous cell cervical carcinoma: the SNAP01 (Studio Neo-Adiuvante Portio) Italian Collaborative Study. *Journal of Clinical Oncology*, Vol.23, No.18, (June 2005), pp. 4137–4145, ISSN 1527-7755

Cai, HB, et al. (2006). Randomized study of preoperative chemotherapy versus primary surgery for stage IB cervical cancer. *The Journal of Obstetrics and Gynaecology Research*, Vol.32, No.3, (June 2006), pp. 315–323, ISSN 1447-0756

Carter, J, et al. (2005). Gynecologic cancer treatment and the impact of cancer-related infertility. *Gynecologic Oncology*, Vol.97, No.1, (April 2005), pp. 90–95, ISSN 0090-8258

Chen, H, et al. (2008). Clinical efficacy of modified preoperative neoadjuvant chemotherapy in the treatment of locally advanced (stage IB2 to IIB) cervical cancer: randomized study. *Gynecologic Oncology*, Vol.110, No.3, (September 2008), pp. 308–315, ISSN 0090-8258

Chiara, S, et al. (1994). Randomized study comparing chemotherapy plus radiotherapy vs. radiotherapy alone in FIGO Stage IIB-III cervical carcinoma. *American Journal of Clinical Oncology*, Vol.17, No.4, (August 1994), pp. 294-297, ISSN 0277-3732

Cibula, D, et al. (2005). Laparoscopic abdominal radical trachelectomy. *Gynecologic Oncology*, Vol.97, No.2, (May 2005), pp. 707–709, ISSN 0090-8258

Covens, A, et al. (2002). How important is removal of the parametrium at surgery for carcinoma of the cervix? *Gynecologic Oncology*, Vol.84, No. 1, (January 2002), pp. 145–149, ISSN 0090-8258

Del Priore, G, et al. (2004). Regarding "First case of a centropelvic recurrence after radical trachelectomy: literature review and implications for the preoperative selection of patients," (92:1002-5) by Morice et al. *Gynecologic Oncology*, Vol.95, No.2, (Nov 2004), pp. 414 ISSN 0090-8258

Dursun, P, et al. (2007). Radical vaginal trachelectomy (Dargent's operation): a critical review of the literature. *European Journal of Surgical Oncology*, Vol.33, No.8, (October 2007), pp. 933-941, ISSN 0748-7983

Eddy GL. (1996). Neoadjuvant chemotherapy before surgery in cervical cancer. *Journal of the National Cancer Institute Monographs*, Vol.21, (1996), pp. 93-99, ISSN 1052-6773

Eddy, GL, et al. (2007). Treatment of ("bulky") stage IB cervical cancer with or without neoadjuvant vincristine and cisplatin prior to radical hysterectomy and pelvic/para-aortic lymphadenectomy: a phase III trial of gynecologic oncology group. *Gynecologic Oncology*, Vol.106, No. , (month 2007), pp. 362-369, ISSN 0090-8258

Friedlander, M, et al. (1983). Cervical carcinoma: a drug-responsive tumour—experience with combined cisplatin, vinblastine, and bleomycin therapy. *Gynecologic Oncology*, Vol.16, No.2, (October 1983), pp. 275-281, ISSN 0090-8258

Friedlander, M, et al. (1984). The integration of chemotherapy into the management of locally advanced cervical cancer: a pilot study. *Gynecologic Oncology*, Vol.19, No.1, (September 1984), pp. 1-7, ISSN 0090-8258

Geisler, JP, et al. (2008). Robotically assisted total laparoscopic radical trachelectomy for fertility sparing in stage Ib1 adenosarcoma of the cervix. *Journal of Laparoendoscopic and Advanced Surgical Techniques*, Vol.18, No.5, (October 2008), pp. 727–729, ISSN 1092-6429

Herod, J, et al. (2000). A randomized, prospective, phase III clinical trial of primary bleomycin, ifosfamide and cisplatin (BIP) chemotherapy followed by radiotherapy versus radiotherapy alone in inoperable cancer of the cervix. *Annals of Oncology*, Vol.11, No.9, (September 2000), pp. 1175-1181, ISSN 0923-7534

Keys, HM, et al. (1999). Cisplatin, radiation, and adjuvant hysterectomy compared with radiation and adjuvant hysterectomy for bulky stage IB cervical carcinoma. *New England Journal of Medicine*, Vol.340, No.15, (April 1999), pp. 1154-1161, ISSN 0028-4793

Kumar, L, et al. (1994). Chemotherapy followed by radiotherapy versus radiotherapy alone in locally advanced cervical cancer: A randomised study. *Gynecologic Oncology*, Vol.54, No.3, (September 1994), pp. 307-315, ISSN 0090-8258

Landoni, F, et al. (1997). Randomised study of radical surgery versus radiotherapy for stage Ib-IIa cervical cancer. *Lancet* Vol.350, No.9077, (August 1997), pp. 535–540, ISSN 0140-6736

Leborgne, F, et al. (1997). Induction chemotherapy and radiotherapy of advanced cancer of the cervix: A pilot study and phase III randomized trial. *International Journal of Radiation Oncology Biology & Physics*, Vol.37, No.2, (January 1997), pp. 343-350, ISSN 0360-3016

Lissoni, AA, et al. (2009). A phase II, randomized trial of neo-adjuvant chemotherapy comparing a three-drug combination of paclitaxel, ifosfamide, and cisplatin (TIP) versus paclitaxel and cisplatin (TP) followed by radical surgery in patients with locally advanced squamous cell cervical carcinoma: the Snap-02 Italian Collaborative Study. *Annals of Oncology*, Vol.20, No.4, (April 2009), pp. 660-665, ISSN 0923-7534

Liu, H, et al. (2008). Pregnancy after neoadjuvant chemotherapy followed by pelvic lymphadenectomy and radical trachelectomy in bulky stage IB1 cervical cancer: A case report. *Australian and New Zealand Journal of Obstetrics and Gynecoogy*, Vol.48, No.5, (October 2008), pp. 517-518, ISSN 0004-8666

Maneo, A, et al. Neoadjuvant chemotherapy and conservative surgery for stage Ib1 cervical cancer. *Gynecologic Oncology*, Vol.111, No.3, (December 2008), pp. 438–443, ISSN 0090-8258

McCormack, M, et al. (2009) A phase II study of weekly neoadjuvant chemotherapy followed by radical chemoradiation for locally advanced cervical cancer, *Proceedings of 2009 ASCO Annual Meeting*, 1527-7755, Florida, May-June 2009.

Morris, M, et al. (1999). Pelvic radiation with concurrent chemotherapy compared with pelvic and para-aortic radiation for high-risk cervical cancer. *New England Journal of Medicine*, Vol.340, No.15, (April 1999), pp. 1137-1143, ISSN 0028-4793

Napolitano, U, et al. (2003). The role of neoadjuvant chemotherapy for squamous cell cervical cancer (Ib-IIIb): a long-term randomized trial. *European Journal of Gynaecological Oncology*, Vol.24, No.1, (2003), pp. 51-59, ISSN 0392-2936

National Cancer Institute. (1999). NCI Issues Clinical Announcement on Cervical Cancer: Chemotherapy Plus Radiation Improves Survival, In: *NEWS*, 20 April 2011, Available from: <http://www.cancer.gov>

Peters, WA, et al. (2000). Concurrent chemotherapy and pelvic radiation therapy compared with pelvic radiation therapy alone as adjuvant therapy after radical surgery in high-risk early-stage cancer of the cervix. *Journal of Clinical Oncology*, Vol.18, No.8, (April 2000), pp. 1606-1613, ISSN 1527-7755

Plante, M, et al. (2004). Vaginal radical trachelectomy: an oncologically safe fertility-preserving surgery. An updated series of 72 cases and review of the literature. *Gynecologic Oncology*, Vol.94, No.3, (September 2004), pp. 614–623, ISSN 0090-8258

Plante, M, et al. (2006). Neoadjuvant chemotherapy followed by vaginal radical trachelectomy in bulky stage Ib1 cervical cancer: case report. *Gynecologic Oncology*, Vol.101, No.2, (May 2006), pp. 367–370, ISSN 0090-8258

Plante M. (2008). Vaginal radical trachelectomy: an update. *Gynecologic Oncology*, Vol.111, Supp.2, (November 2008), pp. S105–S110, ISSN 0090-8258

Rob, L, et al. (2008). A less radical treatment option to the fertility-sparing radical trachelectomy in patients with stage I cervical cancer. *Gynecologic Oncology*, Vol.111, Supp.2, (November 2008), pp. S116–S120, ISSN 0090-8258

Robova, H, et al. (2008). High-dose density chemotherapy followed by simple trachelectomy: full-term pregnancy. *International Journal of Gynecologic Cancer*, Vol.18, No.6, (November-December 2008), pp. 1367–1371, ISSN 1525-1438

Rose, PG, et al. (1999) Concurrent cisplatin-based radiotherapy and chemotherapy for locally advanced cervical cancer. *New England Journal of Medicine*, Vol.340, No.15, (April 1999), pp. 1144-1153, ISSN 0028-4793

Rydzewska, L, et al. Neoadjuvant chemotherapy plus surgery versus surgery for cervical cancer. *Cochrane Database of Systematic Reviews* 2010, Issue 1.Art.No.: CD007406. DOI:10.1002/14651858.CD007406.pub2.

Sardi, J, et al. (1986). Possible new trend in the management of the carcinoma of the cervix uteri. *Gynecologic Oncology*, Vol.25, No.2, (October 1986), pp. 139–149, ISSN 0090-8258

Sardi, J, et al. (1993). Results of a prospective randomized trial with neoadjuvant chemotherapy in stage IB, bulky, squamous carcinoma of the cervix. *Gynecologic Oncology*, Vol.49, No.2, (May 1993), pp. 156–165, ISSN 0090-8258

Sardi, J, et al. (1996). Randomized trial with neoadjuvant chemotherapy in stage IIIB squamous carcinoma cervix uteri: An unexpected therapeutic management. *International Journal of Gynecologic Cancer*, Vol.6, No.2, (March-April 1996), pp. 85-93, ISSN 1525-1438

Sardi, J, et al. (1997). Long-term follow-up of the first randomized trial using neoadjuvant chemotherapy in stage Ib squamous carcinoma of the cervix: the final results. *Gynecologic Oncology*, Vol.67, No.1, (October 1997), pp. 61-69, ISSN 0090-8258

Sardi, J, et al. (1998). Neoadjuvant chemotherapy in cervical carcinoma stage IIB: a randomised controlled trial. *International Journal of Gynecologic Cancer*, Vol.8, No.6, (November-December 1998), pp. 441–450, ISSN 1525-1438

Smith, AL, et al. (2010). Conservative surgery in early-stage cervical cancer: What percentage of patients may be eligible for conization and lymphadenectomy? *Gynecologic Oncology*, Vol.119, No.2, (November 2010), pp. 183–186, ISSN 0090-8258

Souhami, L, et al. (1991). A randomized trial of chemotherapy followed by radiation therapy in stage IIIB carcinoma of the cervix. *Journal of Clinical Oncology*, Vol.9, No.6, (June 1991), pp. 970–977, ISSN 1527-7755

Sundfør, K, et al. (1996). Radiotherapy and neoadjuvant chemotherapy for cervix carcinoma: A randomised multicenter study of sequential cisplatin and 5-fluorouracil and radiotherapy in advanced cervical carcinoma stage IIIB and IVA. *Cancer*, Vol.77, No.11, (June 1996), pp. 2371-2378, ISSN 1097-0142

Tabata, T, et al. (2003). A randomized study of primary bleomycin, vincristine, mitomycin and cisplatin (BOMP) chemotherapy followed by radiotherapy versus radiotherapy alone in stage IIIB and IVA squamous cell carcinoma of the cervix. *Anticancer Research*, Vol.23, No.3C, (May-June 2003), pp. 2885-2890, ISSN 0250-7005

Tattersall, MH, et al. (1992). A randomized trial comparing platinum-based chemotherapy followed by radiotherapy vs. radiotherapy alone in patients with locally advanced cervical cancer. *International Journal of Gynecologic Cancer*, Vol.2, No.5, (September 1992), pp. 244-251, ISSN 1525-1438

Tattersall, MH, et al. (1995). Randomised trial of epirubicin and platinum chemotherapy followed by pelvic radiation in locally advanced cervical cancer. *Journal of Clinical Oncology*, Vol.13, No. , (month 1995), pp. 444-451, ISSN 1527-7755

Tierney, JF, et al. (1999) Can the published data tell us about the effectiveness of neoadjuvant chemotherapy for locally advanced cancer of the uterine cervix? *European Journal of Cancer*. Vol. 35, No. 3, p 406-409, ISSN 0959-8049

Tierney, JF, Neoadjuvant Chemotherapy for Cervical Cancer Meta-Analysis Collaboration (NACCCMA) Collaboration. (2009) Neoadjuvant chemotherapy for locally advanced cervix cancer (Review). *Cochrane Database of Systematic Reviews*. Issue 1. Art. No.:CD001774. DOI: 10.1002/14651858.CD001774.pub2.

Tokuhashi, Y, et al. (1997). Distribution of platinum in human gynecologic tissues and pelvic lymph nodes after administration of cisplatin. *Gynecologic and Obstetric Investigation*, Vol.44, No.4, (1997), pp. 270–274, ISSN 0378-7346

Ungar, L, et al. (2005). Abdominal radical trachelectomy: a fertility-preserving option for women with early cervical cancer. *British Journal of Obstetrics and Gynecology*, Vol.112, No.3, (March 2005), pp. 366–369, ISSN 0306-5456

World Health Organization. (2011). Cancer of the Cervix, In: *Sexual and Reproductive Health*, 19 April 2011, Available from:
<http://www.who.int/reproductivehealth/topics/cancers/en/index.html>

Whitney, CW, et al. (1999). Randomized comparison of fluorouracil plus cisplatin versus hydroxyurea as an adjunct to radiation therapy in stage IIBYIVA carcinoma of the cervix with negative para-aortic lymph nodes: a Gynecologic

Oncology Group and Southwest Oncology Group study. *Journal of Clinical Oncology*, Vol.17, No., (month 1999), pp. 1339-1348, ISSN 1527-7755

8

Percutaneous Pelvic Perfusion with Extracorporeal Chemofiltration for Advanced Uterine Cervical Carcinoma

Takeshi Maruo[1], Satoru Motoyama[2], Shinya Hamana[3], Shigeki Yoshida[4], Masashi Deguchi[4], Mineo Yamasaki[4] and Yanson Ku[5]

[1]*Kobe Children's Hospital and Feto-Maternal Medical Center, Kobe*

[2]*Department of Obstetrics and Gynecology, Aijinkai Chibune General Hospital, Osaka*

[3]*Department of Obstetrics and Gynecology, Akashi Medical Center, Akashi*

[4]*Department of Obstetrics and Gynecology, Kobe University Graduate School of Medicine, Kobe*

[5]*Department of Liver and Transplantation Surgery Kobe University Graduate School of Medicine, Kobe*

Japan

1. Introduction

Advanced stages of uterine cervical cancer, especially those classified as stages IIIa to IVa, are unlikely treated with radical surgery alone. Intra-arterial infusion chemotherapy for advanced uterine cervical cancer has been shown to result in remarkable clinical outcomes because of higher intratumoral concentrations of oncostatics despite minimal adverse effects as compared with those administered systemically (Panici et al. 1991, Vermorken 1993, Kigawa et al. 1996) Scarabelli and his colleagues (1987) described that the intra-arterial infusion as first-line chemotherapy for advanced uterine cervical carcinoma could deliver broadened options and improved radicality of the following conventional treatments such as surgery or radiotherapy, through the immediate tumor response despite the relative low adverse effects. On the contrary, Onishi and his colleagues (Onishi et al. 2000) reported that although intraarterial infusion achieved better local response compared to patients treated with radiotherapy alone, local recurrence and distant metastasis were inevitable in their study group. Studies by Eddy and his colleagues (1995) who used chemotherapy with bleomycin, vincristine, mitomycin and cisplatin followed by radiotherapy in patients with stage IIIb cervical cancer demonstrated a satisfactory response rate but with intolerable toxicity. On the other hand, patients who received intravenous infusion followed by radiotherapy had significantly inferior survival compared with those who received radiotherapy alone (Tattersall et al. 1995). The reason for such discrepancy in the results might be attributed to the insufficient local control of the tumor.

It is generally accepted that the dose escalation of chemotherapy was linked to improved tumor response (Levin and Hryniuk 1987, Levin et al. 1993). Currently, cisplatin has become one of the most effective oncostatics in gynecologic oncology and is believed to demonstrate a potential antitumor effect against squamous cell carcinoma of the cervix (Thigpen et al. 1981,

Ozol and Young 1984). However, higher antitumor effect has been generally accepted to be correlated with higher dose intensity but associated with severe toxicity. To reduce the dose-limiting toxicity and increase the antitumor effect, the authors developed super high-dose intra-arterial cisplatin infusion under percutaneous pelvic perfusion with extracorporeal chemofiltration (PPPEC) to achieve the ultimate use of cisplatin in the neoadjuvant setting for advanced cervical carcinoma (Hamana et al. 2001, Motoyama et al. 2001). The authors have shown that PPPEC system achieved a high-dose cisplatin pelvic perfusion with minimal adverse effects, permitting cisplatin dose escalation with further augmentation of the tumor response. Furthermore, high-dose intra-arterial infusion chemotherapy under PPPEC achieved a high frequency of rapid tumor shrinkage of locally advanced uterine cervical cancer with favorable performance of the subsequent radical surgery (Motoyama et al. 2004).

2. Procedures of percutaneous pelvic perfusion with extracorporeal chemofiltration

2.1 Intra-arterial infusion

Intra-arterial infusion catheters were inserted percutaneously in bilateral internal iliac arteries using Seldinger's techniques via bilateral femoral arteries under fluoroscopic guidance. The tip of the catheter was located close to the uterine artery after ceramic-coil embolization of both superior and inferior gluteal arteries so as to deliver high concentrations of drug in the tumor lesion via the uterine arteries. The other tips of bilateral infusion catheters were connected to an infusion pump.

2.2 Extracoporeal chemofiltration system

For the first course of PPPEC, the right saphenofemoral junction was exposed through a small cut-down incision. Once vascular access established, an activating clotting time longer than 200 seconds was maintained with systemic heparinization. After anticoagulation, the specially designed inferior vena cava (IVC) occlusion balloon catheter (Radiopaque, 60 cm long, 21 French, with a single balloon and three lumens; Sumitomo Bake Corporation., Ohtsu, Japan.) (Ku et al. 1995) was introduced through the right femoral vein and was advanced under fluoroscopic guidance until the tip was beneath the renal vein. The balloon was then inflated with half-strength iodinated contrast at a rate of 4 ml to 6 ml. To determine whether isolation of the IVC was complete, contrast was injected through the drainage lumen under transient occlusion of IVC. Venography taken during this injection showed complete retrograde filling of the entire IVC and confirmed the absence of contrast leak over the isolation balloon (Figure 1). The distal ends of the IVC catheter were connected to the extracorporeal system, including the chemofilter cartridge containing active carbon beads (DHP-1; Kuraray Company, Ltd., Osaka, Japan) and a centrifugal pump (model BP-80; Biomedicus, Inc., Eden Prairie, MN, U.S.A.), as schematically illustrated in Figure 2.

The IVC blood through the balloon catheter was initially directed to the filter-excluded shunt (route A). After hemodynamic stability was verified, the direction of IVC blood flow was switched to the chemofiltration route (route B). After the PPPEC system had been accomplished, super high-dose cisplatin (140-250 mg/m2) alone or cisplatin plus an ordinal dose of pepleomycin (7 mg/m2), mitomycin C (7 mg/m2) and 5-fluorouracil (700 mg/m2) were administered during 30 minutes by dose allocation according to the difference in the bilateral vascularity of the uterine artery, as verified by the previous arteriogram.

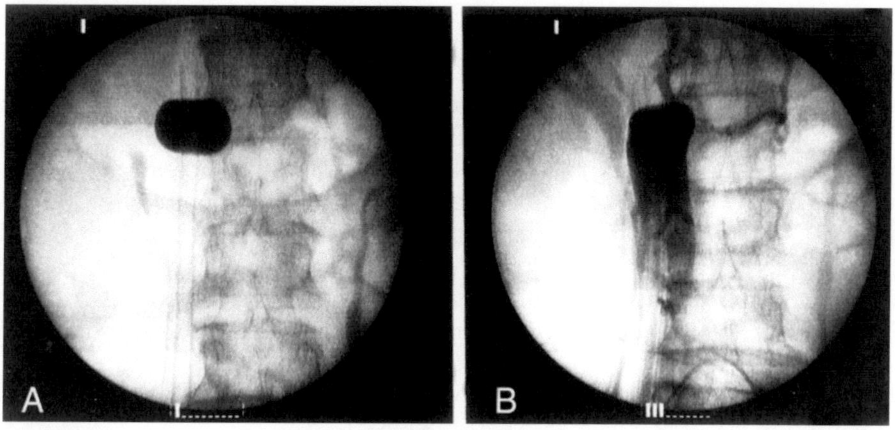

A. Complete IVC occlusion by catheter balloon. **B.** Absence of iodinated contrast leakage above the occluding balloon.

Fig. 1. Roentgenogram and venogram of inferior vena cava (IVC) isolation by catheter balloon.

After PPPEC, the hydration regimen was similar to that of the systemically administered cisplatin for the purpose of reducing renal toxicity. The second course of PPPEC was performed in the same manner via the left saphenofemoral junction, 2 weeks after the first course of PPPEC.

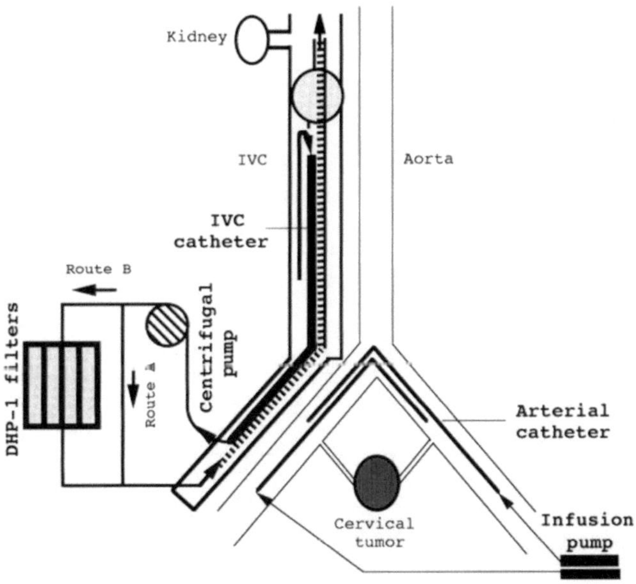

Fig. 2. Diagram of percutaneous pelvic perfusion with extracorporeal chemofiltration system. Tumor-perfusing blood was drained out in the extracorporeal circuit by a centrifugal pump via the drainage channel beneath the balloon in the catheter. After chemofiltration, the blood was directed into the IVC circulation again via the return channel over the balloon in the catheter. The chemofiltration cartridge (DHP-1) contains active carbon beads.

3. Clinical examinations

3.1 Patients

Twenty-three patients admitted to Kobe University Hospital who had uterine cervical cancer stage IIIa to IVa according to the FIGO classification, were included in the present review. None of the patients had severe complications, such as diabetes mellitus, hypertension, renal failure or any other significant co-morbid conditions, and all had a World Health Organization (WHO) performance status (PS) score of 2 or less. All the patients had primary, untreated uterine cervical cancer. Prior to the study, patients were clinically staged based on pelvic examination, and several laboratory examinations, including intravenous pyelography, chest X-ray, cystoscopy, and routine serum chemistries, were performed. Metastasis was detected using a computerized tomography (CT) scan, whereas the localization and the size of cervical tumors were determined using magnetic resonance imaging (MRI) of the abdomen and pelvis.

During the same period of study, the authors had a total of 609 cervical cancer cases managed at our hospital. This includes 109 patients with locally advanced cervical cancer classified as stages IIIa, IIIb, or IVa. Among these 109 patients, 23 consented to PPPEC while the others received radiotherapy alone (17 patients) or conventional therapy (52 patients) consisting of palliative chemotherapy or cytoreductive surgery with or without radiotherapy. Radiotherapy was administered as follows: irradiation to the whole pelvis was 50.4 Gy, center split at 20 Gy, and vaginal vault at 18 Gy.

The mean age of the patients was 56.2±12.0 years. The mean diameter of the cervical tumor was 4.9±1.8 cm. The PS of all patients was zero. Based on FIGO clinical staging, 1 patient was classified as having stage IIIa cancer, 17 patients as having stage IIIb cancer, and 5 patients as having stage IVa cancer. Histologic types included 21 squamous cell carcinoma, 1 adenocarcinoma, and 1 adenosquamous carcinoma. Patients' characteristics are summarized in Table 1.

Age	56.2 ±12.0 y (range: 27-68 y)
Mean diameter of cervical tumor	4.9 ±1.8 cm (range: 4.5 - 12.0 cm)
Performance status (based on WHO)	0
FIGO clinical stage (no. of patients)	
IIIa	1
IIIb	17
IVa	5
Histologic type (no. of patients)	
Squamous cell carcinoma	21
Adenocarcinoma	1
Adenosquamous carcinoma	1

Table 1. Patients' characteristics

Serial blood samples were obtained from prefilter, postfilter, and peripheral blood (radial artery) after the start of cisplatin infusion. Tissue samples were obtained by colposcopic punch biopsies from cervical lesion after the first course of PPPEC and by radical surgery 2 weeks after the second course of PPPEC. Plasma and tissue platinum concentrations were measured by flameless atomic absorption spectrometry (Pera et al. 1979).

3.2 Pharmacokinetics of free platinum in extracorporeal chemofiltration circuit

The time course of mean plasma free-platinum (f-Pt) concentration (n = 3) at each prefilter, postfilter, and peripheral site with various cisplatin doses is shown in Figure 3. The peak plasma concentration (maximum concentration, C_{max}) was noted to be 20 to 30 minutes in each time course, but most of them decayed to less than 1.0 μg/ml at 50 minutes after initiation of the infusion. This is indicative that although the prefilter mean f-Pt C_{max} levels increased in a cisplatin dose-dependent manner (range: 7.2—12.2 μg/ml), the postfilter and peripheral f-Pt C_{max} levels were all in the low range (postfilter range: 2.1—3.6 μg/ml; peripheral range: 1.0—3.8 μg/ml).

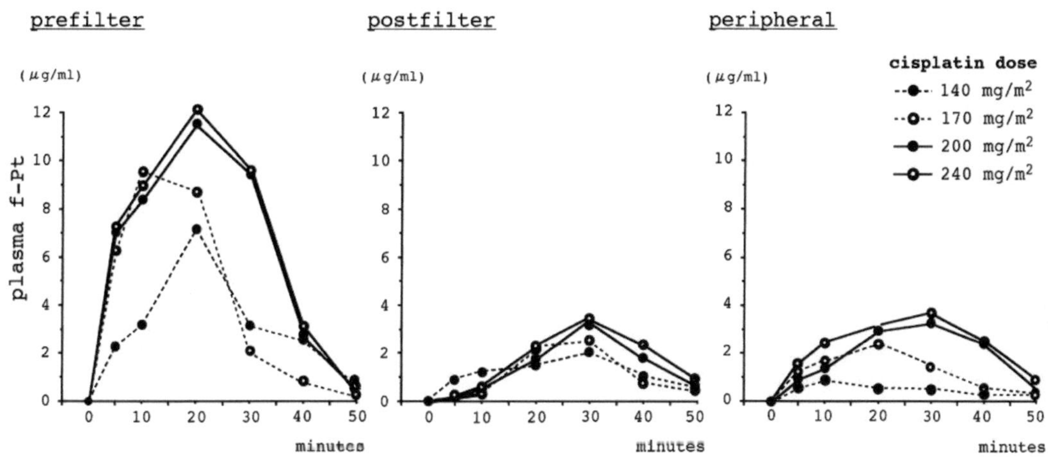

140 mg/m2 (open circle with dashed line), 170 mg/m2 (closed circle with dashed line), 200 mg/m2 (open circle with solid line), 240 mg/m2 (closed circle with solid line).

Fig. 3. Dynamics of plasma free-platinum concentrations at different sites.

3.3 Comparison in pharmacokinetics and tumor response between pppec and conventional arterial infusion (CAI)

The pharmacokinetic study comparing peripheral plasma f-Pt concentrations and area under the concentration-time curve between PPPEC and conventional arterial infusion (CAI) demonstrated that f-Pt C_{max} was 2.1 ± 0.1 μg/ml in PPPEC with cisplatin at a dose of 140 mg/m². This was only a 33% increase in the C_{max} relative to that in CAI (1.5 ± 0.2 μg/ml) with cisplatin at a dose of 70 mg/m², and a 12% increase in the mean area under the concentration–time curve as compared with that in CAI (Figure 4). Conversely, the tumor response rate evaluated after completion of two courses of PPPEC was verified to increase remarkably from 44% with a 70 mg/m^2 cisplatin course to 100% with a 140 mg/m^2 cisplatin course according to cisplatin dose escalation.

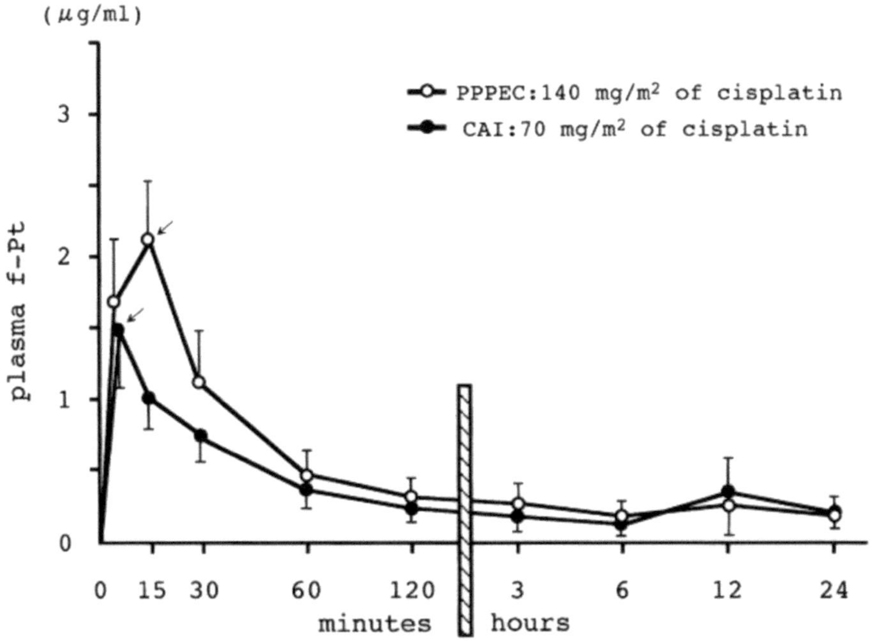

The arrow shows each Cmax. PPPEC, percutaneous pelvic perfusion with extracorporeal chemofiltration; super high-dose intra-arterial cisplatin infusion under percutaneous pelvic perfusion with extracorporeal chemofiltration; CAI, conventional arterial infusion.

Fig. 4. Time course of plasma free-platinum concentrations in peripheral circulation.

3.4 Tissue-platinum concentrations

The mean tissue Pt concentrations obtained by cervical lesion biopsies at 12 hours and 24 hours after the first course of PPPEC are shown in Figure 5A. A dose-dependent increase in the mean tissue Pt concentration was noted. Particularly, the value (18.6 μg/wet · g) in tumor tissue specimens obtained at 24 hours after the first course of PPPEC with cisplatin at a dose of 200 mg/m^2 cisplatin was remarkably higher compared with that with lower doses of cisplatin and with that obtained at 12 hours after PPPEC with the same dose of cisplatin. On the other hand, Figure 5B represents the mean tissue Pt concentration in resected common iliac lymph nodes and cervical tumor tissues obtained by radical surgery. The increase in Pt concentrations in the resected lymph nodes and cervical tumor tissues was distinct, depending on cisplatin dose escalation.

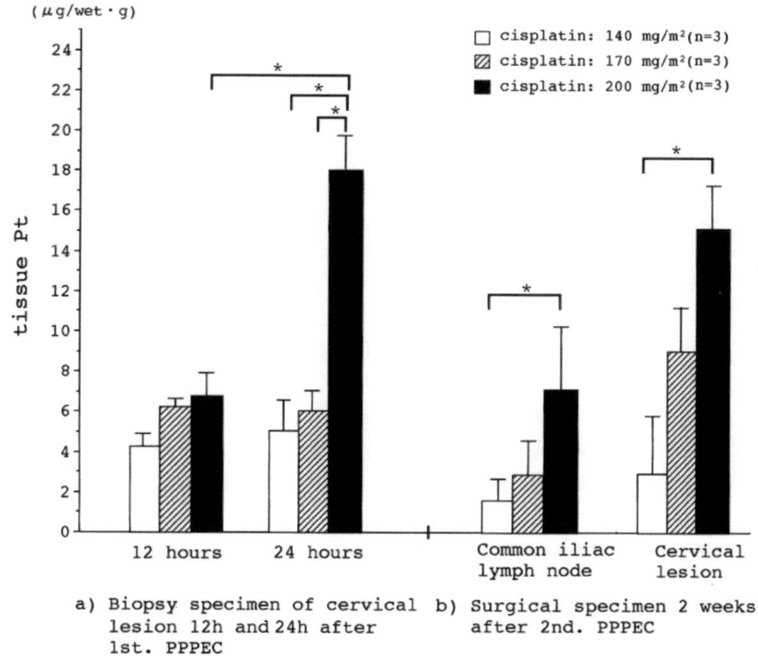

Fig. 5. Tissue platinum concentrations in cervical tumor lesions and resected lymph nodes. Each bar shows the mean tissue Pt concentration in the cervical tumor tissues obtained by biopsies at 12 h and 24 h after the first course of PPPEC **(a)**, and in the surgical specimens and resected common iliac lymph nodes obtained by radical hysterectomy 2 weeks after the second course of PPPEC **(b)**.

3.5 Adverse effects

There was little renal impairment, gastrointestinal toxicity, myelosuppression, and alopecia. Neither neurogenic nor auditory alteration was detected. The other adverse effects connected with PPPEC were mild anemia caused by blood retention in the circuit (~200–300 ml) and hemolysis resulting from destruction by resistance in the circuit. All the adverse effects were less than grade II (Table 2). There were no critical catheter complications in the present study.

Adverse effects	No. of patients (%)
PPPEC related	
Hemolysis/hematuria	0
Thrombocytopenia < 5×10^4/mm³	3 (21.4)
Bleeding	0
Cisplatin related	
Leukopenia <2,000/mm³	2(14.3)
Creatinine >1.5 mg/dl	2(14.3)
Nausea/vomiting	3(21.4)
Alopecia	0

Table 2. Adverse Effects Assessment for PPPEC

3.6 Clinical response

In order to evaluate the tumor response, the volumetric reduction of cervical tumors was calculated by multiplying three spatial axes based on MRI examination. Tumor response was designated as complete response (CR), partial response (PR), minor response (MR) or no response (NR), as previously described (Minagawa et al. 1998). On the other hand, tumor downstaging and clinical response in the vagina, urinary bladder and parametrium were evaluated by colposcopic punch biopsy, cystoscopic examination, drip infusion pyelography, MRI, and gynecologic examination. Tumor downstaging or positive tumor response was considered when the cancer cells in the lesion disappeared or when there was evidence of reduction of parametrial involvement.

The mean volumetric reduction rate was 76% (range: 50%-100%). The tumor response rate evaluated after the second PPPEC were 13% for CR and 74% for PR. The overall tumor response (CR + PR) was 87%. Histopathological effects on the surgical specimens revealed 4% for grade I, 83% for grade II, and 13% for grade III. Tumor downstaging, based on the tumor response and the histologic response reached 83% after the second PPPEC (Table 3).

Tumor reduction % (range)	76 % (range: 50.0-100%)
Tumor response % (no. of patients)	
CR	13% (3 out of 23 patients)
PR	74 % (17 out of 23 patients)
MR + NC	13 %
Histologic effects % (no. of patients)	
G1	4 % (1 out of 23 patients)
G2	83 % (19 out of 23 patients)
G3	13 % (3 patients)
Overall histologic effects	96 % (22 out of 23 patients)
Tumor down-staging % (no. of patients)	83 % (19 patients)

CR, complete response; PR, partial response; MR, minor response; NC, no change

Table 3. Tumor Response after PPPEC

3.7 Surgical performance

Radical surgery was performed on 18 of the 23 patients who had confirmed tumor downstaging. The radical surgery performance rate was 78%. The remaining 5 patients, who had insufficient stage regression (4 cases) and a poor PS despite tumor downstaging (1 case), received radiotherapy. Review of the surgical specimens revealed that 16 of the 18 surgical patients had negative surgical margins, leading to a curative surgery rate of 89%.

Response rate of the involved lesions other than the cervical tumor evaluated after the second PPPEC revealed 89% for the parametrium, 94% for the vagina, and 100% for the urinary bladder. Lymph node metastasis was detected in 9 of the surgical patients and an overall histologic effect in these metastases was 56% (Table 4).

Parameter	Rate in % (no. of patients)
Radical surgery	89 % (18 out of 23 patients)
Curative surgery	89 % (16 out of 18 patients)
Radiotherapy	22% (5 out of 23 patients)
Lesion response	
Parametrium	89 % (16 out of 18 patients)
Vagina	94 % (17 out of 18 patients)
Urinary bladder	100 % (5 out of 5 patients)
Lymph node metastases	50 % (9 out of 18 patients)
G3	0 %
G2	28 % (5 patients)
G1	22 % (4 patients)
Overall histologic effects	56 %

Table 4. Evaluation of radical surgery and surgical specimens after PPPEC

4. Treatment after percutaneous pelvic perfusion with extracorporeal chemofiltration (PPPEC)

Following PPPEC, class III radical hysterectomy based on Rutledge classification was performed on patients who demonstrated tumor downstaging according to FIGO classification. Radiotherapy was useed in patients uncertain for the tumor downstaging or with a poor PS. Adjuvant radiotherapy on the surgical cases was determined based on the histopathologic diagnosis of the surgical specimens. Patients who had pelvic, common iliac or periaortic lymph node metastasis were subjected to periaortic radiation of 40 Gy aside from the whole pelvic and vaginal vault radiation of 18 Gy in patients who had stage IIIa cancer after the second course of PPPEC.

4.1 Clinical outcomes of stage IVa patients

As shown in Table 5, five patients who had confirmed stage IVa cancer with bladder invasion had squamous cell carcinoma. One patient had CR while the other four had PR. All

Case number	1	2	3	4	5
Tumor size (mm)	32	61	28	63	63
Tumor response	PR	PR	CR	PR	PR
Downstaging	Ib	Ib	<Ib	IIb	IIIb
Surgery	+	+	+	+	−
Surgical margin	−	−	−	−	NA
Lymph node metastases	−	+	+	+	NA
Recurrence (months after PPPEC)	−	−	−	11	13
Current status	NED	NED	NED	DOD	DOD

NA, not applicable; NED, no evidence of disease; DOD, died of disease

Table 5. Characteristics of stage IVa patients and their clinical response after PPPEC the stage IVa patients had tumor downstaging. Four patients underwent a class III radical hysterectomy with resultant curative surgery. Three patients had lymph node metastasis and two patients had a recurrence.

4.2 Analysis of recurrent cases

Recurrence was detected in 10 patients (Table 6). Adjuvant therapy administered to these patients consisted of radiotherapy and chemotherapy to those who underwent radical surgery, while chemotherapy was delivered to the rest. The initial stages of the 10 cases were as follows: 8 stage IIIb cancer and 2 stage IVa cancer. Nine of the 10 patients demonstrated lymph node metastasis. The mean time to recurrence was 13.8 months (range: 4-32 months).

	Cases									
Parameters	1	2	3	4	5	6	7	8	9	10
Cell type	SCC	SCC	SCC	SCC	SCC	A	SCC	SCC	SCC	SCC
Surgery	+	+	+	+	−	+	+	+	−	−
S. margins	−	+	+	−	NA	−	−	−	NA	NA
LN mets	+	−	+	+	+	+	+	+	+	+
Adj therapy	RCT	RCT	RCT	RCT	CT	RCT	RCT	RCT	CT	CT
Rec sites	l	p	p	p	p	p	ud	ud	p	p
Rec (months)	16	12	11	8	13	10	11	32	4	11

A, adenocarcinoma; Adj therapy, adjuvant therapy; CT, chemotherapy; l, lungs; LN mets, lymph node metastases; NA, not applicable; p, pelvis; RCT, radiotherapy and chemotherapy; Rec (months), evidence of recurrence in months after PPPEC; Rec sites, areas of recurrence; SCC, squamous cell carcinoma; ud, undetectable.

Table 6. Evaluation of recurrent cases

4.3 Evaluation of survival

As far as the survival of the patients who received two courses of PPPEC is concerned, the 5-year progression-free survival was similar among those who underwent radical surgery (47%) and those who underwent radiotherapy (50%) after PPPEC. The 5-year progression-free survival (47%) in the PPPEC group was higher to that of patients who received radiotherapy alone (28%) at the authors institution (Kobe University Hospital). Furthermore, patients who received PPPEC showed an improvement in the 5-year survival rate (74%) compared with that of a similar patient group who received radiotherapy alone at our hospital (58%) or those who received conventional therapy, which includes those who had palliative chemotherapy or cytoreductive surgery with or without radiotherapy (43%) (Figure 6).

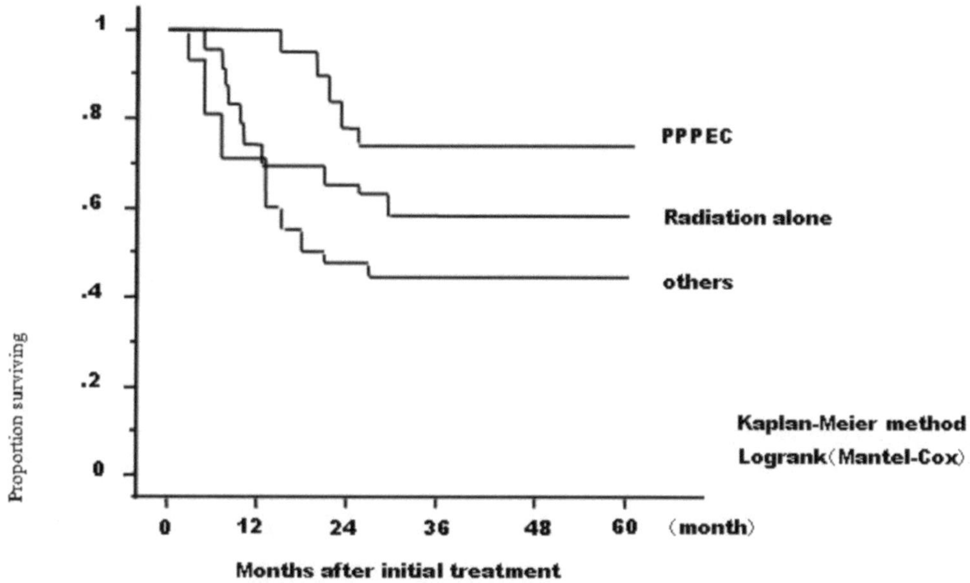

Fig. 6. Survival rate of patients comparing the different treatments at authors' institution. Patients who received PPPEC showed an improvement of the 5-year survival rate (74%) compared with that of similar patient group who received radiotherapy alone (58%) or those who received conventional therapy (43%). Survival was compared by the Kaplan-Meier method.

5. Discussion

The use of PPPEC demonstrated a significant increase in tissue Pt-concentrations in patients receiving at a dose of 200 mg/m^2 cisplatin at a time or more than 400 mg/m^2 cisplatin in total compared with those receiving cisplatin at a dose of 140 mg/m^2 at a time or 280 mg/m^2 cisplatin in total. It might be crucial for tumor cell kill that high intratumoral tissue Pt concentrations must be achieved throughout the entire tumor. Providing insight into this concept, the dose allocation of cisplatin administered in PPPEC was decided according to the vascular disparity among bilateral uterine arteries (Kohno et al. 1993). Because of the high reduction rate of f-Pt by DHP-1 filters, the amount of f-Pt passing into the peripheral circulation was remarkably decreased; therefore, the dose-limiting toxicities, especially nephrotoxicity, were limited and tolerated.

The mean tissue Pt concentration in common iliac lymph nodes after administration of cisplatin at a dose of 400 mg/m^2 was 7.4 μg/wet · g, which was higher than the minimal concentration (3.4 μg/wet · g) for tumor cell kill (Jaffe et al. 1983), but was lower than the satisfactory concentration (17.0 μg/wet · g) for total tumor cell kill. This may be responsible for the ineffective control of lymph node metastases. Because tissue Pt concentrations in pelvic lymph nodes correlated with the distance from the cervix, it seems that antitumor effect in the pelvic lymph nodes, particularly distant lymph nodes, such as common iliac and para-aortic nodes, may be inferior to that in cervical tumor lesions.

In this review, the results of 23 patients with an initial diagnosis of uterine cervical cancer stage IIIa to IVa treated with high-dose cisplatin or high-dose cisplatin plus ordinal doses of pepleomycin, mitomycin C and 5-fluorouracil administered in two courses at a 2-week interval by means of PPPEC were presented. The reduction of extensive parametrial involvement and complete regression of bladder invasion after the second course of PPPEC made radical hysterectomy possible in these patients. After the performance of PPPEC, radical surgery or radiotherapy were performed. In advanced stages of uterine cervical cancer, radical hysterectomy is generally associated with surgical difficulties; hence, the use of vessel-sealing system, electrocautery system or argon beam coagulation is advocated. Therefore, the prognosis of patients who have stage IIIb or IVa uterine cervical cancer based on the present therapeutic strategy with PPPEC was better compared with that of conventional therapy. Our findings were congruent to published reports demonstrating that the use of intra-arterial infusion was beneficial to patients with advanced uterine cervical cancer (Minegawa et al. 1998, Sugiyama et al. 1998, Fujiwaki et al. 1999, Nagata et al. 2000).

The existence of lymph node metastasis is a poor prognostic factor in patients with cervical cancer (Terada et al. 1988, Tinga et al. 1992). Patients with locally advanced uterine cervical cancer have a high incidence of lymph node metastasis. In the patients treated with PPPEC, the rate of overall histologic effects in metastatic lymph nodes barely reached 56%, a value which was less compared with the overall histologic effects in the cervical tumor (96%). This could be attributed to the decline in the chemodrug concentrations at areas distant from the infusion site. Intra-arterial infusion chemotherapy might have less antitumor effect in the pelvic lymph nodes than in the cervical tumor lesions. In order to improve the long-term prognosis of locally advanced uterine cervical cancer, it is necessary to increase tumoricidal chemodrug concentrations in periaortic lymph nodes, or the pelvic lymph nodes at least (Burke et al. 1987). To achieve a satisfactory antitumor effect in periaortic lymph nodes, higher doses of cisplatin, an effective combination with other oncostatic agents, or a novel drug delivery system will be required (Park et al. 1995, Leone et al. 1996).

Up to the present time, with 63 months of median follow-up time, the 5- year survival rate for patients treated with PPPEC is superior to that of patients who received the conventional mode of treatment consisting of palliative surgery or chemotherapy and radiotherapy at the authors' institution (Kobe University Hospital, Kobe, Japan). Furthermore, the 5-year progression-free survival and 5-year survival in the PPPEC group are higher than those of patients who received radiotherapy alone at authors' institution. This prompted the authors to use the PPPEC system in the management of patients who have locally advanced uterine cervical cancer. Although the 5-year progression free survival in those patients who received radical surgery or radiation therapy after PPPEC is similar, several clinical and pathological factors have been implicated to be of prognostic significance as far as progression-free survival and prognosis are concerned. These are as follows: Gynecologic Oncology Group PS (0-2), tumor size, tumor growth pattern (exophytic vs. barrel), histologic type, tumor grade and age at study entry (Key et al. 2003). Further research should be directed to the identification of suitable chemotherapeutic agents, defining clinical indications, and development of technical modification to make it more generally applicable.

6. Conclusion

The clinical results described in the present review suggest that PPPEC has a therapeutic advantage because of prompt tumor downstaging of locally advanced uterine cervical cancer with minimal adverse effects, thereby facilitating more options and radicality of the subsequent main therapy. This further leads to an improvement of the long-term survival for patients with locally advanced uterine cervical cancer. A prospective randomized trial will clarify the optimal mode of initial therapy for patients with stages IIIa - IVa uterine cervical cancer.

7. Acknowledgment

The authors would like to thank the staff members of the Department of Liver and Transplantation Surgery of Kobe University Graduate School of Medicine, Kobe, Japan for their dedicated collaboration to establish the PPPEC system for advanced uterine cervical cancer. This study was supported by the Grant-in-Aid for Scientific Research 15390506 from the Japanese Ministry of Education, Culture, Sports, Science and Technology.

8. References

Burke TW, Hoskins WJ, Heller PB, et al. Prognostic factors associated with radical hysterectomy failure. Gynecol Oncol 1987; 26: 153-159.

Eddy GL, Manetta A, Alvarez RD, Williams L, Creasman WT. Neoadjuvant chemotherapy with vincristine and cisplatin followed by radical hysterectomy and pelvic lymphadenectomy for FIGO stage IB bulky cervical cancer: a Gynecologic Oncology Group pilot study. Gynecol Oncol 1995;57:412-6.

Fujiwaki R, Maede Y, Ohnishi Y, et al. Prognosis of patients with stage IIIb-IVa squamous cell carcinoma of the cervix following intra-arterial neoadjuvant chemotherapy. J Exp Clin Cancer Res 1999;18:143-6.

Hamana S, Motoyama S, Maruo T. et al, Super high-dose intraarterial cisplatin infusion under percutaneous pelvic perfusion with extracorporeal chemofiltration for advanced uterine cervical carcinoma: I. Analysis for pharmacokinetics, tumor response, and toxicity of platinum. Am J Clin Oncol 2001;24:241-6.

Jaffe N, Knapp J, Chuang VP, et al. Osteosarcoma: intra-arterial treatment of the primary tumor with cis-diammine-dichloroplatinum II (CDP). Angiographic, pathologic, and pharmacologic studies. Cancer 1983; 51: 402–7.

Keys HM, Bundy BN, Stehman FB, et al. Radiation therapy with and without extrafascial hysterectomy for bulky stage Ib cervical carcinoma: a randomized trial of the Gynecologic Oncology Group. Gynecol Oncol 2003;89:343-353.

Kigawa J, Minagawa Y, Ishihara H, et al. The role of neoadjuvant intraarterial infusion chemotherapy with cisplatin and bleomycin for locally advanced cervical cancer. Am J Clin Oncol 1996; 19: 255-259.

Kohno Y, Iwanari O, Kitano M. Prognostic importance of histologic vascular density in cervical cancer treated with hypertensive intraarterial chemotherapy. Cancer 1993; 72: 2394–400.

Ku Y, Fukumoto T, Iwasaki T, et al. Clinical pilot study on high-dose intraarterial chemotherapy with direct hemoperfusion under hepatic venous isolation in patients with advanced hepatocellular carcinoma. Surgery 1995; 117: 510–9.

Leone B, Vallejo C, Perez J, et al. Ifosfamide and cisplatin as neoadjuvant chemotherapy for advanced cervical cancer. Am J Clin Oncol 1996; 19:132-135.

Levin L, Hryniuk WM. Dose-intensity analysis of chemotherapy of advanced ovarian cancer. J Clin Oncol 1987; 5: 756–67.

Levin L, Simon R, Hryniuk WM. Importance of multi-agent chemotherapy regimens in ovarian carcinoma. J Natl Cancer Inst 1993; 85: 1732–42.

Minagawa Y, Kigawa J, Irie T, et al. Radical surgery following neoadjuvant chemotherapy for patients with stage IIIB cervical cancer. Ann Surg Oncol 1998;5:539-43.

Motoyama S, Hamana S, Ku Y, et al. Neoadjuvant high-dose intraarterial infusion chemotherapy under percutaneous pelvic perfusion with extracorporeal chemofiltration in patients with stages IIIa - Iva cervical cancer. Gynecolgic Oncology 2004,; 95: 576-582

Motoyama S, Hamana S, Ku Y, et al. Super high-dose intraarterial cisplatin infusion under percutaneous pelvic perfusion with extracorporeal chemofiltration for advanced uterine cervical carcinoma: II. Its impact on clinical response and subsequent surgery. Am J Clin Oncol 2001;24:247-50.

Nagata Y, Araki N, Kimura H, et al. Neoadjuvant chemotherapy by transcatheter arterial infusion method for uterine cervical cancer. J Vasc Interv Radiol 2000;11:313-9.

Onishi H, Yamaguchi M, Kuriyama K, Tsukamoto T, Ishigame K, Ichikawa T, Aoki S, Yoshikawa T, Araki T, Nambu A, Araki T, Hashi A, Yasumizu T, Hoshi K, Ito H. Effect of concurrent intra-arterial infusion of platinum drugs for patients with stage III or IV uterine cervical cancer treated with radical radiation therapy. Cancer J Sci Am 2000;6:40-5.

Ozol RF, Young RC. Chemotherapy of ovarian cancer. Semin Oncol 1984; 11: 251–63.

Panici PB, Greggi S, Scambia G, et al. High-dose cisplatin and bleomycin neoadjuvant chemotherapy plus radical surgery in locally advanced cervical carcinoma: a preliminary report. Gynecol Oncol 1991; 41: 212–6.

Park S, Kim B, Kim J, et al. Phase I/II study of neoadjuvant intraarterial chemotherapy with mitomycin-C, vincristine, and cisplatin in patients with stage IIb bulky cervical cancer.Cancer1995;76:814-823.

Pera MF, Harder HC. Analysis for platinum in biological material by flameless atomic absorption spectrometry. Clin Chem 1979; 73: 1245–9.

Scarabelli C, Tumolo S, Paoli A, et al. Intermittent pelvic arterial infusion with peptichemio, doxorubucin, and cisplatin for locally advanced and recurrent carcinoma of the uterine cervix. Cancer 1987; 60: 25–30.

Sugiyama T, Nishida T, Hasuo Y, et al. Neoadjuvant intraarterial chemotherapy followed by radical hysterectomy and/or radiotherapy for locally advanced cervical cancer. Gynecol Oncol 1998;69:130-6.

Tattersall MH, Lorvidhaya V, Vootiprux V, Cheirsilpa A, Wong F, Azhar T, Lee HP, Kang SB, Manalo A, Yen MS, Kampono N, Aziz F. Randomized trial of epirubicin and cisplatin chemotherapy followed by pelvic radiation in locally advanced cervical cancer. Cervical Cancer Study Group of the Asian Oceanian Clinical Oncology Association. J Clin Oncol 1995;13:444-51.

Terada KY, Morley GW, Roberts JA. Stage Ib cancer of the cervix with lymph node metastases. Gynecol Oncol 1988;31:389-395.

Thigpen T, Shingleton H, Homesley H, et al. Cis-platinum in treatment of advanced or recurrent squamous cell carcinoma of the cervix: a phase II study of the Gynecologic Oncology Group. Cancer 1981; 48: 899–903.

Tinga DJ, Bouma J, Aalders JG. Patients with squamous cell versus adeno(squamous) cancer of the cervix, what factor determine the prognosis?. Int Gynecol Cancer 1992;2: 83-91.

Vermorken JB. The role of chemotherapy in squamous cell carcinoma of the uterine cervix: a review. Int J Gynecol Cancer 1993; 3: 129–42.

9

Neoadjuvant Treatment for Oesophago-Gastric Cancer

John E. Anderson and Jo-Etienne Abela
Department of Surgery, Royal Alexandra Hospital Paisley, Scotland
United Kingdom

1. Introduction

In the United Kingdom, oesophageal cancer ranks as the ninth most common cancer with a rising incidence of 13 per 100,000 head of population. Some two-thirds of all oesophageal lesions are adenocarcinomas, the rest are squamous cell carcinomas. The incidence of stomach cancer is similar but a decline has been registered over the past two decades. For both conditions the age at presentation is 60 years or more in over two-thirds of patients. Tumours of the oesophago-gastric junction have received detailed attention over the past years. This is in part because surgical excision through a single operative field may not be possible. Moreover, for this subset of lesions, a rising incidence and worse survival have been registered.

Oesophago-gastric malignancies carry a poor prognosis especially when diagnosed at an advanced stage outside screening programmes. In Western countries, this is reflected as overall five year-survival rates ranging from 5 to below 20%. Over the years, treatment has evolved into a multi-modality strategy which is best formulated and overseen in a multidisciplinary setting. The treatment of an individual patient will depend on accurate and reliable tumour staging, assessment of the patient's fitness for radical surgical and/or oncological treatment, the level of expertise available locally and, of course, the patient's informed decisions. In a typical surgical unit in the United Kingdom, resection rates will not usually surpass 20%.

After radical surgery with curative intent the median disease free survival is of the order of two years with 50% of cases developing metastases and/or recurrence in the first year. These disheartening figures offer the rationale for the addition of further oncological treatment to radical surgery. Neoadjuvant chemotherapy and/or radiotherapy is administered before surgery with the aim of shrinking the primary tumour and theoretically ablating micro-metastases and reducing the risk of haematogenous and lymphatic dissemination. This treatment, however, has the potential for toxicity and complications and must be used carefully in patients with co-morbidity. There are concerns that pre-operative treatment may influence the patient's ability to withstand the surgical insult and the percentage of patients who are fit enough to complete post-surgical treatment regimens is also diminished.

This chapter will review the main influential randomised trials employing neoadjuvant treatment for these cancers. It will also comment on the other randomised and non-randomised series published in the literature focusing on the effect of treatment on resectability, peri-operative morbidity and mortality, resection specimen pathological stage and completeness of excision and longer-term outcomes. Finally, future prospects will be explored.

2. Neoadjuvant radiotherapy for oesophageal cancer

Preoperative radiotherapy in oesophageal cancer patients aims to reduce tumour size, decrease the extent of localised microscopic residual disease and lower the risk of tumour dissemination at the time of surgery. The first published study suggesting that such treatment may improve survival for this group of patients was by Kakyama et al in 1967. The study reported a 5 year survival rate of 37.5% for the group receiving preoperative radiotherapy compared with 19.1% 5 year survival rate in the surgery alone arm. The criticisms of the study are that it was retrospective with no statistical analysis of the data.

During the 1980's and early 1990's five randomised controlled trials were published comparing neoadjuvant radiotherapy and surgery alone (Launois et al 1981, Gignoux et al 1987, Wang et al 1989, Arnott et al 1992 and Nygaard et al 1992). All these studies except for Arnott et al were restricted to treating squamous cell carcinoma. Radiation doses ranged from 20Gy to 40Gy and were given over a period of eight to twenty eight days. A summary of the five trials is shown in Table 1.

Study	Tumour histology	Treatment	n	Percentage of patients alive at 5 years
Launois et al 1981	SCC	Surgery alone	57	11.5
		Pre-op radiotherapy + Surgery	67	9.5
Gignoux et al 1987	SCC	Surgery alone	102	11
		Pre-op radiotherapy + Surgery	106	10
Wang et al 1989	SCC	Surgery alone	102	30
		Pre-op radiotherapy + Surgery	104	35
Arnott et al 1992	SCC & Adeno	Surgery alone	86	17
		Pre-op radiotherapy + Surgery	90	9
Nygaard et al 1992	SCC	Surgery alone	41	9
		Pre-op radiotherapy + Surgery	48	21

Table 1. A summary of neoadjuvant radiotherapy studies. SCC - squamous cell carcinoma. Adeno - adenocarcinoma.

None of the trials proved any significant improvement in 5 year survival. However, Nygaard et al 1992 did report 3-year survival rates of 20% in those patients receiving preoperative radiotherapy compared to 5% in the surgery alone arm. This improved survival was only achieved after pooling data from the radiotherapy group with patients receiving preoperative chemo-radiotherapy and did not prove to be statistically significant.

Each of the five trials mentioned contained relatively small numbers of patients. Therefore in order to investigate any small benefit afforded by preoperative radiotherapy, data from all 1147 patients were used in a meta-analysis published by Arnott et al 1998. This study again showed there was no clear evidence that preoperative radiotherapy improves the survival of patients with potentially resectable oesophageal cancer [hazard ratio (HR) 0.89; (95% CI 0.78 -1.01); p=0.062].

To date there have been no new studies published relating to neoadjuvant radiotherapy (Cochrane Review, Arnott et al 2010).

3. Neoadjuvant chemotherapy for oesophageal and gastric cancer

Chemotherapy aims to downstage tumours and remove distant micro metastasises. There have been many randomised controlled trials comparing overall survival of oesophageal cancer patients receiving neoadjuvant chemotherapy followed by surgery with surgery alone (Roth et al 1988, Nygaard et al 1992, Schlag et al 1992, Maipang 1994, Law 1997, Kelsen 1998, Acona 2001 and The UK Medical Research Council (MRC) trial 2002. The two largest of these studies are by Kelsen et al 1998 and the MRC trial of 2002.

Kelsen et al enrolled 440 patients with resectable oesophageal cancer that included squamous cell carcinoma, adenocarcinomas and undifferentiated tumours. The patients were randomised into two groups.

The surgery alone group numbered 227 patients who had primary surgery. The chemotherapy arm of the trial consisted of 213 patients. Both underwent the same surgical procedure. Surgical mortality was similar in each group, 10% in the chemotherapy arm and 13% in surgery alone group.

The patients in the chemotherapy arm received three cycles of cisplatin and fluorouracil before surgery. 71% of patients completed all three cycles. 7% of patients showed a complete clinical regression while 12% achieved a partial regression. Complete responses (T0N0M0) were found in 2.5% of patients.

Following chemotherapy 133 patients went on to have a R0 resection. This sub group was due to receive two post-operative cycles of chemotherapy, however, only 32% completed both courses due to patient or physician choice.

Overall median survival in the surgery alone group was 16.1 months compared to 14.9 months in the chemotherapy group (p=0.53). Two year survival was 37% and 35% respectively (p=0.74). There was no difference in outcome between patients with adenocarcinoma and squamous cell carcinoma. Among patients whose resection was curative, there was no significant difference in survival between those who did and those who did not undergo chemotherapy (median survival, 27.4 and 25 months, respectively). Kelsen et al concluded that neoadjuvant chemotherapy did not improve survival in oesophageal cancer. It must be noted that the operative mortality in this study is higher than would be deemed acceptable at present (less than 5%).

Kelsen et al 2007 published an update on their 1998 paper in which they looked at the longer term survival of the same group of patients. This again showed no difference in overall survival between patients receiving preoperative chemotherapy compared to those receiving surgery alone although patients with objective tumour regression after preoperative chemotherapy did have an improved survival. The paper also evaluated failure patterns on the basis of completeness of resection, concluding that only R0 resection results in substantial long term survival irrespective of whether neoadjuvant chemotherapy is given.

Like Kelsen et al the MRC study was a multi-centre trial recruiting patients suffering from either adenocarcinoma or squamous cell carcinoma of the oesophagus. 802 patients took part and were randomised into two groups, surgery alone n=402 and preoperative chemotherapy plus surgery n=400. Two cycles of chemotherapy were given using cisplatin and fluorouracil. Unlike Kelsen's study, the MRC trial allowed clinicians to give patients preoperative radiotherapy (25-32.5Gy). Nine percent of patients in both groups received radiotherapy.

Of the 400 patients assigned to the chemotherapy arm, 372 received chemotherapy, 350 completed two cycles while 22 patients only completed one. Pathological data from the resected specimens showed that patients who received preoperative chemotherapy had smaller tumours (p=0.0001) that extended less frequently into surrounding tissue and showed less lymph node involvement than tumours in the surgery alone group. Nodes at any site were involved in 195 (58%) of the chemotherapy group and 216 (68%) of the surgery alone patients (p=0.009).

Median survival in the chemotherapy group was 16.8 months compared with 13.3 months in the surgery alone group. Two year survival rates were 43% compared with 34%, respectively. There was no evidence to suggest that the effect of chemotherapy varied in accordance with histology. The MRC trial concluded that overall survival was better in the neoadjuvant chemotherapy group than the surgery alone group (HR 0.79; 95% CI 0.67–0.93; p=0.004) with an estimated reduction in risk of death of 21%.

Critics of the MRC study suggest that the inclusion of patients receiving preoperative radiotherapy as well as neoadjuvant chemotherapy may be the cause for the improved survival in the chemotherapy group. However, the estimate of treatment effect on overall survival was not altered by removal of those patients from the analysis who received preoperative radiotherapy; hazard ratio for the 728 patients (364 CS, 364 S) who did not receive radiotherapy was 0.78 (95% CI 0.66–0.93; p=0.005). In the chemotherapy group compared with the surgery alone group, more patients were alive without residual or recurrent disease (p<0.0001)

In 2009 the long term results of the MRC 2002 trial were published. This paper confirmed that survival benefit was maintained in the chemotherapy group with a hazard ratio of 0.84 (95% CI, 0.72 to 0.98; p =0 .03) which in absolute terms is a 5-year survival of 23.0% for chemotherapy group compared with 17.1% for surgery alone patients. The study also showed that the treatment effect is consistent in both adenocarcinoma and squamous cell carcinoma (Allum et al 2009).

As well as the MRC 2002 and Kelsen study six other smaller randomised control trials have compared survival between oesophageal cancer patients receiving surgery alone or neoadjuvant chemotherapy plus surgery. These additional studies are listed in Table 2 and all contain small numbers of participants.

Study	CS, number of patients	S, number of patients
Roth et al 1988	19	20
Nygaard et al 1992	56	25
Schlag et al 1992	22	24
Maipang et al 1994	24	22
Law et al 1997	74	73
Kelsen 1998	233	234
Ancona et al 01	48	48
MRC 02	400	402
Total	876	848

Table 2. Randomised control trials comparing surgery alone (S) vs neoadjuvant chemotherapy plus surgery (CS) for the treatment of resectable oesophageal cancer.

Combining the data from all eight studies in a meta-analysis would increase the ability to detect an improved survival rate. Furthermore any benefit from preoperative chemotherapy relating to the specific histological subtypes could be more effectively elucidated. Gebski et al 2007 undertook such a meta-analysis pooling data from 1724 patients. The results showed an overall benefit of giving preoperative chemotherapy (HR 0.9; 95% CI 0.81-1.00; p=0.05), equating to a survival benefit of 7% at 2 years. The treatment effect of neoadjuvant chemotherapy relative to tumour cell type indicated that patients with squamous cell carcinoma gained no benefit from preoperative chemotherapy (hazard ratio for mortality 0.88 (95% CI 0.75-1.03; p=0.12). However, quite the opposite was the case for those with adenocarcinoma, who gained a significant benefit from neoadjuvant chemotherapy (hazard ratio for mortality 0.78 :95% CI 0.64-0.95: p=0.014).

Further evidence that neoadjuvant chemotherapy improves survival for patients with adenocarcinoma comes in the form of the MRC MAGIC Trial (Cunningham et al 2006) which evaluated the survival benefits of giving preoperative epirubicin, cisplatin, and infused fluorouracil (ECF) in patients with gastric and oesophagogastric adenocarcenomas.

In brief, the study recruited 503 patients with resectable adenocarcinoma of the stomach, oesophagogastric junction or lower oesophagus. Of the 503 patients approximately 26% had a tumour of the lower oesophagus or gastro-oesophageal junction. The patients were randomised to receive either preoperative chemotherapy plus surgery n= 250 or surgery alone n=253. Three cycles of ECF were given preoperatively to the chemotherapy group followed by three further cycles postoperatively. Only 41.6% of the group completed all six cycles.

Pathological examination of the resected specimens confirmed significantly smaller tumour diameters in the chemotherapy group compared with the surgery alone group (p<0.001). The chemotherapy patients also had a higher proportion of T1 and T2 tumours than the surgery group (p=0.002) while those patients with gastric cancer showed a significant trend to less advanced nodal disease (p=0.01) which suggests tumour shrinkage or 'down staging' within the chemotherapy group.

On final analysis the chemotherapy group had a significantly higher likelihood of progression-free survival (HR 0.66; 95%CI 0.53 to 0.81; p<0.001) and of overall survival (HR 0.75; 95% CI 0.60 to 0.93; p = 0.009) which translates into 5 year survival rates of 36.3% for the chemotherapy group and 23% for the surgery alone group. Importantly there was no clear evidence of heterogeneity of treatment effect according to the site of the primary tumour, age group, sex, or the WHO performance status. These results lead to the trial concluding that preoperative ECF chemotherapy improves overall and progression-free survival among patients with resectable adenocarcinoma of the stomach, lower esophagus, or gastroesophageal junction, as compared with surgery alone.

Li et al 2010 performed a meta-analysis of 14 trials of neoadjuvant chemotherapy for gastric cancer (including of course the MAGIC trial). This study distils some very important aspects of the rationale for preoperative treatment and clearly reports some conclusions based on large numbers of patients. A total of 2271 patients (1054 in the neoadjuvant group and 1217 in the surgery only group) were analysed with a median follow-up period of 54 months. Table 3 outlines the main conclusions.

Parameter	Number of studies	Effect (CS vs S)
Overall survival at 3 years	12	48.1% vs 46.9%, favouring CS NNT - 84
Progression free survival at 3 years	3	41.1% vs 27.5%, favouring CS NNT - 8
Tumour downstaging	6	49.9% vs 37.5% for T0-2 favouring CS NNT - 9
R0 resection rate	8	75.2% vs 69.9%, favouring CS
Perioperative mortality	3	5.4% vs 4.6%, equivalent
Subgroup analyses	n/a	Effect on overall survival higher for T3 and T4 lesions Effects higher in Western studies Monotherapy inferior to multiple drug regimens IV route better than others

Table 3. Conclusions from the meta-analysis of neoadjuvant chemotherapy for gastric cancer by Li et al 2010. CS - neoadjuvant, S - surgery only, n/a not applicable, NNT - numbers needed to treat, IV - intravenous administration.

4. Neoadjuvant chemo-radiotherapy for oesophageal cancer

Neoadjuvant chemo-radiotherapy aims to downstage tumours preoperatively and reduce the risk of both local and distant metastatic recurrence. There has been great interest in this area with nine randomised control trials comparing overall survival between patients receiving neoadjuvant chemo-radiotherapy plus surgery (CRTS) and surgery alone (S) in oesophageal cancer patients. Table 6 summarises the treatment regimens while Table 7 shows the overall mortality estimates for each trial.

As shown in Tables 4 the numbers of patients taking part in each chemo-radiotherapy trial is relatively small. Treatment regimens also differ with radiation doses ranging from 20 to 50.4 Gy given either concurrently with the chemotherapy or sequentially which would reduce radiosensatisation of the tumour. The type of chemotherapeutic agents administered also varies. However, in the majority of trials, this is in the form of cisplatin (20-100mg/m^2) and 5-fluorouracil (300-1000mg/m^2).

Trial	Cell Type	CRTS n	S n	CRT Treatment	Sequential or Concurent radiotherapy	Hazard Ratio (95% CI)
Nygaard et al 1992	SCC	53	25	Cisplatin, Bleomycin & 35Gy	Sequential	0.76 (0.45-1.28)
Apinop et al 1994	SCC	35	34	Cisplatin, 5FU & 40Gy	Concurrent	0.80 (0.48-1.34)
Le Prise et al 1994	SCC	41	41	Cisplatin, 5FU & 20Gy	Sequential	0.85 (0.50-1.46)
Walsh et al 1996	Adeno	48	50	Cisplatin, 5FU & 40Gy	Concurrent	0.58 (0.38-0.88)
Bosset et al 1997	SCC	148	148	Cisplatin & 37 Gy	Sequential	0.96 (0.73-1.27)
Urba et al 2001	Adeno & SCC	50	50	Cisplatin, 5FU & 45Gy	Concurrent	0.74 (0.48-1.12)
Lee et al 2004	SCC	51	50	Cisplatin, 5FU & 45.6Gy	Concurrent	0.88 (0.48-1.62)
Burmeister et al 2005	Adeno & SCC	128	128	Cisplatin, 5FU & 35Gy	Concurrent	0.94 (0.70-1.26)
Tepper et al 2008	Adeno & SCC	30	26	Cisplatin, 5FU & 50.4Gy	Concurrent	0.40 (0.18-0.87)
Walsh et al 1995,unpublished	SCC	29	32	Cisplatin, 5FU & 40Gy	Concurrent	0.74 (0.46-1.18)
Total		623	586			0.81 (0.70-0.93)

Table 4. Summary of treatment given in chemo-radiotherapy trials & overall mortality estimates for neoadjuvant chemo-radiotherapy compared to surgery alone. SCC- Squamous cell carcinoma, Adeno - Adenocarcinoma, CRTS - Chemo-radiotherapy+Surgery, S -Surgery alone, CRT – Chemo-radiotherapy

Although most of the trials suggest there is benefit from giving preoperative chemo-radiotherapy, only two show a significant benefit in terms of overall mortality when compared to surgery alone. These studies are those by Walsh et al 1996 (HR 0.58;95% CI 0.38-0.88) who only enrolled adenocarcinoma patients and Tepper et al 2008 (HR 0.40; 95% CI 0.18-0.87) who included approximately 25% squamous cell carcinoma patients.

In order to shed more light on the effect of chemo-radiotherapy two recent meta-analyses have been published Gebski et al (2007) and Jin et al (2009).

Gebski et al using the pooled data showed that there was a relative reduction in mortality for patients receiving neoadjuvant chemo-radiotherapy (HR 0.81; 95% CI 0.70–0.93; p=0.002)

and that there was no evidence of heterogeneity between the trials or any temporal effect. Gebski et al. went on to look at the survival benefit of chemo-radiotherapy for the different tumour cell types. Patients with adenocarcinoma were shown to benefit (HR 0.75; 95% CI 0.59–0.95; p=0.02) while those with squamous cell carcinoma receiving sequential radiotherapy gained no survival advantage (HR 0.9; 95% CI 0.72-1.03; p=0.18.) However, when radiotherapy was administered concurrently a significant survival benefit was seen in squamous cell carcinoma patients (HR 0.76; 95%CI 0.59-0.98; p=0.04).
Jin et al 2009 using the same data as Gebski et al (plus the addition of a trial by Natsugoe et al 2006 containing 55 patients) also concluded that oesophageal cancer patients gain a survival benefit from receiving neoadjuvant chemotherapy Odds Ratio (OR) 1.78 (95% CI 1.20-2.66, p = 0.004) for 3 year survival. The paper goes on to state that there is no survival benefit from chemo-radiotherapy for those patients with squamous cell carcinoma (OR 1.34; 95% CI 0.98-1.82; p = 0.07) for 3-year survival implying only adenocarcinoma patients benefit. This should be treated with caution as odds ratios have been superseded by hazard ratios as a more reliable method of survival analysis. Furthermore, Jin et al 2009 suggest that the p value of 0.04 for the hazard ratio relating to concurrent chemo-radiotherapy providing survival benefit for SCC patients in Gebski et al meta-analysis is not significant. However, an important point made by Jin et al is that the post-operative mortality of chemo-radiotherapy patients is significantly higher than those receiving surgery alone (OR: 1.68, 95% CI: 1.03-2.73, p = 0.04). This point was also noted in the meta-analysis by Fiorica et al (2004).

5. Conclusion

To date, no randomised control trial has shown any survival benefit from neoadjuvant radiotherapy in the treatment of resectable oesophageal cancer. A number of trials have suggested preoperative chemotherapy could improve survival (Roth et al 1988, Law et al 1997, Ancona et al 2001 & MRC 2002) However, only the MRC 2002 and MRC MAGIC trial 2006 (only 26% of which had lower oesophageal/gastro-oesophageal junction tumours) showed a small improvement that was statistically significant. For chemo-radiotherapy, the studies by Walsh et al (1996) and Tepper et al (2008) are the only two trials to show a significant survival benefit.
All the trials investigating neoadjuvant chemotherapy or chemo-radiotherapy were small in size, often lacking the power necessary to detect small differences between groups. In order to detect a small yet worthwhile benefit from these different treatment modalities, data have been pooled for meta-analysis. The most comprehensive of these by Gebski et al (2007) showed an overall survival benefit from neoadjuvant chemo-radiotherapy of 13% at two years and a benefit of 7% at two years from preoperative chemotherapy. When looking at histological subtypes; chemo-radiotherapy improved survival for both adenocarcinoma and squamous cell carcinoma patients; chemotherapy also improved survival in those with adenocarcinoma however, no benefit was shown for patients with squamous cell carcinoma. Although chemo-radiotherapy has been shown to provide the greatest survival benefit, it has been associated with a higher post-operative mortality (Fiorica et al 2004 & Jin et al 2008). As a consequence, clinicians are still divided as to which treatment would be best for their patients.
In this chapter, the majority of trials discussed have employed cisplatin and 5-FU. However, the doses and radiation given to those patients receiving chemoradiotherapy have varied, which makes comparisons between trials more difficult. All the randomised control trials were designed over a decade ago. Since then, new chemotherapeutic agents have become

available and the delivery of radiotherapy has also advanced. In recent years the use of taxanes, when given concurrently with radiotherapy in the treatment of non-small cell lung cancer, have shown potential (Choy et al 1998, 2000 & Lau 2001). In a phase II trial, Van Meerten et al (2006) used Paclitaxel and Carboplatin with concurrent radiotherapy (total dose 41.4Gy) in oesophageal cancer patients with encouraging results. The CROSS trial uses the same chemo-radiotherapy regime in a phase III randomised control trial comparing neoadjuvant chemo-radiotherapy followed by surgery with surgery alone for surgically resectable oesophageal adenocarcinoma and squamous cell carcinoma (Van Meijl et al 2008).

After the encouraging results of both the MRC 2002 and MAGIC trials further investigation of neoadjuvant chemotherapy to treat oesophageal cancer in the form of the OE05 trial are on-going. OE05 is a randomised control trial comparing standard noeadjuvant chemotherapy (2 cycles of cisplatin + 5FU) with neoadjuvant ECX (4 cycles of Epirubicin, Cisplatin and Capecitabine) (OE05 clinical protocol 2008). The results of both trials are keenly awaited.

The major drawback with chemotherapy and chemo-radiotherapy lies in that both treatments are non-specific for the tumour or metastases they are targeting. A significant amount of non-malignant tissue is injured by both forms of treatment. In an attempt to fine tune the delivery of radiotherapy brachytherapy has been used in the palliative treatment of patients with advanced luminal oesophageal cancer. Overall survival at one year was 19.4% (Sur et al 1998). More recently, immunotherapy in the form of tumor-infiltrating lymphocytes (TILs), tumour vaccines and adoptive T-cell immunotherapy, which specifically targets tumour cell surface antigens using a chimeric immune receptor have been developed. Specific targeting would reduce damage of non-malignant tissue, could have the ability to down stage tumours preoperatively, mop up any residual micro metastases following surgery and might be an alternative neoadjuvant treatment in the future. A number of small preliminary trials have sown the possible potential of an immunotherapy approach however, larger clinical trials are needed.

In summary neoadjuvant chemotherapy and chemo-radiotherapy have both shown a significant benefit to survival of oesophageal cancer patients with resectable disease. Chemo-radiotherapy appears more effective, however, is associated with a higher postoperative mortality than preoperative chemotherapy. Further large scale randomised control trials using new chemotherapeutic agents are on the horizon and new treatments such as immunotherapy which have the ability to specifically target only malignant tissue may provide further improvement in survival in these patients.

6. References

Allum, W. H.; Stenning, S. P. Bancewicz, J. Clark, P. I. & Langley, R. E. (2009) Long-Term results of a randomized trial of surgery with or without preoperative chemotherapy in esophageal cancer *Journal of Clinical Oncology* 27: 5062-7

Ancona, E. Ruol, A. Santi, S. Merigliano, S. Sileni, V. C. Koussis, H. Zaninotto, G. Bonavina, L. & Peracchia, A. (2001) Only pathologic complete response to neoadjuvant chemotherapy improves significantly the long term survival of patients with resectable esophageal squamous cell carcinoma: final report of a randomized, controlled trial of preoperative chemotherapy versus surgery alone. *Cancer* 91: 2165-2174

Apinop, C.; Puttisak, P. & Preecha, N. (1994) A prospective study of combined therapy in esophageal cancer *Hepatogastroenterology* 41: 391-393

Arnott, S. J.; Duncan, W. Kerr, G. R.; Walbaum, P. R.; Cameron, E.; Jack, W. J. L. & MacKillop, W. J. (1992) Low dose preoperative radiotherapy for carcinoma of the oesophagus: Results of a randomized clinical trial. *Radiotherapy & Oncology* 24: 108–113

Arnott, S. J.; Duncan, W. Gignoux, M. Girling, D. J. Hansen, H. S. Launois, B. Nygaard, K. Parmar, M. K. Roussel, A. Spiliopoulos, G. Stewart, L. A. Tierney, J. F. Mei, W. & Rugang, Z. (1998) Preoperative radiotherapy in esophageal carcinoma: a meta-analysis using individual patient data (Oesophageal cancer collaborative group) *International Journal of Radiation Oncology • Biology • Physics* 41(3):579-83

Arnott, S.J.; Duncan, W. Gignoux, M. Girling, D. Hansen, H. Launois, B. Nygaard, K. Parmar, M. K. B. Rousell, A. Spiliopoulos, G. Stewart, L. Tierney, J. Wang, M. & Rhugang, Z. Oeosphageal Cancer Collaborative Group (2010) Preoperative radiotherapy for esophageal carcinoma (Review) *The Cochrane Library* Issue 11: Wiley

Bosset, J. F.; Gignoux, M. Triboulet, J. P. Tiret, E. Mantion, G. Elias, D. Lozach, P. Ollier, J. C. Pavy, J. J. Mercier, M. & Sahmoud, T. (1997) Chemoradiotherapy followed by surgery compared with surgery alone in squamous-cell cancer of the esophagus *New England Journal of Medicine* 337: 161-167

Burmeister, B. H.; Smithers, B. M. Gebski, V. Fitzgerald, L. Simes, R. J. Devitt, P. Ackland, S. Gotley, D. C. Joseph, D. Millar, J. North, J. Walpole, E. T. Denham, J. W. (2005) Surgery alone versus chemoradiotherapy followed by surgery for resectable cancer of the oesophagus: a randomised controlled phase III trial *The Lancet Oncology* 6: 659-668

Choy, H.; Akerley, W. Safran, H. Graziano, S. Chung, C. Williams, T. Cole, B. & Kennedy, T. (1998) Multiinstitutional phase II trial of paclitaxel, carboplatin, and concurrent radiation therapy for locally advanced non-small-cell lung cancer. *Journal of Clinical Oncology* 16: 3316-3322

Choy, H.; Devore, R. F. III Hande, K. R. Porter, L. L. Rosenblatt, P. Yunus, F. Schlabach, L. Smith, C. Shyr, Y. & Johnson, D. H. (2000) A phase II study of paclitaxel, carboplatin, and hyperfractionated radiation therapy for locally advanced inoperable non-small-cell lung cancer (a Vanderbilt Cancer Center Affiliate Network Study) *International Journal of Radiation Oncology • Biology • Physics* 47:931-937

Cunningham, D.; Allum, W. H. Stenning, S. P. Thompson, J. N. Van de Velde, C. J. Nicolson, M. Scarffe, J. H. Lofts, F. J. Falk, S. J. Iveson, T. J. Smith, D. B. Langley, R. E. Verma, M. Weeden, S. & Chua, Y. J. MAGIC Trial Participants. (2006) Perioperative Chemotherapy versus Surgery Alone for Resectable Gastroesophageal Cancer *New England Journal of Medicine* 355: 11-20

Fiorica, F.; Di Bona, D. Schepis, F. Licata. A, Shahied, L. Venturi, A. Falchi, A. M. Craxì, A. & Cammà, C. (2004) Preoperative chemoradiotherapy for oesophageal cancer: a systematic review and meta-analysis *Gut* 53: 925-30

Gebski, V.; Burmeister, B. Smithers, B. M. Foo, K. Zalcberg, J. Simes, J. Australasian Gastro-Intestinal Trials Group (2007) Survival benefits from neoadjuvant chemoradiotherapy or chemotherapy in oesophageal carcinoma: a meta-analysis *The Lancet Oncology* 8: 226-34

Gignoux, M.; Roussel, A. Paillot, B. Gillet, M. Schlag, P. Dalesio, O. Buyse, M. & Duez, N. (1988) The value of preoperative radiotherapy in esophageal cancer: Results of a study by the EORTC. *Recent Results in Cancer Research* 110: 1–13

Jin, H. L.; Zhu, H. Ling, T. S. Zhang, H. J. & Shi, R. H. (2009) Neoadjuvant chemoradiotherapy for resectable esophageal carcinoma: A meta-analysis *World Journal of Gastroenterology* 15: 5983-91

Kakyama, K.; Orihato, H. & Yamaguchi K. (1967) Surgical treatment combined with preoperative concentrated irradiation for oesophageal cancer. *Cancer* 20: 778-788

Kelsen, D. P.; Winter, K. A. Gunderson, L. L. Mortimer, J. Estes, N. C. Haller, D. G. Ajani, J. A. Kocha, W. Minsky, B. D. Roth, J. A. & Willett, C.G.; Radiation Therapy Oncology Group; USA Intergroup. (2007) Long-Term Results of RTOG Trial 8911 (USA Intergroup 113): A Random Assignment Trial Comparison of Chemotherapy Followed by Surgery Compared With Surgery Alone for Esophageal Cancer *Journal of Clinical Oncology* 25 3719-25

Kelsen, D.P.; Ginsberg, R. Pajak, T.F. Sheahan, D. G. Gunderson, L. Mortimer, J. Estes, N. Haller, D. G. Ajani, J. Kocha, W. Minsky, B. D. & Roth, J. A. (1998) Chemotherapy followed by surgery compared with surgery alone for localized esophageal cancer. *New England Journal of Medicine* 339: 1979-1984

Lau, D.; Leigh, B. Gandara, D. Edelman, M. Morgan, R. Israel, V. Lara, P. Wilder, R. Ryu, J. & Doroshow, J. (2001) Twice-weekly paclitaxel and weekly carboplatin with concurrent thoracic radiation followed by carboplatin/paclitaxel consolidation for stage III non-small-cell lung cancer: a California Cancer Consortium phase II trial *Journal of Clinical Oncology* 19: 442-447

Launois, B.; Delarue, D. Campion, J. P. & Kerbaol, M. Preoperative radiotherapy for carcinoma of the esophagus *Surgery, Gynecology & Obstetrics* 153:690–692

Law, S.; Fok, M. Chow, S. Chu, K. M. & Wong, J. (1997)Preoperative chemotherapy versus surgical therapy alone for squamous cellcarcinoma of the esophagus: a prospective randomized trial. *Journal of Thoracic & Cardiovascular Surgery* 114: 210-217

Lee, J. L.; Park, S. I. Kim, S. B. Jung, H. Y. Lee, G. H. Kim, J. H. Song, H. Y. Cho, K.J. Kim, W. K. Lee, J. S. Kim, S. H. Min, Y. I. (2004) A single institutional phase III trial of preoperative chemotherapy with hyperfractionation radiotherapy plus surgery versus surgery alone for resectable esophageal squamous cell carcinoma. *Annals of Oncology* 15: 947-954

Le Prise, E.; Etienne, P.L. Meunier, B. Maddern, G. Ben Hassel, M. Gedouin, D. Boutin, D. Campion, J. P. & Launois, B. (1994) A randomized study of chemotherapy, radiation therapy, and surgery versus surgery for localized squamous cell carcinoma of the esophagus *Cancer* 73: 1779-1784

Li W.; Qin J., Sun Y.H., Liu T.S. (2010) Neoadjuvant chemotherapy for advanced gastric cancer: a meta-analysis. *World Journal of Gastroenterology* 16: 5621-5628.

Maipang, T.; Vasinanukorn, P. Petpichetchian, C. Chamroonkul, S. Geater, A. Chansawwaang, S. Kuapanich, R. Panjapiyakul, C. Watanaarepornchai, S. & Punperk, S. (1994) Induction chemotherapy in the treatment of patients with carcinoma of the esophagus. *Journal of Surgical Oncology* 56: 191-197

Medical Research Council Oesophageal Cancer Working Group. (2002) Surgical resection with or without preoperative chemotherapy in oesophageal cancer: a randomised controlled trial. *Lancet* 359: 1727-1733

Medical Research Council OE05 A randomised controlled trial comparing standard chemotherapy followed by resection versus ECX chemotherapy followed by resection in patients with resectable adenocarcinoma of the oesophagus clinical protocol version 5 (31st July 2008) *MRC Clinical Trials Unit web page* http://www.ctu.mrc.ac.uk/plugins/StudyDisplay/protocols/OE05Protocol Version531stJuly2008.pdf

Natsugoe, S.; Okumura, H. Matsumoto, M. Uchikado, Y. Setoyama, T. Yokomakura, N. Ishigami, S. Owaki, T. & Aikou, T. (2006) Randomized controlled study on preoperative chemoradiotherapy followed by surgery versus surgery alone for esophageal squamous cell cancer in a single institution *Diseases of the Esophagus* 19: 468-472

Nygaard, K.; Hagen, S. Hansen, H. S. Hatlevoll, R. Hultborn, R. Jakobsen, A. Mantyla, M. Modig, H. Munck-Wikland, E. Rosengren, B. Tausjø, J. & Elgen, K. (1992) Pre-operative radiotherapy prolongs survival in operable esophageal carcinoma: A randomized, multicenter study of preoperative radiotherapy and chemotherapy. The second Scandinavian trial in esophageal cancer. *World Journal of Surgery* 16:1104 –1110

Roth, J. A.; Pass, H. I. Flanagan, M. M. Graeber, G. M. Rosenberg, J. C. & Steinberg, S. (1988) Randomized clinical trial of preoperative and postoperative adjuvant chemotherapy with cisplatin, vindesine, and bleomycin for carcinoma of the esophagus. *Journal of Thoracic & Cardiovascular Surgery* 96: 242-8

Schlag, P. M. (1992) Randomized trial of preoperative chemotherapy for squamous cell cancer of the esophagus. *Archives of Surgery* 127: 1446-1450

Sur, R. K. Donde, B. Levin, V. C. & Mannell, A. (1998) Fractionated high dose rate intraluminal brachytherapy in palliation of advanced esophageal cancer *International Journal of Radiation Oncology • Biology • Physics* 40: 447-53

Tepper, J.; Krasna, M. J. Niedzwiecki, D. Hollis, D. Reed, C. E. Goldberg, R. Kiel, K. Willett, C. Sugarbaker, D. & Mayer, R. (2008) Phase III trial of trimodality therapy with cisplatin, fluorouracil, radiotherapy, and surgery compared with surgery alone for esophageal cancer: CALGB 9781 *Journal of Clinical Oncology* 26: 1086-1092

Urba, S. G.; Orringer, M. B. Turrisi, A. Iannettoni, M. Forastiere, A. & Strawderman, M. (2001) Randomized trial of preoperative chemoradiation versus surgery alone in patients with locoregional esophageal carcinoma. *Journal of Clinical Oncology* 19: 305-313

van Heijl, M.; van Lanschot, J. J. Koppert, L. B. van Berge, Henegouwen, M. I. Muller, K. Steyerberg, E. W. van Dekken, H. Wijnhoven, B. P. Tilanus, H. W. Richel, D. J. Busch, O. R. Bartelsman, J. F. Koning, C. C. Offerhaus, G. J. & van der Gaast, A. (2008) Neoadjuvant chemoradiation followed by surgery versus surgery alone for patients with adenocarcinoma or squamous cell carcinoma of the esophagus (CROSS) *Bio Med Central Surgery* 8:21

van Meerten, E. Muller, K. Tilanus, H. W. Siersema, P. D. Eijkenboom, W. M. van Dekken, H. Tran, T. C. & van der Gaast, A. (2006) Neoadjuvant concurrent chemoradiation with weekly paclitaxel and carboplatin for patients with oesophageal cancer: a phase II study *British Journal of Cancer* 94: 1389-94

Walsh T. (1995) The role of multimodality therapy in improving survival: a prospective randomised trial. In: Predicting, defining and improving outcomes for oesophageal carcinoma [MD thesis]. Dublin: Trinity College, University of Dublin, 124 - 50

Walsh, T. N.; Noonan, N. Hollywood, D. Kelly, A. Keeling, N. & Hennessy, T. P. (1996) A comparison of multimodal therapy and surgery for esophageal adenocarcinoma *New England Journal of Medicine* 335: 462-467

Wang, M.; Gu, X. Z. Yin, W. B. Huang, G. J. Wang, L. J. & Zhang, D. W. (1989) Randomized clinical trial on the combination of preoperative irradiation and surgery in the treatment of esophageal carcinoma: Report on 206 patients. *International Journal of Radiation Oncology • Biology • Physics* 16:325–327

10

Developments in Neoadjuvant Chemotherapy and Radiotherapy in Rectal Cancer

Sofia Conde[1], Margarida Borrego[2] and Anabela Sá[2]
[1]*Portuguese Oncology Institute, Porto*
[2]*Coimbra University Hospitals*
Portugal

1. Introduction

The treatment of rectal cancer has evolved dramatically through the last three decades. Until the 1970's and 1980's, surgery was often the only therapeutic modality employed in the treatment of rectal cancer patients. However, local recurrence with surgery alone was significant resulting in patient morbidity and death (Gunderson & Sosin, 1974; Rich et al., 1983). Some studies have demonstrated that adjuvant chemotherapy and radiotherapy (RT) improved local relapse and survival in patients with tumors extending into the perirectal fat (T3) or with involvement of mesorectal or pelvic lymph nodes (N1-3) (Gastrointestinal Tumor Study Group, 1985; National Institutes of Health Consensus Conference, 1990; Wolmark et al, 2000).

Neoadjuvant chemoradiotherapy has become the standard of care for stages II and III rectal cancer since the CAO/ARO/AIO trial (Sauer et al, 2004). Ever since, efforts have been made in order to discover which drug or combination of drugs have better results in terms of local recurrence and survival.

In this chapter we will give an overview of the history of neoadjuvant chemotherapy and radiotherapy in rectal cancer, the current standards of care as well as ongoing trials in the neoadjuvant setting for locally advanced rectal cancer.

2. Neoadjuvant radiotherapy for rectal cancer

Before the advent of total mesorectal excision surgery, only the Swedish rectal cancer trial and two meta-analyses showed a survival advantage with neoadjuvant radiation therapy (Cammá et al, 2007; Colorectal Cancer Collaborative Group, 2001). The Swedish trial randomly assigned 1168 patients to undergo preoperative RT (25 Gy delivered in 5 fraction in 1 week) followed by surgery within one week or to have surgery alone. The preoperative arm had reduced rates of local recurrence and improved survival among patients with resectable rectal cancer (Swedish Rectal Cancer Trial, 1997). These results were confirmed in a recent update of this trial, with a median follow-up time of 13 years (Folkesson et al, 2005).

Total mesorectal excision (TME) is now the standard of care for rectal cancer surgery, permitting en bloc removal of intact tumor with its lymphatic and vascular supply resulting in a negative circumferential margin and lower local relapse rates. In this setting, two large studies have explored the role of preoperative RT and demonstrated their superiority.

The Dutch Colorectal Cancer Group randomly assigned 1861 patients with rectal cancer either to preoperative RT (5 Gy x 5) followed by TME or to TME alone. They concluded that short-term preoperative radiotherapy reduces the risk of local recurrence at 2 years (2.4% *vs* 8.2%, $p<0.001$) in patients with rectal cancer who undergo a TME. However, neoadjuvant RT did not have any impact on distant relapse or overall survival (Kapiteijn et al, 2001). These results were confirmed on a long-term follow-up study of 6 years (Peeters et al, 2007).
The Medical Research Council (MRC) CR07 and National Cancer Institute of Canada (NCIC) Clinical Trials Group (CTG) C016 trial was a multicentre (1350 patients from 80 centers in 4 countries) randomized controlled trial comparing short-course preoperative radiotherapy (25 Gy in 5 fractions) with selective postoperative chemoradiotherapy (45 Gy in 25 fractions with concurrent 5-Fluorouracil) for patients with involvement of the circumferential resection margin after TME (Sebag-Montefiore et al, 2009). They reported a reduction of 61% in the relative risk of local recurrence for patients receiving preoperative radiotherapy ($p<0.0001$), an absolute difference at 3-years local recurrence rate of 6.2% (4.4% *vs* 10.6%), a relative improvement in disease-free survival of 24% for patients receiving preoperative radiotherapy ($p = 0.013$) and an absolute difference at 3 years of 6% (77.5% *vs* 71.5%). Overall survival (OS) did not differ between the groups ($p = 0.40$).
Therefore, neoadjuvant radiotherapy has proved to result in better local control than surgery ± adjuvant therapy in locally advanced rectal cancer. The impact on survival has not been clear.

3. Neoadjuvant chemoradiation for rectal cancer

The administration of chemotherapy in combination with radiotherapy can have an additive effect, in which there is no interaction between the treatment modalities and each strategy is separately effective. More promising is a combination in which a synergistic effect is achieved. The main chemotherapeutic agents used in chemoradiotherapeutic combinations for rectal cancer are 5-fluorouracil (5-FU) and oral fluoropyrimidines. The main goals of chemoradiation are the reduction of local and distant recurrences in order to improve survival. It was in this context that in the last decades there have been many studies which have associated diverse chemotherapeutic agents to radiotherapy.

3.1 5-FU plus radiotherapy

Currently, chemoradiation using 5-fluorouracil (5-FU) as a radiosensitizer is considered the common approach for rectal cancer in the neoadjuvant setting. There are a number of mechanisms by which 5-FU could increase radiation sensitivity at the cellular level. First is through the killing of S-phase cells which are relatively radioresistant. 5-FU has also a sensitizing effect related to enzyme thymidylate synthase inhibition and the ability to damage DNA. The primary toxicities of 5-FU include gastrointestinal symptoms including diarrhea, myelosupression, inflammation of mucosae, including the eyes, nose and urinary tract, neurotoxicity at high-dose levels, and rare cardiac toxicity (Zhu & Willett, 2003).
The CAO/ARO/AIO trial (Sauer et al, 2004) compared preoperative with postoperative chemoradiotherapy for locally advanced rectal cancer. In this randomized clinical trial preoperative treatment consisted of 50.4 Gy delivered in fractions of 1.80 Gy/day, 5 days per week, and 5-FU given in a 120 hour continuous intravenous infusion at a dose of 1000 mg/m^2 of body surface area per day during the first and fifth weeks of radiotherapy. Surgery was performed 6 weeks after completion of chemoradiotherapy. One month after

surgery, 4 cycles of 5-FU (500 mg/m^2/d) were given. Chemoradiotherapy was identical in the postoperative treatment group except for the delivery of a boost of 5.4 Gy. They concluded that preoperative chemoradiotherapy improved local control (5-year cumulative incidence of local relapse: 6% *vs* 13%, $p = 0.006$) and was associated with reduced toxicity (27% *vs* 40%, $p = 0.001$) but did not improve overall survival (76% *vs* 74%, $p = 0.80$). Significant tumor downstaging was seen after preoperative combined-modality treatment with an 8% pathologic complete response (pCR) rate. Posttrial review showed that sphincter-saving surgeries were more likely to occur in the neoadjuvant chemoradiation group than in the adjuvant group (39% *vs* 19%, $p = 0.004$).

Despite the lack of survival advantage, these findings have set neoadjuvant chemoradiation as the new standard of care in the United States and in Europe in the treatment of rectal cancer.

Recently, European trials have further evaluated the role of concurrent 5-FU-based chemotherapy with radiation therapy in the neoadjuvant treatment of rectal cancer.

A large phase III French study, Fédération Francophone de Cancérologie Digestive (FFCD) 9203, randomized patients with stage II/III rectal cancer to receive RT alone (45 Gy in 25 fractions) or 5-FU/leucovorin (LV) with RT (FU/LV 350/20 mg/m^2/d on days 1 to 5 and 29 to 33 of RT). Patients in both arms subsequently underwent surgery and four cycles of 5-FU/LV. The preoperative chemoradiation arm showed a significant improvement in pathologic complete response (pCR) rate (11.4% *vs* 3.6%, $p < 0.05$) and local relapse rate (8.1 *vs* 16.5%, $p < 0.05$). The 5-year survival in both arms was 67% (Gerard et al, 2006).

Another large phase III study, European Organisation for Research and Treatment of Cancer (EORTC) 22921, randomized patients with stage II/III rectal cancer to receive neoadjuvant RT alone (45 Gy in 25 fractions) *vs* RT with bolus 5-FU/LV (350/20 mg/m^2/d during the first and fifth weeks of preoperative RT), with a subsequent randomization to postsurgical (3 to 10 weeks after chemoradiation) 5-FU/LV chemotherapy or no postsurgical chemotherapy. The study demonstrated no significant difference in overall survival between the groups that received chemotherapy preoperatively and those who received it postoperatively. The 5-year cumulative incidence rates for local relapse were 8.7%, 9.6%, and 7.6% in the groups receiving chemotherapy preoperatively, postoperatively, or both, respectively, and 17.1% in the group that did not receive chemotherapy ($p = 0.002$). The authors concluded that in patients with rectal cancer who receive preoperative radiotherapy, adding 5-FU–based chemotherapy either preoperatively or postoperatively conferred a significant advantage in terms of local control (Bosset et al, 2005).

3.2 Oral fluoropyrimidines plus radiotherapy

Preoperative RT with continuous i.v. 5-FU infusion has the biologic advantage of prolonging exposure of tumor cells to 5-FU and improving antitumor activity. However, its disadvantages include the requirement of central venous access with potential complications, such as bleeding, thrombosis, infection and pneumothorax (Grem, 1997). Most patients receiving chemotherapy prefer oral therapies to intravenous regimens because of their possibility to receive treatment without attending clinics, to continue daily activities and to maintain a relatively normal lifestyle. There is evidence that, with regular patient education and monitoring, adequate patient compliance to oral medications can be achieved, although issues of compliance and safety remain a concern (Lee et al, 1992).

Oral chemotherapy mimics the pharmacokinetics of continuous 5-FU infusion and avoids technical barriers of i.v. infusion with the advantage of convenience. Oral fluoropyrimidines such as UFT or capecitabine, constitute an attractive alternative.

Although there are some studies comparing infusional preoperative chemoradiotherapy (5-FU) with oral neoadjuvant chemoradiotherapy either with capecitabine or UFT (De la Torre et al, 2008; Kim et al, 2007), there is not yet a single randomized study comparing the results of both of these modalities of oral neoadjuvant chemotherapy along with radiotherapy.

3.2.1 Capecitabine plus radiotherapy

Capecitabine is an oral fluoropyrimidine carbamate prodrug of 5-FU designed to generate 5-flurouracil (5-FU) preferentially in tumor cells (Pentheroudakis & Twelves, 2002), as concentration of the key enzyme thymidine phosphorylase is higher in tumor cells compared with normal tissue. In preclinical studies, irradiation with thymidine phosphorylase was found to be upregulated in tumor tissue resulting in a selective synergistic effect of capecitabine on radiotherapy (Schuller et al, 2000; Sawada et al, 1999; Miwa et al, 1998). Capecitabine is administered daily to mimic a continuous infusion of 5-FU (De Bruin et al, 2008). This continuous regimen is likely to have a more constant cytotoxic action, thereby limiting tumor regrowth. The side-effect profile of capecitabine is similar to that observed when 5-FU is given as a protracted infusion and consists mainly in diarrhea. The dose-limiting toxicity is the hand–foot syndrome, occurring as the capecitabine dose reaches 1000 mg/m^2 twice daily. Other toxicities were generally mild to moderate (Van Cutsem et al, 2001; Hoff et al, 2001).

A phase I study on rectal cancer defined the recommended dose of capecitabine to be 825 mg/m^2 twice daily, administered 7 days/week during a conventional RT period of about 6 weeks for preoperative therapy in locally advanced rectal cancer (Dunst et al, 2002).

Some phase II studies confirmed that capecitabine is an adequate substitute for continuous infusional 5-FU in preoperative chemoradiation regimens with regard to the favorable toxicity profile, considerable downstaging effect and pathologic complete response on the tumor, and could increase the possibility of sphincter preservation in distal rectal cancer (Dunst et al, 2004; Kim et al, 2005; De Paoli et al, 2006; Krishnan et al, 2006).

The randomized phase III NSABP-R04 study is currently comparing capecitabine/RT to 5-FU/RT (with and without concurrent oxaliplatin). This will help determine if capecitabine can substitute for 5-FU in the neoadjuvant treatment of rectal cancer. The primary aim of the study is to compare the rate of local-regional relapse in the two groups. Co-primary end points are pCR and progression-free survival (PFS).

In conclusion, neoadjuvant radiotherapy concomitant to capecitabine has proved so far to be well tolerated and is an adequate substitute for continuous infusion of 5-FU.A smaller phase III trial is underway in Germany to compare adjuvant capecitabine chemoradiation versus 5-FU chemoradiation in patients with rectal cancer. PETACC is conducting a neoadjuvant/adjuvant rectal cancer study comparing capecitabine single agent *versus* capecitabine-oxaliplatin combination.

3.2.2 UFT plus radiotherapy

UFT is an oral combination of uracil and tegafur in a fixed 1:4 molar ratio (Hoff et al, 1998). Tegafur is a prodrug converted to 5-FU by the hepatic microsomal system following intestinal absorption. Uracil competitively inhibits dihydropyrimidine dehydrogenase, the chief catabolic enzyme of 5-FU, which results in elevated and maintained concentrations of 5-FU for a prolonged period and thus simulates a continuous infusion of 5-FU to improve the absorption and bioavailability of tegafur (Ho et al, 1998; Sulkes et al, 1998; Hirata et al, 1993).

In preclinical experiments, leucovorin (LV) has been combined with UFT in an attempt to enhance antitumor activity (Okabe et al, 1997). In patients with advanced colorectal cancer, the combination of UFT and oral LV produced objective response rates ranging from 25% to 42% (Pazdur et al, 1999). Preliminary results from two large randomized studies in patients with metastatic colorectal cancer suggested that patients treated with UFT/LV and those receiving bolus intravenous 5-FU/LV may have an equivalent response and survival rate (Pazdur et al, 1999; Carmichael et al, 1999). In the adjuvant setting Japanese investigators compared postoperative UFT to surgery alone; UFT led to a significantly improved 4-year disease-free survival, particularly in patients with rectal cancer (Nakazato et al, 1997). Like infusional 5-FU, UFT is generally well tolerated, with diarrhea, nausea, and anorexia being the most frequent adverse effects. In reported trials, grade 3 or 4 diarrhea occurred in 4% to 21% of patients (Ho et al, 1998; Pazdur et al, 1999; Carmichael et al, 1999). UFT is not associated with significant myelosuppression, mucositis, hand-foot syndrome, or alopecia.

Pharmacokinetic studies have shown that 5-FU plasma levels in patients receiving protracted infusions of 5-FU are similar to those found in patients receiving oral UFT, although peak levels of 5-FU are higher with UFT (Ho et al, 1998). There are a large number of patients who have received UFT plus oral LV as adjuvant chemotherapy or to treat metastatic disease, however, there is less data on the use of UFT/LV with radiation therapy in patients with rectal cancer.

In the phase I study by Hoff et al. (Hoff et al, 2000), 15 patients with resectable stage II/III rectal cancer were treated with escalating doses of UFT (250 - 400 mg/m^2/day) together with a fixed dose of LV (90 mg/day). UFT was taken in three equal doses per day, 5 days/week for the duration of a 5-week course of preoperative RT (1.8 Gy/day administered to the pelvis; total dose of 45 Gy). The maximum tolerated dose (MTD) was UFT 350 mg/m^2/day.

A lower MTD for UFT of 240 mg/m2/day was defined in the phase I study by Pfeffer et al. (Pfeffer et al, 2004). UFT was taken with LV 30 mg/day for 4 weeks and RT (1.8 Gy/day, 5 days/week for 5 weeks; total dose of 45 Gy) was delivered using a three-field technique.

The phase II studies have attempted to improve on the regimens used in the dose-finding studies. Wang et al. combined a dose-intense RT schedule (45 Gy in 4 weeks) with two courses of UFT at lower doses 200 mg/m^2/day on days 1–28 in cycle 1 and 250 mg/m^2/day in cycle 2 (postradiotherapy) with LV in an attempt to minimize side-effects and maintain systemic treatment during the postradiation period. This approach was effective, with high rates of downstaging (75%), pCR (25%) and sphincter preservation (55%); OS and PFS rates at 3 years (92% and 76%, respectively) were excellent. Transient grade 3/4 adverse events were rare (Wang et al, 2005).

In a large phase II study by Fernández-Martos et al, 94 patients with T3–4 tumors received a higher dose of UFT (400 mg/m^2/day) without LV, together with RT 5 days/week for 5 weeks (total dose 45 Gy; 1.8 Gy/day). After surgery, four cycles of adjuvant 5-FU (Mayo regimen) were administered to most patients (76%). Treatment was well tolerated and pCR occurred in 15% of patients (Fernández-Martos et al, 2004).

Different dose regimens were also evaluated. Feliu et al evaluated a regimen with higher doses of UFT but they had a higher toxicity profile (Feliu et al, 2002). Kundel et al studied a combination of lower doses of UFT + LV with a similar tolerability profile but slightly reduced efficacy (Kundel et al, 2007).

In a phase III study UFT/LV has been compared with bolus 5-FU/LV in preoperative chemoradiotherapy for locally advanced rectal cancer. Of 155 patients, pCR rate was 13%

in both arms, although more patients in the UFT group had tumor downstaging (59% *vs* 43%; $p = 0.04$). Although the study was not powered to exclude clinically significant differences between the groups, outcomes in the UFT group did not differ from those in the 5-FU group. Most notable, however, was the difference in the tolerability profiles, with 5-FU/LV group showing more severe leucopenia compared with the UFT group (De la Torre et al, 2008).

The National Cancer Center of Korea has implemented a pilot study to evaluate a higher dose of enteric-coated tegafur/uracil (400 mg/m^2/d) plus LV (90 mg/d) for 7 days a week during 50.4 Gy pelvic RT and concluded that this scheme has showed favorable efficacy (pCR rate 22.2%) and toxicity profiles. A phase II trial is ongoing to test this treatment (Kim et al, 2009).

In conclusion, UFT/LV neoadjuvant treatment concomitant to radiotherapy has proved to be well tolerated with good results in terms of treatment response compared to 5-FU based preoperative schedules. However, there is a lack of randomized trials comparing these both oral fluoropyrimidines in the neoadjuvant setting concomitant to radiotherapy in rectal cancer as well as randomized trials comparing them to 5-FU regimens.

3.3 Oxaliplatin-based combination regimens

Significant interest has arisen in the past several years in developing combinations of 5-FU, oxaliplatin, and RT in the neoadjuvant treatment of rectal cancer. This interest has been supported by the systemic synergistic activity between oxaliplatin and fluoropyrimidines and the added radiation-sensitizing activity of oxaliplatin (de Gramont et al, 2000; Goldberg et al, 2004). The mechanism of radiation sensitization appeared to be through cell-cycle perturbations. It remains controversial whether oxaliplatin should be delivered before or after radiation to maximize its radiosensitizing activity. The main toxicities described are hematologic toxicity (neutropenia, trombocitopenia), nausea and/or vomiting, diarrhea, mucositis and neurologic toxicity which is dose limiting.

3.3.1 Oxaliplatin/5-FU plus radiotherapy

The Cancer and Leukemia Group B (CALGB) investigated a combination of escalating weekly doses of oxaliplatin in combination with continuous-infusion 5-FU at 200 mg/m^2/d and RT at 1.8 Gy/fraction for a total of 50.4 Gy in a phase I/II study. The recommended phase II dose of oxaliplatin in this combination was identified as 60 mg/m^2/wk (in 6 doses). Although 25% of patients had a pCR, this treatment was associated with an excessive rate (38%) of grade 3/4 diarrhea (Ryan et al, 2006).

The Studio Terapia Adiuvante Retto (STAR)-01 randomized phase III trial investigated the effect of adding oxaliplatin to preoperative FU-based pelvic chemoradiation in patients with locally advanced rectal cancer. Randomization was between infused 5-FU (225 mg/m^2/day) concomitant to external-beam pelvic RT (50.4 Gy in 28 daily fractions) or the same regimen plus weekly oxaliplatin (60 mg/m^2 x 6). They concluded that the addition of weekly oxaliplatin to standard FU-based preoperative chemoradiation significantly increased toxicity without affecting local tumor response. The reduced pathologic M+ rate suggested a potential effect on distant micrometastases. However, longer follow-up is needed to assess the impact on efficacy endpoints (Aschele et al, 2009).

The randomized NSABP-R04 trial is currently addressing the value of adding oxaliplatin to 5-FU radiation therapy.

3.3.2 Oxaliplatin/capecitabine plus radiotherapy

Capecitabine/oxaliplatin combinations have demonstrated efficacy and tolerability comparable to that of 5-FU/oxaliplatin in the first-line treatment of metastatic colorectal cancer. Several studies have investigated the combination of capecitabine, oxaliplatin, and radiation in the neoadjuvant treatment of rectal cancer in hopes of improving both local and systemic disease control.

In a phase I/II study, daily capecitabine (including weekends) was combined with a fixed dose of oxaliplatin at 130 mg/m^2 on days 1 and 29 concurrently with RT 45 Gy (25 fractions) in patients with borderline or unresectable rectal cancer. The MTD of capecitabine in this combination was 650 mg/m^2 twice daily. A total of 96 patients were enrolled and there was a pCR in 19% of patients and only 22% experienced grade 3/4 adverse events, the most common being gastrointestinal (Glynne-Jones et al, 2006).

Roedel et al conducted a phase II neoadjuvant study of capecitabine and oxaliplatin (XELOX) plus radiation in 110 patients with locally advanced rectal cancer. The regimen consisted of capecitabine at 825 mg/m^2 twice daily on days 1 to 14 and 22 to 35 along with oxaliplatin 50 mg/m^2 on days 1, 8, 22, and 29, plus RT (50.4 Gy in 28 fractions). Grade 3 toxicity, mainly diarrhea, occurred in 14% of patients. Of the resected specimens 15% showed a pCR (Roedel et al, 2006).

The Capecitabine Oxaliplatin Radiotherapy and Excision (CORE) study investigated a variant regimen of capecitabine twice daily on Mondays through Fridays and weekly oxaliplatin at 50 mg/m^2 concurrently with radiation at 45 Gy in patients with threatened or positive circumferential margins by magnetic resonance imaging. Initial results from this multicenter phase II study showed an R0 resection rate of 67% and a pCR rate of 13% (Rutten et al, 2006).

Other researchers have investigated a capecitabine/oxaliplatin regimen similar to the one used in the CORE study (Machiels et al, 2005; Alonso et al, 2007; Ofner et al, 2007; Carlomagno et al, 2007; Salimichokami et al, 2006). These studies were associated with pCR rates of 14% to 24%, tumor-downstaging rates of 52% to 78%, and grade 3/4 diarrhea rates of 8% to 30%.

The current recommended dose for capecitabine given twice daily on radiation days with weekly oxaliplatin and RT (1.8 Gy × 25–28 fractions) is 825 mg/m^2 twice daily and 50 mg/m^2 weekly for capecitabine and oxaliplatin, respectively.

The recommended doses of capecitabine, oxaliplatin, and radiation therapy may tend to be lower in the United States than in Europe, because higher rates of toxicity have been reported in the US for capecitabine monotherapy or capecitabine/oxaliplatin combinations (Haller et al, 2006). The exact etiology for the discrepancy in toxicity at equal capecitabine dosing may be related to increased folic acid supplementation in the American diet. It is prudent at this time to consider 725 mg/m^2 twice daily dosing for capecitabine in combination with weekly oxaliplatin (50 mg/m^2) and RT (50.4 Gy) in the US until further safety data become available from NSABP-R04. The 825 mg/m^2 dose level of capecitabine combined with a similar oxaliplatin/RT regimen is clearly tolerable and feasible in Europe.

The phase III trial ACCORD 12/0405 - Prodige 2 randomly assigned patients to receive 5 weeks of RT 45Gy/25 fractions with concurrent capecitabine 800 mg/m^2 twice daily 5 days/week (CAP45) or RT 50Gy/25 fractions with same dose of capecitabine plus oxaliplatin 50 mg/m^2 once weekly (CAPOX50). More preoperative grade 3 to 4 toxicity occurred in the CAPOX50 group (25% *vs* 1%, $p<0.001$). The ypCR rate was 13.9% with CAP45 and 19.2% with CAPOX50 ($p = 0.09$). In this trial, a benefit of Oxaliplatin was not demonstrated and they concluded that this drug should not be used with concurrent irradiation (Gerard et al, 2010).

A large phase III pan-European trial (PETACC-6) comparing capecitabine and oxaliplatin chemoradiation with capecitabine chemoradiation alone as neoadjuvant treatment in T3/4 N1/2 patients is in development.

3.3.3 Oxaliplatin/UFT plus radiotherapy

Patients in a phase I/II study by Aschele et al. received weekly oxaliplatin (60 mg/m^2/day), escalating doses of UFT (200 - 350 mg/m^2/day, 5 days/week) and LV (90 mg/day, fixed dose) during RT (total dose 50.4 Gy). Nine patients had a major down-staging (ypT0-2 pN0) with 4 pCRs (2 of them among the 6 patients treated at the highest dose level). The authors concluded that oral UFT may replace infusional 5-FU in combination with weekly oxaliplatin and standard pelvic radiotherapy with low toxicity and promising activity. The recommended dose for further studies is 350 mg/m^2/day (Aschele et al, 2009).

Preliminary results from a phase II study by Fernández-Martos et al. demonstrated that UFT 400 mg/m^2/day, taken 5 days/week for 5 weeks and oxaliplatin 85 mg/m^2 on days 1, 15 and 29 can be administered safely with radiotherapy (50 Gy total) to patients with locally advanced rectal cancer. A pCR rate of 15% was observed (Fernández-Martos et al, 2005).

3.4 Irinotecan-based combination regimens

The addition of the topoisomerase-I inhibitor irinotecan to 5-FU significantly improves response rates, median time to progression and overall survival compared with 5-FU/LV alone in patients with metastatic colorectal cancer. Preclinical studies have demonstrated irinotecan to be a potent radiosensitising agent in human lung tumour xenografts and colorectal cancer. Irinotecan may potentiate radiation by attaching to the DNA-topoisomerase I adducts in sites of DNA single strand breaks. Alternatively, fractionated radiotherapy could synchronise the tumor cell population in the S phase of the cell cycle, where cells are more sensitive to irinotecan chemotherapy. The major dose limiting toxicity of combining irinotecan with 5-FU and radiation was diarrhea. The rate of severe neutropenia did not appear to be increased.

Given its systemic and radiosensitizing activities, irinotecan has been incorporated in the neoadjuvant treatment of rectal cancer.

3.4.1 Irinotecan/5-FU plus radiotherapy

In a phase I/II study, Mitchell et al evaluated a weekly irinotecan regimen in combination with 5-FU and concurrent pelvic radiation. Patients with primary or recurrent clinical stage T3/4 adenocarcinoma of the rectum received escalating doses of weekly irinotecan (30 to 50 mg/m^2) in combination with continuous-infusion 5-FU and concurrent RT (50.4 Gy). The MTD in this study was identified as irinotecan at 50 mg/m^2 in combination with 5-FU at 225 mg/m^2/d on radiation days. pCR rate was 24% (Mitchell, 2000).

In another irinotecan-based neoadjuvant trial, 37 patients were treated with irinotecan at 50 mg/m2/wk and continuous-infusion 5-FU (250 mg/m^2/d, days 1–43) concurrently with RT (50.4 Gy in 28 fractions). The pCR rate was 22%, tumor-downstaging rate was 75%, and PFS at 40 months was 73% (Klautke et al, 2005).

A phase II trial (Mohiuddin et al, 2006) evaluated 5-FU plus hyperfractionated RT in comparison with standard RT combined with infusional 5-FU and weekly irinotecan. The Irinotecan arm consisted of 5-FU (225 mg/m^2/d Mondays through Fridays) plus irinotecan (50 mg/m^2/wk) and conventional RT (50.4 Gy for T3 and 54 Gy for T4). The tumor-downstaging rate was 78% and pCR rate was 28%.

A modest pCR rate (14%) was described in another study (Navarro et al, 2006) of continuous-infusion 5-FU (225 mg/m^2/d), irinotecan (50 mg/m^2/wk), and concurrent RT (45 Gy).

Irinotecan was also investigated on a daily × 5 schedule in combination with a standard-bolus 5-FU/LV-plus-RT regimen. A total of 59 patients were treated with RT (45 Gy), 5-FU/LV (350/20 mg/m^2/d) on days 1 to 5 and 29 to 33, and escalating doses of irinotecan (6, 8, 10, 12, 14, 16, 18, and 20 mg/m^2/d) on days 1 to 5 and 29 to 33. Irinotecan at 18 mg/m^2 was selected as the recommended dose for future studies. A pCR was observed in 24% patients and tumor downstaging in 41% of patients (Glynne-Jones et al, 2007).

The above studies incorporating irinotecan with 5-FU and radiation appear to show promising results, as seen in the pCR rate and the number of patients who eventually had successful surgery. Nonetheless, toxicity (mainly diarrhea) is of concern.

3.4.2 Irinotecan/capecitabine plus radiotherapy

The combination of irinotecan, capecitabine and radiation therapy has been investigated in the neoadjuvant treatment of rectal cancer.

In a phase I study, Hofheinz et al evaluated a weekly regimen of Irinotecan in combination with twice-daily capecitabine and radiation therapy. The recommended regimen from this study consisted of capecitabine at 500 mg/m^2 twice daily in combination with weekly Irinotecan at 50 mg/m^2/wk plus RT (50.4 Gy in 28 fractions). An interesting pCR rate of 21% was seen (Hofheinz et al, 2005).

A phase II study further evaluated the safety and efficacy of these dose levels in 36 patients. A pCR was seen in 15% of patients, tumor downstaging in 55% and grade 3/4 diarrhea in 11% of patients (Willeke, 2007).

In another phase I/II study, Klautke et al investigated a regimen of weekly Irinotecan at 40 mg/m^2 in combination with escalating doses of capecitabine twice daily and concurrent RT (50.4 Gy). The maximum tolerated dose was confirmed at the 750 mg/m^2 capecitabine dose level. Pathologic complete response was achieved in15%, while pathologic downstaging was seen in 62% of patients (Klautke et al, 2006).

No adequately powered head-to-head studies have compared irinotecan- or oxaliplatin-based neoadjuvant chemoradiation studies. In a small neoadjuvant randomized phase II study, similar downstaging was seen for both capecitabine/oxaliplatin– and capecitabine/irinotecan-based neoadjuvant radiation. The irinotecan-based combination was associated with increased diarrhea and chemoradiation-induced fibrosis (Privitera et al, 2006).

Although preliminary, the current findings indicate that combinations of capecitabine and weekly irinotecan are feasible in this setting.

3.4.3 Irinotecan/UFT plus radiotherapy

Preliminary results from a Japanese phase I trial in which UFT (300 mg/m^2/day, 5 days/week) was combined with concurrent weekly irinotecan (starting at 30 mg/m^2) and RT (2 Gy/day, 40–50 Gy total) resulted in an excess of grade 3 diarrhea (Yasui et al, 2006).

3.5 Bevacizumab-based chemoradiation

Vascular endothelial growth factor (VEGF) mRNA and protein expression is markedly upregulated in metastatic colon and rectal cancer and is associated with disease progression and inferior survival. VEGF blockade serves as a potent and nontoxic enhancer of radiation therapy. It can reduce tumor vascular permeability and tumor interstitial pressure, thus enhancing delivery of large molecules to tumors. Life-threatening toxicities seen to date have included hemorrhage and thrombosis. Less severe toxicities include proteinuria, hypertension, fever, chills, rash, headache, infection, epistaxis and mouth ulceration.

Based on the improved outcome of the addition of bevacizumab with 5-FU/LV–based regimens in the metastatic setting and the synergy with radiation therapy in preclinical models, there is a strong rationale for combining antiangiogenic therapy with neoadjuvant chemoradiation therapy in patients with rectal cancer.

3.5.1 Bevacizumab/5-fu plus radiotherapy

The safety of bevacizumab in the neoadjuvant chemoradiation setting was established in a phase I/II study. A total of 22 patients received bevacizumab (5 or 10 mg/kg) every 2 weeks, continuous-infusion 5-FU (225 $mg/m^2/24$ h), and RT (50.4 Gy), followed by surgery in 7 to 9 weeks. Two of the five patients in the cohort receiving bevacizumab at 10 mg/Kg with 5-FU plus RT experienced grade 3/4 dose-limiting diarrhea and colitis during treatment. This regimen showed significant downstaging (55%) with a 22% pCR rate. Bevacizumab at 5 mg/kg every 2 weeks in combination with RT plus 5-FU yielded promising results and did not show any dose-limiting toxicity or perioperative morbidity/mortality (Willett et al, 2007).

3.5.2 Bevacizumab/capecitabine plus radiotherpy

Crane et al reported the preliminary results of a phase II trial in patients with T3/T4 or node-positive rectal cancer receiving preoperative RT (50.4 Gy), every-other-week bevacizumab (5 mg/kg for three doses starting concurrently with RT), and capecitabine (900 mg/m^2 orally twice a day on RT days only), followed by surgery. No grade 3 toxicity was observed. Five patients (29%) achieved a pCR (Crane et al, 2007).

Torino et al presented the results of a phase II study of neoadjuvant antiangiogenic therapy (intravenous infusion of bevacizumab 5 mg/Kg each two weeks for 4 courses, the first administration 2 weeks before chemoradiotherapy) combined with capecitabine (825 mg/m^2 twice daily) and RT (50.4 Gy / 28 fractions) in patients with locally advanced rectal cancer. The authors concluded this is a feasible and safe regimen with a tumor downstaging rate of 6.9%, a pCR rate of 9.3% and conservative surgery in 72.5% patients (Torino et al, 2008).

3.5.3 Bevacizumab plus xeliri/-xelox plus radiotherapy

Bevacizumab was also evaluated with capecitabine and either oxaliplatin or irinotecan in a pilot feasibility study. A total of 11 patients with advanced rectal cancer received bevacizumab (5 mg/Kg) every 2 weeks with capecitabine (1000 mg/m^2 twice daily on days 1 to 14 before the chemoradiation phase and then 825 mg/m^2 twice daily during RT on days 22 to 55) plus irinotecan at 180 mg/m^2 (XELIRI) or oxaliplatin at 130 mg/m^2 (XELOX) on days 1, 22, 43, and concurrent radiotherapy (54 Gy). Surgery was carried out 8 weeks after the completion of chemoradiation. Only one patient had grade 3 diarrhea and was unable to complete the planned chemotherapy. In combination with XELIRI/-XELOX plus RT, bevacizumab neither increased the treatment toxicity profile nor provoked any surgical delay or modifications (Privitera et al, 2007).

Another phase I trial from the Duke University evaluated the combination of concurrent capecitabine, oxaliplatin, and bevacizumab in patients with stage II–IV rectal cancer. A total of 11 patients were treated with escalating doses of capecitabine, oxaliplatin, and a fixed dose of bevacizumab (15 mg/Kg on day 1 and 10 mg/Kg on days 8 and 22). At dose level 1, patients were treated with oxaliplatin at 50 mg/m^2 weekly, capecitabine at 625 mg/m^2 twice daily, and concurrent RT (50.4 Gy) without dose-limiting toxicity. At dose level 2 (capecitabine, 825 mg/m^2 twice a day), two patients had dose-limiting toxicities of diarrhea and tenesmus-type symptoms. The recommended phase II dose was bevacizumab at 15 mg/Kg on day 1 and 10 mg/Kg on days 8 and 22, oxaliplatin at 50 mg/m^2 weekly, and capecitabine at 625 mg/m^2 twice a day on radiation days (Czito et al, 2007).

These studies suggest that the addition of bevacizumab to chemoradiation is safe and feasible in the neoadjuvant treatment of rectal cancer. Larger studies are needed to investigate whether the addition of this agent results in additional benefits in terms of tumor downstaging or disease-free survival.

3.6 Cetuximab plus chemoradiation

Cetuximab is a chimeric monoclonal antibody targeting the epidermal growth factor receptor (EGFR). EGFR is expressed in 25% to 75% of colorectal cancer and its overexpression has been associated with poor prognosis and increased risk for metastasis. This agent has significant clinical activity in metastatic colorectal cancer, both as monotherapy or in combination with irinotecan.

Cetuximab has a long-life and a convenient weekly dosing schedule. It is generally well tolerated with acne-like rash and nail changes being the most common side effects.

3.6.1 Cetuximab/5-FU plus radiotherapy

A pilot study conducted at Memorial Sloan-Kettering Cancer Center investigated the safety of cetuximab in combination with standard neoadjuvant 5-FU and RT in patients with locally advanced or locally recurrent rectal cancer. A total of 20 patients received cetuximab at 400 mg/m^2 on day 1 followed by 250 mg/m^2/wk × 4, continuous-infusion 5-FU at 225 mg/m^2/d over 5.5 weeks, and concurrent pelvic RT (50.4 Gy). Of the 20 patients enrolled, 12% of patients had a pCR. Grade 3 diarrhea was seen in 10% of patients (Chung, 2006).

3.6.2 Cetuximab/capecitabine plus radiotherapy

A Belgian phase I/II trial evaluated a regimen of cetuximab, capecitabine, and RT in 40 patients with endoscopically staged locally advanced rectal cancer. Patients were treated with a loading dose of cetuximab at 400 mg/m^2 the first week followed by 250 mg/m^2/wk × 5, escalating doses of capecitabine twice daily, and concurrent RT (45 Gy in 25 fractions). The recommended regimen consisted of capecitabine, 825 mg/m^2 twice daily, in combination with cetuximab and RT. This dose level was investigated in 30 patients. Only 2 patients (5%) experienced a pCR. Grade 3 diarrhea occurred in 15% of patients (Machiels, 2007).

3.6.3 Cetuximab/capecitabine/oxaliplatin plus radiotherapy

Cetuximab was also investigated in combination with oxaliplatin, capecitabine, and concurrent RT. Rodel et al conducted a phase I/II trial of cetuximab (400 mg/m^2 loading dose followed by 250 mg/m²/wk × 5), oxaliplatin 50 mg/m² weekly, escalating doses of capecitabine (days 1 to 14 and days 22 to 35), and RT (50.4 Gy). The phase II dose was identified at a capecitabine dose level of 1650 mg/m²/d on days 1 to 14 and 22 to 35. A total of 48 patients were enrolled on the phase II trial. Tumor downstaging was observed in 47% patients with pCR in 9% patients. Grade 3-4 diarrhea was seen in 19% patients. This combination is feasible and safe and the addition of cetuximab did not compromise chemotherapy doses and did not lead to higher toxicity. However, the addition of cetuximab produced a relatively low rate of pathologic responses and underachieved the assumptions. Further preclinical and clinical research is necessary to clarify the mechanism and define the reason of this phenomenon (Rödel, 2007).

3.6.4 Cetuximab/irinotecan/capecitabine plus radiotherapy

Cetuximab has been similarly investigated in Irinotecan-based neoadjuvant rectal cancer trials. A German phase I trial investigated a combination of cetuximab, irinotecan, and capecitabine in 20 patients with rectal cancer. Cetuximab was given weekly (400 mg/m² loading dose followed by 250 mg/m² on days 8, 15, 22, and 29) and escalating doses of irinotecan and capecitabine with pelvic RT (50.4 Gy). Irinotecan at 40 mg/m² and capecitabine at 500 mg/m² twice daily were determined as the recommended doses for future studies. About 7% of patients with T3 disease and 80% with T2 disease achieved a pCR (Hofheinz, 2006).
Larger phase II trials are ongoing.

4. Short course *vs* long course radiotherapy

As mentioned above, randomized trials have demonstrated superior local control, lower toxicity and better compliance of radiotherapy or radiochemotherapy administered before rather than after surgery. Similar long-term survival, local control and late morbidity have been reported for both these methods in non-comparative studies.
The benefit of the short-course schedule is a lower rate of early toxicity than with chemoradiation. It is less expensive and more convenient, especially in centers with a long waiting list. On the other hand, the use of high doses per fraction raises concern about late toxicity.
Conventionally fractionated chemoradiation might be better than the short course radiation schedule at reducing local recurrences as well as permitting better sphincter preservation because tumor bulk is reduced before surgery. However, there is no firm evidence to support this. In Europe, there is still much debate about the two different approaches to preoperative therapy.
Bujko et al have randomly assigned 312 patients to receive either preoperative irradiation (25 Gy / 5 fractions) and surgery within 7 days or chemoradiation (50.4 Gy / 28 fraction with bolus 5-FU and LV) and surgery 4-6 weeks later. Early toxicity was higher in the chemoradiation group (18.2% *vs* 3.2%, $p<0.001$). After a median follow-up of 48 months, there were no differences on 4-year OS (67.2% *vs* 66.2%, $p = 0.960$), disease free survival (58.4% *vs* 55.6, $p = 0,820$), local recurrence (9% *vs* 14.2%, $p = 0.170$) or severe late toxicity (10.1% *vs* 7.1%, $p = 0.360$) (Bujko, 2006).
The intergroup trial (TROG, AGITG, CSSANZ, RACS) also randomized patients either to short course radiotherapy (25 Gy in 5 fractions in 1 week, followed by surgery the following week, and 6 courses of postoperative chemotherapy) or long course chemoradiotherapy

(pelvic RT 50.4 Gy, 1.8 Gy/fraction, in 5.5 weeks, continuous infusion 5-FU 225 mg/m^2/day during RT, followed by surgery in 4 to 6 weeks, and 4 courses of postoperative chemotherapy). Each course of postoperative chemotherapy was to be 5-FU 425 mg/m^2 and folinic acid 20 mg/m^2 for 5 days. There was no clear evidence for a difference between short course radiotherapy and long course chemoradiotherapy in terms of 3-year local recurrence rates (7.5% vs 4.4%, p = 0.24). Distant recurrence (5-year distant recurrence-free rates were 72% *vs* 69%, $p = 0.85$) and OS rates (5-years OS were 74% *vs* 70%, $p = 0.56$) were similar. Both provided good local control. Late toxicity rates were not substantially different between arms (RTOG grade 3-4: 7.6% *vs* 8.8%; $p = 0.84$) (Ngan, 2010).

The Stockholm III trial addressed issues regarding the fractionation of radiotherapy and timing of surgery for rectal cancer. They randomized patients into 3 groups: Group 1 - short-course RT (5 x 5Gy) and surgery within 1 week; Group 2 - short-course RT (5 x 5Gy) and surgery after 4-8 weeks; Group 3 – long-course RT (25 x 2Gy) and surgery after 4-8 weeks. Severe acute toxicity was low, irrespective of fractionation. Short-course radiotherapy with immediate surgery had a tendency towards more postoperative complications, but only if surgery was delayed beyond 10 days after the start of radiotherapy (Pettersson, 2010).

The Berlin Cancer Society is recruiting patients for a multi-centre randomized study either to short-course radiotherapy (25 Gy / 5 fractions) + TME surgery within 5 days or radiochemotherapy (50.4 Gy / 28 fractions with continuous infusion 5-FU) + TME surgery 4-6 weeks later. All patients received adjuvant chemotherapy (12 weeks continuous infusion 5-FU) (Siegel, 2010).

5. Prognostic factors for responders to chemoradiation

The predictive factors for response to neoadjuvant chemoradiotherapy in rectal cancer have not been well characterized. A better understanding of predictive factors eventually may lead to the development of risk-adapted treatment strategies, such as more aggressive preoperative regimens, in patients who are less likely to respond to standard preoperative therapy.

The role of tumor markers, CEA and CA19.9, in rectal cancer is still in debate. In 2006 Yoon-ah Park et al showed that elevated pretreatment CEA levels (>5ng/ml) were associated with poor tumor response to preoperative chemoradiation (Park, 2006). Das et al (Das, 2007) concluded that CEA level (>2.5 ng/ml) resulted in significantly lower pCR rates ($p = 0.015$).

The most commonly reported early endpoint is the rate of pCR. It appears to be associated in some non randomized studies with improvement in PFS (Janjan, 2001; Valentini; 2002). It has been shown in one randomized trial that time interval between RT and surgery influences the degree of downstaging, with 10% of patients operated within 2 weeks of RT experiencing pathological downstaging compared to 26% of patients operated 6-8 weeks after RT ($p = 0.005$) (Francois, 1999). Many studies have shown that neoadjuvant chemoradiotherapy significantly increases the rate of pCR, as well as nodal and tumor downstaging.

The most recent published article (Maas, 2010) evaluating the long-term outcome in patients with a pCR after chemoradiotherapy for rectal cancer concluded that patients with pCR have better long-term outcome than those who did not. They stated that pCR might be indicative of a prognostically favourable biological tumor profile with lower propensity for local or distant recurrence and improved survival.

The Gastro-Intestinal Working Group of the Italian Association of Radiation Oncology analyzed retrospectively 566 patients with LARC achieving pCR after neoadjuvant therapy and they verified that this favorable group of patients had a very low rate of local recurrence (1.2%) and a favorable clinical outcome independent of the neoadjuvant chemotherapy schedule used, achieving a 5-year PFS of 84.7% and 5-year OS of 91.6%. In such a group of patients, the use of postoperative chemotherapy could be very debatable. Conversely, the subset of patients older than 60 years, with cStage III and treated with a radiation dose of 45 Gy or less experienced a relatively worse prognosis, even after achieving ypCR. The prognosis of the high-risk group of patients compares with the outcome of a non-selected population (Capirci, 2008).

Some other studies (Kim, 2006; Fernandez-Martos, 2004; Rodel, 2005; García-Aguilar, 2003). also showed excellent oncologic outcomes in patients with pCR. Valentini et al (Valentini, 2002) have demonstrated that, after preoperative chemoradiotherapy, clinical response and tumor and nodal pathologic downstaging have a close correlation with improved outcome. Indeed, patients with tumor downstaging had a 5-year local control of 87.8%, a PFS of 73.1% and an OS of 82.9%, while those who had not tumor downstaging had a local control of 70.5%, a PFS of 47.2% and an OS of 60.9%. Those patients with nodal downstaging also had better 5-year local control (84.3%), PFS (67.1%) and OS (74.3%) than those who did not have nodal downstaging (72%, 42.2% and 56.1%, respectively).

On the other hand, Salvatore Pucciarelli et al have not found statistically significant differences for PFS and OS on comparing the actuarial survival curves of patients with different tumor responses to preoperative treatment, whether evaluated as tumor regression grade or as pTNM stage (Pucciarelli, 2004).

It was in this context that we developed a single-institute study to evaluate the therapeutic response and impact on survival of preoperative RT, alone or combined with chemotherapy, in patients with locally advanced rectal cancer. We studied 132 patients treated preoperatively either with RT alone, RT and concomitant oral chemotherapy (capecitabine or UFT+LV) or RT and concomitant chemotherapy with 5-FU in continuous infusion. Patients were then submitted to adjuvant chemotherapy. In our study we verified that the combination of chemotherapy to RT significantly increased the tumor response, especially the nodal downstaging, at the expense of a higher but manageable toxicity (majority grade 1-2 toxicities). It also allowed a higher complete surgical resection without increasing postoperative complications rate. Tumor downstaging was superior (p = 0.224) in patients treated with chemoradiotherapy (CAP/UFT-LV + RT: 47.7%; 5-FU + RT: 52.4%) than in patients of the RT arm (26.7%). Nodal downstaging was significantly better (p = 0.008) in CAP/UFT-LV + RT group comparing to RT group and 5-FU+RT group (82.1% *vs* 54.5% and 54.8%, respectively). The neoadjuvant chemoradiotherapy groups had better pCR (CAP/UFT-LV + RT GROUP: 16.9%; 5-FU + RT GROUP: 11.9%) compared to the RT arm (0%) (p = 0.207). We registered a locoregional control of 95%, the global 3- and 5-year PFS was 75% and 68%, respectively, the global 3- and 5-year OS was 88% and 80%, respectively. Both 5-year OS (84% *vs* 59%, p = 0.038) and PFS (69% *vs* 55%, p = 0.05) were significantly higher in patients treated with neoadjuvant chemoradiation than in the RT group. We have also found a better PFS in those patients who had pCR (100% *vs* 62%, p = 0.023). When considering only those patients cT3-4 who had downstaging to ypT0-2, we found a significantly better locoregional control (100% *vs* 89, p = 0.027), PFS (88% *vs* 43%, p = 0.003) and OS (89% *vs* 77%, p = 0.048). Adjuvant chemotherapy had no impact on locoregional control, PFS or on OS (Conde, 2010).

6. Conclusions

Neoadjuvant therapy is widely accepted as the current standard of care for locally advanced rectal cancer and has evolved from the use of preoperative radiation alone to wider use of preoperative combined chemoradiation. Downstaging of disease has been significantly improved and pCR which was historically below 10% with preoperative radiation alone, now range from 15-30% with preoperative chemoradiation. In a number of studies pCR following neoadjuvant therapy appears to be a strong surrogate for effectiveness of treatment with lower local recurrence of disease and improved sphincter preservation and survival of patients. While the availability of new chemotherapeutic drugs (oxaliplatin, irinotecan) and molecular targeted agents (bevacizumab, cetuximab) holds a great deal of promise, we have seen that in many cancers, more drugs or more intensive regimens are not always as successful as we would have hoped. Early results in phase II trials appear to have a pCR plateaued at 20-30%. The use of multi-drug combinations increased toxicity of treatment hence resulting in a suboptimal therapeutic ratio.

The historical problem of high local pelvic recurrence following surgery (20-30%) no longer is a cause of poor survival in patients (<10%). The problem remains the persistent high rate of distant metastasis (30-35%) in this disease. New paradigms in neoadjuvant therapy are therefore needed to further improve results of treatment. Although we have not been successful in developing new agents that are effective radiation sensitizers in rectal cancer, this is still a very worthwhile goal, and innovations in biologics and nanoparticles could be of major importance (Mohiuddin M., et al, 2009).

7. References

Alonso V., Lambea J., Salud A., et al. (2007). Preoperative chemoradiotherapy with Capecitabine and Oxaliplatin in locally advanced rectal carcinoma: A phase II trial (abstract 4044). *J Clin Oncol*, Vol. 25, No. 18S, (2007), pp. 174-179.

Aschele C., Pinto C., Cordio S., et al. (2009). Preoperative fluorouracil (FU)-based chemoradiation with and without weekly Oxaliplatin in locally advanced rectal cancer: Pathologic response analysis of the Studio Terapia Adiuvante Retto (STAR)-01 randomized phase III trial. *J Clin Oncol*, Vol. 27 No.18S, (2009) (suppl; abstr CRA4008).

Aschele C., Vitali M., Caroti C., et al. (2009). A phase I study of Uracil/Tegafur (UFT) and oral Leucovorin (LV) + weekly Oxaliplatin (OXA) and preoperative radiotherapy (RT) in locally advanced rectal cancer (LARC). ASCO 2009 (Abstr 409).

Bosset J., Calais G., Mineur L., et al. (2005). Enhanced tumorocidal effect of chemotherapy with preoperative radiotherapy for rectal cancer: preliminary results EORTC 22921. *J Clin Oncol*, Vol. 23, (2005), pp. 5620-5627.

Bujko K., Nowacki M.P., Nasierowska-Guttmejer A., et al. (2006). Long-term results of a randomized trial comparing preoperative short course radiotherapy with preoperative conventionally fractionated chemoradiation for rectal cancer; *Br J Surg*, Vol. 93, (2006), pp. 1215-1223.

Cammá C., Giunta M., Fiorica F., et al. (2000). Preoperative Radiotherapy for resectable rectal cancer. A meta-analysis. *JAMA*, Vol. 284, (2000), pp. 1008-1015.

Capirci C., Valentini V., Cionini L., et al. (2008). Prognostic value of pathologic complete response after neoadjuvant therapy in locally advanced rectal cancer: long-term analysis of 566 ypCR patients. *Int J Radiat Oncol Biol Phys*, Vol.72, No. 1, (2008), pp. 99-107.

Carlomagno C., Ferrante A., Solla R., et al. (2007). Preoperative chemoradiation therapy with Capecitabine (CAP) and Oxaliplatin (OX) in locally advanced rectal cancer (LARC): A phase II study (abstract 301). *Gastrointestinal Cancers Symposium*, (Jan 2007), pp. 19-21.

Carmichael J., Popiela T., Radstone D., et al. (1999). Randomized comparative study of ORZELt (oral Uracil/Tegafur (UFT™) plus Leucovorin (LV)) versus parenteral 5-fluorouracil (5-FU) in patients with metastatic colorectal cancer. *Proc Am Soc Clin Oncol*, Vol. 18, No. 264a, (1999), (abstr 1015)

Chung K.Y., Minsky B., Schrag D., et al. Phase I trial of preoperative Cetuximab with concurrent continuous infusion 5-fluorouracil and pelvic radiation in patients with local-regionally advanced rectal cancer (abstract 3560). *J Clin Oncol*, Vol. 24, No. 18S, (2006), pp. 161-169.

Colorectal Cancer Collaborative Group. (2001). Adjuvant radiotherapy for rectal cancer: a systematic overview of 8507 patients from 22 randomised trials. *Lancet*, Vol. 358, (2001), pp. 1291-1304.

Conde S., Borrego M., Teixeira T., et al. (2010). Impact of neoadjuvant chemoradiation on pathologic response and survival of patients with locally advanced rectal cancer. *Rep Pract Oncol Radiother*, Vol. 15, (2010), pp. 51-59.

Crane C., Eng C., Chang G., et al. (2007). Preliminary results of a phase II trial concurrent Bevacizumab with neoadjuvant Capecitabine based chemoradiation for locally advanced rectal cancer (abstract SS-10). *Oncology*, Vol. 5 (suppl 2), No.4, (2007).

Czito B.G., Bendell J.C., Willett C.G., et al. (2007). Bevacizumab, Oxaliplatin, and Capecitabine with radiation therapy in rectal cancer: Phase I trial results. *Int J Radiat Oncol Biol Phys*, Vol. 68, (2007), pp. 472-478.

Das P., Skibber J.M., Rodriguez-Bigas M.A., et al. (2007). Predictors of tumor response and downstaging in patients who receive preoperative chemoradiation for rectal cancer. *Cancer*, Vol. 109, (2007), pp. 1750-17555.

De Bruin A.F., Nuyttens J.J., Ferenschild F.T., et al. Preoperative chemoradiation with Capecitabine in locally advanced rectal cancer. *Netherl J Medicine*, Vol. 66, (2008), pp. 71-76.

de Gramont A., Figer A., Seymour M., et al. (2000) Leucovorin and fluorouracil with or without Oxaliplatin as first-line treatment in advanced colorectal cancer. *J Clin Oncol*, Vol. 18, (2000), pp. 2938-2947.

De la Torre A., Garcia-Berrocal M.I., Arias F., et al. (2008). Preoperative chemoradiatiotherapy for rectal cancer: randomized trial comparing oral Uracil and Tegafur and oral Leucovorin vs. intravenous 5-fluorouracil and Leucovorin. *Int J Radiat Oncol Phys*, Vol. 70, (2008), pp. 102-110.

De Paoli A., Chiara S., Luppi G., et al. (2006). Capecitabine in combination with preoperative radiation therapy in locally advanced, resectable, rectal cancer: a multicentric phase II study. *Ann Oncol*, Vol. 17, (2006), pp. 246-251.

Dunst J., Reese T., Sutter T. et al. (2002). Phase I trial evaluating the concurrent combination of radiotherapy and Capecitabine in rectal cancer. *J Clin Oncol*, Vol. 20, No. 19, (2002), pp. 3983-3991.

Dunst J., Reese T., Debus J. et al. (2004). Phase-II-study of preoperative chemoradiation with Capecitabine in rectal cancer. *Proc Am Soc Clin Oncol*, Vol. 23, (2004), pp. 260 (Abstr 3559).

Feliu J., Calvilio J., Escribano A. et al. (2002). Neoadjuvant therapy of rectal carcinoma with UFT–Leucovorin plus radiotherapy. *Ann Oncol*, Vol. 13, (2002), pp. 730–736.

Fernandez-Martos C., Aparicio J., Bosch C. et al. (2004). Preoperative Uracil, Tegafur, and concomitant radiotherapy in operable rectal cancer: a phase II multicenter study with 3 years' follow-up. *J Clin Oncol*, Vol. 22, (2004), pp. 3016–3022.

Fernandez-Martos C., Bosch C., Aparicio J. et al. Oxaliplatin, Uracil/Tegafur (UFT) and radiotherapy in operable rectal cancer. Preliminary results of a multicenter phase II study. *J Clin Oncol*, Vol 23 (16 Suppl) (Abstr 3648), (2005).

Folkesson J., Birgisson H., Pahlman L., et al. (2005). Swedish rectal cancer trial: long lasting benefits from radiotherapy on survival and local recurrence rate; *J Clin Oncol*, Vol. 23, (2005), pp. 5644-5650.

Francois Y., Nemoz C., Baulieux J., et al. (1999). Influence of the interval between radiation therapy and surgery on downstaging and rate of sphincter sparing surgery for rectal cancer: the Lyon R90-01 randomized trial. *J Clin Oncol*, Vol. 17, (1999), pp. 2396-2402.

García-Aguilar J., de Anda E.H., Sirivongs P. et al. (2003). A pathologic complete response to preoperative chemoradiation is associated with lower local recurrence and improved survival in rectal cancer patients treated by mesorectal excision. Dis *Colon Rectum*, (2003), pp. 298-304.

Gastrointestinal Tumor Study Group. (1985). Prolongation of the disease-free interval in surgically treated rectal carcinoma. *N Eng J Med*, Vol. 312, (1985), pp. 1465-1472.

Gérard J.P., Conroy T., Bonnetain F., et al. (2006). Preoperative radiotherapy with or without concurrent fluorouracil and Leucovorin in T3-4 rectal cancers: Results of FFCD 9203. *J Clin Oncol*, Vol. 24, (2006), pp. 4620-4625.

Gérard J.P., Azria D., Gourgou-Bourgade S., et al. (2010). Comparison of Two Neoadjuvant Chemoraditherapy Regimens for Locally Advanced Rectal Cancer: Results of the Phase III Trial ACCORD 12/0405-Prodige 2. *J Clin Oncol*, Vol. 28, (2010), pp. 1638-44.

Glynne-Jones R., Sebag-Montefiore D., Maughan T.S., et al. (2006). A phase I dose escalation study of continuous oral Capecitabine in combination with Oxaliplatin and pelvic radiation (XELOX-RT) in patients with locally advanced rectal cancer. *Ann Oncol*, Vol. 17, (2006), pp. 50-56.

Glynne-Jones R., Falk S., Maughan T.S., et al. (2007). A phase I/II study of Irinotecan when added to 5-fluorouracil and Leucovorin and pelvic radiation in locally advanced rectal cancer: A Colorectal Clinical Oncology Group Study. *Br J Cancer*, Vol. 96, (2007), p. 551-558.

Goldberg R.M., Sargent D.J., Morton R.F., et al. (2004). A randomized controlled trial of fluorouracil plus Leucovorin, Irinotecan, and Oxaliplatin combinations in patients with previously untreated metastatic colorectal cancer. *J Clin Oncol*, Vol. 22, (2004), pp. 23-30.

Grem J.L. (1997). Systemic treatment options in advanced colorectal cancer: perspectives on combination 5-fluorouracil plus Leucovorin. *Semin Oncol*, Vol. 24(Suppl. 18), (1997), pp. 8-18.

Gunderson L.L., Sosin H. (1974). Areas of failure found at reoperation (second or symptomatic look) following "curative surgery" for adenocarcninoma of the rectum. Clinicopathologic correlation and implications for adjuvant therapy. *Cancer*, Vol. 34, (1974), pp. 1278-1292.

Haller D.G., Cassidy J., Clarke S., et al. (2006). Tolerability of fluoropyrimidines appears to differ by region (abstract 3514). *J Clin Oncol*, Vol. 24, No. 18S, (2006), pp. 149.

Hirata K., Sasaki K., Yamamitsu S., et al. (1993). A comparison of 5-fluorouracil concentration of 5-fluorouracil drip infusion versus oral UFT in plasma of same patients. *Jpn J Cancer Chemother*, Vol. 20, (1993), pp. 1409-1411.

Ho D.H., Pazdur R., Covington W. et al. (1998). Comparison of 5-fluorouracil pharmacokinetics in patients receiving continuous 5-fluorouracil infusion and oral Uracil plus N1-(2'-tetrahydrofuryl)-5-fluorouracil. *Clin Cancer Res*, Vol. 4, (1998), pp. 2085–2088.

Hoff P.M., Pazdur R., Benner S.E., et al. (1998). UFT and Leucovorin: A review of its clinical development and therapeutic potential in the oral treatment of cancer. Anticancer *Drugs*, Vol. 9, (1998), pp. 479-490.

Hoff P.M., Janjan N., Saad E.D. et al. (2000). Phase I study of preoperative oral Uracil and Tegafur plus Leucovorin and radiation therapy in rectal cancer. *J Clin Oncol*, Vol. 18, (2000), pp. 3529–3534.

Hoff P.M., Ansari R., Batist G., et al. (2001). Comparison of oral Capecitabine versus intravenous fluorouracil plus Leucovorin as firstline treatment in 605 patients with metastatic colorectal cancer: Results of a randomized phase III study. *J Clin Oncol*, Vol. 19, (2001), pp. 2282–2292.

Hofheinz R.D., von Gerstenberg-Helldorf B., Wenz F., et al. (2005). Phase I trial of Capecitabine and weekly Irinotecan in combination with radiotherapy for neoadjuvant therapy of rectal cancer. *J Clin Oncol*, Vol. 23, (2005), pp. 1350-1357.

Hofheinz R.D., Horisberger K., Woernle C., et al. (2006). Phase I trial of Cetuximab in combination with Capecitabine, weekly Irinotecan, and radiotherapy as neoadjuvant therapy for rectal cancer. *Int J Radiat Oncol Biol Phys*, Vol. 66, (2006), pp. 1384-1390.

Janjan N.A., Crane C., Feig B.W., Cleary K. et al. (2001). Improved overall survival among responders to preoperative chemoradiation for locally advanced rectal cancer. *Am J Clin Oncol*, Vol. 24, (2001), pp. 107–112.

Kapiteijn E., Marijnen C.A.M., Nagtegaal I.D., et al. (2001). Preoperative radiotherapy combined with total mesorectal excision for resectable rectal cancer; *N Engl J Med*, Vol. 345, No 9, (2001), pp. 638-646.

Kim J.C., Kim T.W., Kim J.H., et al. (2005). Preoperative concurrent radiotherapy with Capecitabine before total mesorectal excision in locally advanced rectal cancer; *Int J Radiat Oncol Biol Phys*, Vol. 63, No 2, (2005), pp. 346-353.

Kim N.K., Baik S.H., Seong J.S., et al. (2006). Oncologic outcomes after neoadjuvant chemoradiation followed by curative resection with tumor-specific mesorectal excision for fixed locally advanced rectal cancer: Impact of postirradiated pathologic downstaging on local recurrence and survival. *Ann Surg*, Vol. 244, No 6, (2006), pp. 1024-30.

Kim D.Y., Jung K.H., Kim T.H., et al. (2007). Comparison of 5-Fluorouracil/Leucovorin and Capecitabine in preoperative chemoradiotherapy for locally advanced rectal cancer. *Int J Radiat Oncol Biol Phys*, Vol. 67, (2007), pp. 378-384.

Kim S.Y., Hong S.Y., Kim D.Y., et al. (2009). A pilot study of neoadjuvant chemoradiation with higher dose enteric-coated Tegafur/Uracil plus Leucovorin for locally advanced rectal cancer. *ECCO/ESMO 2009* (poster).

Klautke G., Feyerherd P., Ludwig K., et al. (2005). Intensified concurrent chemoradiotherapy with 5-fluorouracil and Irinotecan as neoadjuvant treatment in patients with locally advanced rectal cancer. *Br J Cancer*, Vol. 92, (2005), pp. 1215-1220.

Klautke G., Kuchenmeister U., Foitzik T., et al. (2006). Concurrent chemoradiation with Capecitabine and weekly Irinotecan as preoperative treatment for rectal cancer: Results from a phase I/II study. *Br J Cancer*, Vol. 94, (2006), pp. 976-981.

Krishnan S., Janjan N.A., Skibber J.M., et al. (2006). Phase II study of Capecitabine (Xeloda®) and concomitant boost radiotherapy in patients with locally advanced rectal cancer; *Int J Radiat Oncol Biol Phys*, Vol. 66, No. 3, (2006), pp. 762-771.

Kundel Y., Brenner B., Symon Z. et al. (2007). A phase II study of oral UFT and Leucovorin concurrently with pelvic irradiation as neoadjuvant chemoradiation for rectal cancer. *Anticancer Res*, Vol. 27, (2007), pp. 2877–2880.

Lee C.R., Nicholson P.W., Souhami R.L., et al. (1992). Patient compliance with oral chemotherapy as assessed by a novel oral technique; *J Clin Oncol*, Vol. 10, (1992), pp. 1007-1013.

Maas M., Nelemans P.J., Valentini V., et al. (2010). Long-term outcome in patients with a pathological complete response after chemoradiation for rectal cancer: a pooled analysis of individual patient data. *Lancet Oncol*, Vol. 11, No. 9, (2010), pp. 835-44.

Machiels J.P., Duck L., Honhon B., et al. (2005). Phase II study of preoperative Oxaliplatin, Capecitabine and external beam radiotherapy in patients with rectal cancer: The RadiOxCape study. *Ann Oncol*, Vol. 16, (2005), pp. 1898-1905.

Machiels J.P., Sempoux C., Scalliet P., et al. (2007). Phase I/II study of preoperative Cetuximab, Capecitabine, and external beam radiotherapy in patients with rectal cancer. *Ann Oncol*, Vol. 18, (2007), pp. 738-744.

Mitchell E.P. (2000). Irinotecan in preoperative combined-modality therapy for locally advanced rectal cancer. *Oncology*, Vol. 14, (2000), pp. 56-59.

Miwa M., Ura M., Nishida M., et al. (1998). Design of a novel oral fluoropyrimidine carbamate, Capecitabine, which generates 5-fluorouracil selectively in tumours by enzymes concentrated in human liver and cancer tissue. *Eur J Cancer*, Vol. 34, (1998), pp. 1274-81.

Mohiuddin M., Winter K., Mitchell E., et al. (2006). Randomized phase II study of neoadjuvant combined-modality chemoradiation for distal rectal cancer: Radiation Therapy Oncology Group Trial 0012. *J Clin Oncol*, Vol. 24, (2006), pp. 650-655.

Mohiuddin M., Mohiuddin M., Marks J., et al. (2009). Future directions in neoadjuvant therapy of rectal cancer: Maximizing pathological complete response rates. *Cancer Treatment Reviews*, Vol. 35, (2009), pp. 547-52.

Nakazato H., Koike A., Saji S., et al. (1997). Efficacy of oral UFT as adjuvant chemotherapy to curative resection of colorectal cancer: A prospective randomized clinical trial. *Proc Am Soc Clin Oncol*, Vol. 16, (1997), pp. 279a (abstr 990).

National Institutes of Health Consensus Conference. Adjuvant therapy for patients with colon and rectal cancer. *J Am Med Assoc*, Vol. 264, (1990), pp. 1444–1450.

Navarro M., Dotor E., Rivera F., et al. (2006). A Phase II study of preoperative radiotherapy and concomitant weekly Irinotecan in combination with protracted venous infusion 5-fluorouracil, for resectable locally advanced rectal cancer. *Int J Radiat Oncol Biol Phys*, Vol. 66, (2006), pp. 201-205.

Ngan S., Fisher R., Goldstein D., et al. (2010). A randomized trial comparing local recurrence (LR) rates between short-course (SC) and long-course (LC) preoperative radiotherapy (RT) for clinical T3 rectal cancer: An intergroup trial (TROG, AGITG, CSSANZ, RACS); *J Clin Oncol*, Vol. 28, (2010), pp. 15s (suppl; abstr 3509).

Ofner D., de Vries A., Thaler J., et al. (2007). Preoperative Oxaliplatin (O), Capecitabine (X), and external beam radiotherapy (RT) in patients (pts) with newly diagnosed, primary operable, locally advanced rectal cancer (LARC) (abstract 14527). *J Clin Oncol*, Vol. 25, No. 18S, (2007), pp. 627.

Okabe H., Toko T., Saito H., et al. (1997). Augmentation of the chemotherapeutic effectiveness of UFT, a combination of Tegafur [1-(2-tetrahydrofuryl)-5-fluorouracil] with uracil, by oral 1-Leucovorin. *Anticancer Res*, Vol. 17, (1997), pp. 157-164.

Park Y., Sohn S., Seong J., et al. (2006). Serum CEA as a predictor for the response to preoperative chemoradiation in rectal cancer. J. Surg. *Oncol*, Vol. 93, (2006), pp. 145-150.

Pazdur R., Douillard J.Y., Skillings J.R., et al. (1999). Multicenter phase III study of 5-fluorouracil (5-FU) or UFT™ in combination with Leucovorin (LV) in patients with metastatic colorectal cancer. *Proc Am Soc Clin Oncol*, Vol. 18, (1999), pp. 263 (abstr 1009).

Peeters K.C.N.J., Marijnen C.A.M., Nagtegaal I.D., et al. (2007). The TME Trial after a median follow-up of 6 years: increased local control but no survival benefit in irradiated patients with resectable rectal carcinoma; *Ann Surgery*, Vol. 246, No. 5, (2007), pp. 693-701.

Pentheroudakis G., Twelves C. (2002). The rational development of Capecitabine from the laboratory to the clinic. *Anticancer Res*, Vol. 22, (2002), pp. 3589–3596.

Pettersson D., Cedermark B., Holm T., et al. (2010). Interim analysis of the Stockholm III trial of preoperative radiotherapy regimens for rectal cancer; *Br J Surg*, Vol. 97, No. 4, (2010), pp. 580-587.

Pfeffer M.R., Kundel Y., Zehavi M. et al. (2004). A phase I study of oral UFT given concomitantly with standard preoperative radiotherapy for rectal cancer. *Isr Med Assoc J*, Vol. 6, (2004), pp. 595–598.

Privitera G., Spatola C., Acquaviva G., et al. (2007). Addition of Bevacizumab (Beva) to xeliri/xelox chemoradiotherapy in neoadjuvant setting for patients (pts) with locally advanced rectal cancer (LARC): A feasibility study. *J Clin Oncol*, Vol. 25, No. 18S, (2007), pp. 631 (abstract 14583).

Privitera G., Spatola C., Acquaviva G., et al. (2006). Neoadjuvant XELOX vs XELIRI in combination with concomitant boost 3D-conformal radiotherapy in locally advanced rectal cancer (LARC) (abstract 3570). *J Clin Oncol*, Vol. 24, No. 18S, (2006), pp. 163.

Pucciarelli S., Toppan P., Friso M.L. et al. (2004). Complete pathologic response following preoperative chemoradiation therapy for middle to lower rectal cancer is not a prognostic factor for a better outcome. *Dis Colon Rectum*, Vol. 47, (2004), pp. 1798-1807.

Rich T., Gunderson L.L., Lew R., et al. (1983). Patterns of recurrence of rectal cancer after potencially curative surgery. *Cancer*, Vol. 52, (1983), pp. 1317-1329.

Rodel C., Martus P., Papadoupolos T., et al. (2005). Prognostic significance of tumor regression after preoperative chemoradiotherapy for rectal cancer. *J Clin Oncol*, Vol. 23, (2005), pp. 8688-8696.

Rodel C., Arnold D., Hipp M., et al. (2007). Phase I-II Trial of Cetuximab, Capecitabine, Oxaliplatin, and radiotherapy as preoperative treatment in rectal cancer. *Int J Radiat Oncol Biol Phys*, Vol. 70, (2007), pp. 1081-1086.

Roedel C., Arnold D., Hipp M., et al. (2006). Multicenter phase II trial of preoperative radiotherapy with concurrent and adjuvant Capecitabine and Oxaliplatin in locally advanced rectal cancer; German Rectal Cancer Study Group. *Gastrointestinal Cancers Symposium*, (2006), (abstract 349).

Rutten H., Sebag-Montefiore D., Glynne-Jones R., et al. (2006). Capecitabine, Oxaliplatin, radiotherapy, and excision (CORE) in patients with MRI-defined locally advanced rectal adenocarcinoma: Results of an international multicenter phase II study. *J Clin Oncol*, Vol. 24, No. 18S, (2006), pp. 153 (abstract 3528).

Ryan D.P., Niedzwiecki D., Hollis D., et al. (2006). Phase I/II study of preoperative Oxaliplatin, Fluorouracil, and external-beam radiation therapy in patients with locally advanced rectal cancer: Cancer and Leukemia Group B 89901. *J Clin Oncol*, Vol. 24, (2006), pp. 2557-2562.

Salimichokami M., Vafai M., Derakhshani S., et al. (2006). Phase-2 study of neoadjuvant chemoradiation in locally advanced rectal adenocarcinoma: The Radio-Xelox study. *J Clin Oncol*, Vol. 24, No. 18S, (2006), pp. 620(abstract 13549).

Sauer R., Becker H., Hohenberger W., et al. (2004). Preoperative versus postoperative chemoradiotherapy for rectal cancer. *N Eng J Med*, Vol. 351, (2004), pp. 1731–1740.

Sawada N., Ishikawa T., Sekiguchi F., et al. (1999). X-ray irradiation induces thymidine phosphorylase and enhances the efficacy of Capecitabine (Xeloda) in human cancer xenografts. *Clin Cancer Res*, Vol. 5, (1999), pp. 2948-2953.

Schuller J., Cassidy J., Dumont E., et al. (2000). Preferential activation of Capecitabine in tumor following oral administration to colorectal cancer patients. *Cancer Chemother Pharmacol*, Vol. 45, (2000), pp. 291-297.

Segab-Montefiore D., Stephens R.J., Steele R., et al. (2009). Preoperative radiotherapy versus selective postoperative Chemoradiotherapy in patients with rectal cancer (MRC CR07 and NCIC-CTG C016): a multicentre, randomized trial. *Lancet*, Vol. 373, (2009), pp. 811-820.

Siegel R., Burock S., Wernecke K., et al. (2009). Preoperative short-course radiotherapy versus combined radiochemotherapy in locally advanced rectal cancer: a multi-centre prospectively randomized study of the Berlin Cancer Society - Study protocol; *BMC Cancer*, Vol. 9, (2009), pp. 50.

Sulkes A., Benner S.E., Canetta R.M. (1998). Uracil-ftorafur: An oral fluoropyrimidine active in colorectal cancer. *J Clin Oncol*, Vol. 16, (1998), pp. 3461–3475.

Swedish Rectal Cancer Trial. (1997). Improved survival with preoperative radiotherapy in resectable rectal cancer. *N Engl J Med*, Vol. 336, (1997), pp. 980-987.

Torino F., Cascinu S., Ciardiello F. et al. (2008). A Phase II Study of Neoadjuvant Antiangiogenic Therapy Combined With Capecitabine (C) and Radiotherapy (RT) in Patients with Locally Advanced Rectal Cancer (LARC). *ESMO 2008* (abstract 418P)

Valentini V., Coco C., Picciocchi A., et al. (2002). Does downstaging predict improved outcome after preoperative chemoradiation for extraperitoneal locally advanced rectal cancer? A long-term analysis of 165 patients. *Int J Radiat Oncol Biol Phys*, Vol. 53, (2002), pp. 664–674.

Van Cutsem E., Twelves C., Cassidy J., et al. (2001). Oral Capecitabine compared with intravenous fluorouracil plus Leucovorin in patients with metastatic colorectal cancer: Results of a large phase III study. *J Clin Oncol*, Vol. 19, (2001), pp. 4097–4106.

Wang L.W., Yang S.H., Lin J.K., et al. (2005). Pre-operative chemoradiotherapy with oral Tegafur–Uracil and Leucovorin for rectal cancer. *J Surg Oncol*, Vol. 89, (2005), pp. 256–263.

Willeke F., Horisberger K., Kraus-Tiefenbacher U., et al. (2007). A phase II study of Capecitabine and Irinotecan in combination with concurrent pelvic radiotherapy (CapIri-RT) as neoadjuvant treatment of locally advanced rectal cancer. Br J Cancer, Vol. 96, (2007), pp. 912-917.

Willett C., Duda D., Boucher Y., et al. (2007). Phase I/II study of neoadjuvant Bevacizumab with radiation therapy and 5-fluorouracil in patients with rectal cancer: initial results. J Clin Oncol, Vol. 25, No. 18S, (2007), pp. 173(abstract 4041).

Wolmark N., Wieand H.S., Hyams D.M., et al. (2000). Randomizes trial of postoperative adjuvant chemotherapy with or without radiotherapy for carcinoma of the rectum: National Surgical Adjuvant Breast and Bowel Project Protocol R-02; J Natl Cancer Inst, Vol. 92, (2000), pp. 388-396.

Yasui M., Ikeda M., Sekimoto M., et al. (2006). Preliminary results of phase I trial of oral Uracil/Tegafur (UFT), Leucovorin plus Irinotecan and radiation therapy for patients with locally recurrent rectal cancer. World J Surg Oncol, Vol. 4, (2006), pp. 83.

Zhu A.X., Willett C.G. (2003). Chemotherapeutic and biologic agents as radiosensitizers in rectal cancer; Semin Rad Oncol, Vol. 13, No. 4, (2003), pp. 454-458.

11

Neoadjuvant Chemotherapy for Colorectal Liver Metastases

Pamela C. Hebbard, Yarrow J. McConnell and Oliver F. Bathe
University of Calgary
Canada

1. Introduction

Over the last decade, since the development of improved systemic agents for colorectal cancer, there has been increasing exploration of the use of neoadjuvant strategies for colorectal liver metastases (CRLM). In some cases, upfront chemotherapy enables downsizing, in order to enhance resectability. In other cases, neoadjuvant chemotherapy is a means to expedite delivery of systemic therapy and perhaps also to select patients for subsequent treatments.

2. Surgical management of colorectal liver metastases

Since the 1980s, hepatectomy has been increasingly performed for patients with liver-only metastases from colorectal cancer. The first large series were published in the 1990s, demonstrating 5-year survival of 25-40% for patients who underwent R0 resections. These compared favorably with the 0-5% survival rates for patients with technically resectable disease who did not undergo resection, or who had positive margins at resection (R1 or R2) (Scheele & Altendorf-Hofmann, 1999). The patients included in these early series where a highly select group, mostly with solitary lesions less than 5 cm in diameter. However, from these data the initial guiding principles of surgery for CRLM were developed: a) exclusion of patients with any extra-hepatic metastases; b) removal of all detectable liver metastases while providing sufficient residual liver volume for postoperative function; and c) achievement of negative margins (R0 resection; Fong et al., 1997).

With advancements in preoperative staging, surgical techniques, and multimodality treatment since that time, this definition of resectability has been greatly expanded. Current approaches extend the possibility of surgical resection to patients with CRLM involving: both lobes of the liver; large/multiple lesions requiring extended hepatectomies; and extra-hepatic sites, particularly pulmonary (Yang et al., 2010). For practical purposes, the only remaining limits on the definition of "resectable" are the achievement of negative margins, preservation of adequate remnant liver (minimum 20% with a healthy liver) with vascular and biliary inflow/outflow, and capacity of the patient to tolerate the planned, often multimodality, treatment (Charnsangavej et al., 2006; Nordlinger et al., 2009).

Even with these expanded resection criteria and increasingly aggressive surgical strategies, survival rates have continued to improve. Recent large series report 5-year overall survival of 53 - 58% and 5-year recurrence-free survival of 28 - 36% (Abdalla et al., 2004; Choti et al., 2002; Fernandez et al., 2004; Figueras et al., 2001; Pawlik et al., 2005). These series are predominantly from highly specialized institutions. Studies of national administrative databases, over the same time period, report a more modest 5-year overall survival of 22 - 33% following hepatectomy (Cummings et al., 2007; Robertson et al., 2009; Wang et al., 2007). In all studies, whether single centre or population based, the great majority of patients undergoing surgery also received preoperative and/or postoperative chemotherapy. The integration of medical and surgical therapies, with advances in each, and improvements in our ability to effectively and safely combine modalities, has undoubtedly contributed to the observed improvement, or at least stability, of survival rates despite the inclusion of patients with increasingly advanced disease.

Although the presence of extra-hepatic metastases continues to be associated with worse overall survival, aggressive multi-site resection strategies, in combination with chemotherapy, have achieved 5-year survival rates of 19 - 28% at specialty centres (Adam et al., 2011; Carpizo & D'Angelica, 2009; Figueras et al., 2007). Surgical candidates with multi-site metastases are often treated with several cycles of chemotherapy and then resected, often with multiple operations, if they show stable or responsive disease. Those with only pulmonary extra-hepatic metastases are the most commonly treated in this fashion but emerging data suggests that indicators of tumor biology and total number of metastatic sites are stronger predictors of survival than the actual sites of metastatic disease, assuming that complete resection can be achieved (Adam et al., 2011).

Prior to resection of liver metastases, patients undergo detailed radiographic examination of the liver by either CT or MRI. In many centres, PET-CT imaging is obtained on all patients with potentially resectable liver lesions. The addition of PET imaging has been shown to alter management in 10-30% of patients, usually by the detection of previously unknown extra-hepatic lesions (Charnsangavej et al., 2006). With all types of imaging, evaluation by an experienced hepatobiliary radiologist is an important part of surgical, chemotherapeutic, and other treatment planning.

Patients with synchronous liver metastases at the time of their primary tumor diagnosis require individualized decision-making regarding surgery and any neoadjuvant chemotherapy. In the case of an obstructing primary tumor or a patient with significant anemia, a surgical approach to address the primary tumour is usually required prior to consideration of chemotherapy and/or resection of CRLM. In asymptomatic patients, staged or combined resections of the primary and metastatic lesions can be considered, with similar perioperative outcomes and survival in large retrospective series (de Haas et al., 2010; Lyass et al., 2001; Martin et al., 2009). One clinical trial is currently accruing patients in an attempt to address this question prospectively (Rennes University Hospital, 2009). Decision-making regarding the surgical approach depends on the complexity of each part of the surgery, the surgeons' experience, the patient's ability to tolerate lengthy and complex surgery, and logistical factors (Charnsangavej et al., 2006). Neoadjuvant chemotherapy is now frequently offered to these patients. Overall, survival appears to be similar between the various approaches, although no prospective trials have considered this question (Brouquet et al., 2010).

In patients with bilobar CRLM or in whom resection of all lesions would leave an insufficient future liver remnant (FLR), several surgical and interventional techniques are available to convert the patient to a resectable state. Hypertrophy of the FLR can be achieved by ligating or embolizing the portal vein feeding the diseased lobe(s) of the liver (Figure 1). If on repeat imaging, 4 - 6 weeks following portal vein embolization (PVE), the FLR has adequately hypertrophied, patients can undergo extended hepatectomy with perioperative

A

B

C

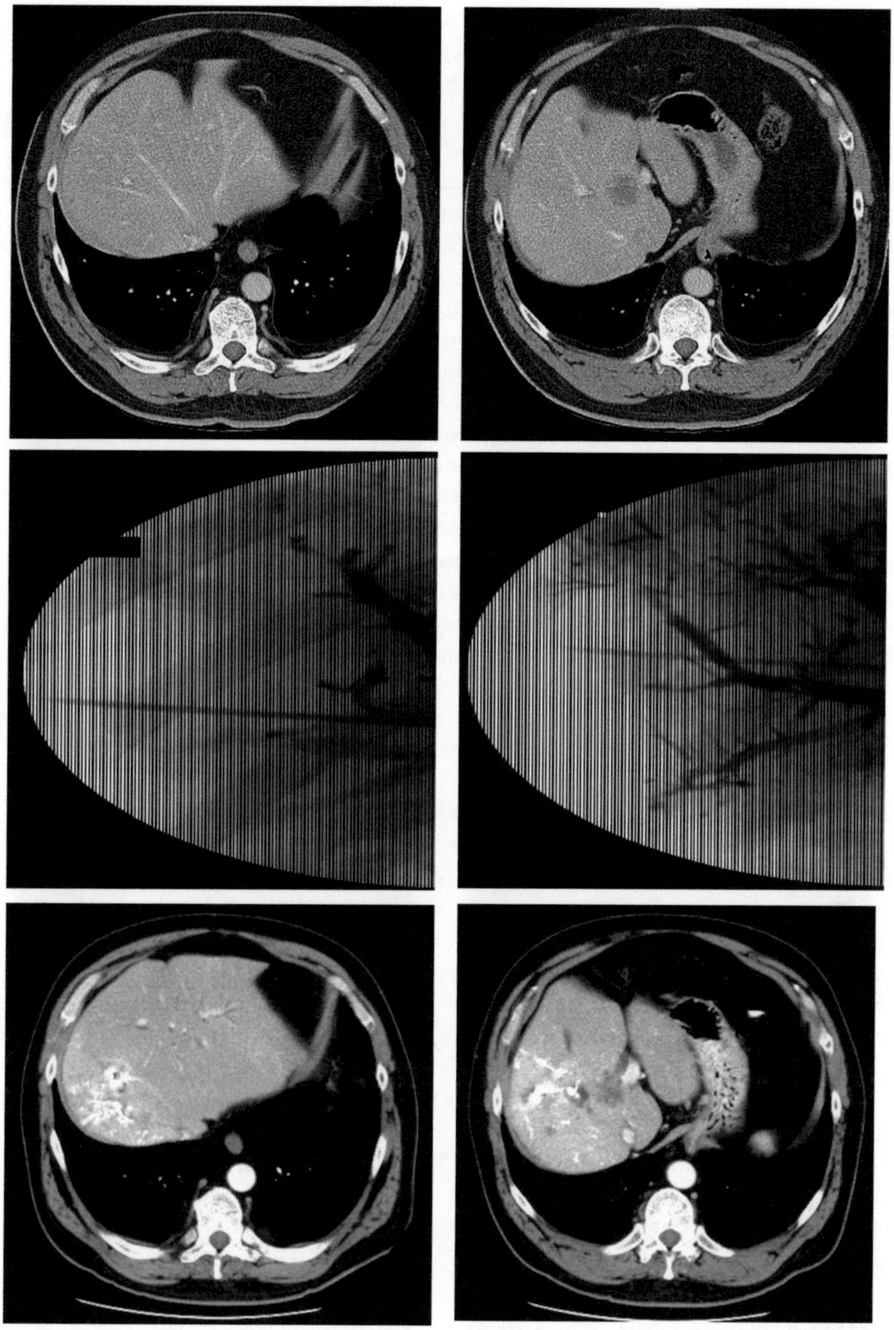

Fig. 1. Portal vein embolization is used to induce hypertrophy of the liver remnant. The lobe or segments containing the liver metastases (and to be resected) is embolized, if it is anticipated that the remaining liver will be too small to provide adequate functional hepatic reserve (A, B). After 4 – 6 weeks, the non-embolized segments of liver will hypertrophy (C), allowing an extensive liver resection with a greater margin of safety.

outcomes and long-term survival similar to that in patients who did not require PVE (Abdalla et al., 2006; Yang et al., 2010). One contraindication to PVE is the presence of lesion(s) in the FLR, due to the risk of progression with hypertrophy. In these cases, a staged approach to resection may be possible. At the initial operation, the lesion(s) in the FLR are resected and the portal vein to the remainder of the diseased liver is ligated. If the patient recovers well and sufficient hypertrophy is achieved, a second laparotomy with extended hepatectomy is undertaken 6 - 12 weeks later. Perioperative morbidity and long-term survival with this approach appears to be similar to that of patients with a similar burden of disease who achieve complete resection with a single hepatectomy (Chun et al., 2007; Wicherts et al., 2008; Yang et al., 2010). The administration of chemotherapy has been successfully implemented with all of these approaches - preoperatively, between staged operations, and postoperatively. The relative contribution of surgical and chemotherapeutic components of these complex management algorithms is unknown. However, as in the more straightforward clinical scenarios discussed in detail below, any evidence of disease progression while on chemotherapy is usually cause for re-evaluation of any further surgical intervention.

When complete surgical resection cannot be achieved, even with the use of adjuncts such as PVE and staged hepatectomies, radiofrequency ablation (RFA) can be used in conjunction with hepatectomy. When compared head-to-head for single lesions, RFA has a significantly higher recurrence rate and is inferior to resection (Aloia et al., 2006a). However, in the era of modern chemotherapy, patients with multiple lesions treated with a combination of resection and RFA, long-term survival rates similar to those of patients with complete resection have been achieved (Nikfarjam et al., 2009). This suggests that in patients with CRLM that are stable or regressing on chemotherapy, but which remain technically unresectable, an approach that includes resection and RFA may be considered.

The final surgical scenario worth noting in the context of CRLM is the patient with synchronous disease who stabilizes or responds to neoadjuvant chemotherapy but whose liver disease remains unresectable. These patients may have an extended survival and the question often arises whether there is value in resecting their primary lesion. Data supporting a survival benefit from such a resection come from series that pre-date modern chemotherapy (Cook et al., 2005; Ruo et al., 2003). With the prolonged survival offered by current chemotherapy regimens, any added benefit is more likely to be related to prevention of local morbidity. The likelihood of developing obstruction and/or pain from local invasion appears to be greatest in patients with rectosigmoid lesions. Therefore, prophylactic resection, particularly when it can be achieved with minimal morbidity, is likely of benefit in this group of patients (Scheer et al., 2008). In all others, the chance of requiring emergent palliative surgery appears to be minimal and decisions regarding resection are made on an individual basis (Cellini et al., 2010).

In general, the surgical management of CRLM is becoming more complicated and more aggressive. Partly, this is due to technical advances in hepatobiliary surgery. Perhaps of greater import is the development of newer systemic agents with greater activity against metastatic colorectal cancer.

3. Systemic agents used for metastatic colorectal cancer

Modern chemotherapy for metastatic colorectal cancer is typically a multi-drug regimen. Doublet regimens of a fluoropyrimidine combined with either oxaliplatin or irinotecan are highly effective in metastatic and adjuvant colorectal cancer. The addition of a targeted biologic agent further increases response rates in appropriate metastatic patients (Compton et al., 2008; Douillard et al., 2010; Folprecht et al, 2010).

Fluorouracil is a pyrimidine analog developed in the 1950s. It functions to interrupt DNA synthesis by inhibiting DNA methylation. Fluorouracil can be given in an intravenous form, 5-FU, or orally via capecitabine, which is subsequently metabolized to an active molecule. When given in IV formulation, fluorouracil is commonly combined with the folate derivative, leucovorin, to enhance its function.

Irinotecan (also known as CPT-11) was approved for use in metastatic colorectal cancer in the mid-1990s. It is an inhibitor of topoisomerase I, a complex that reduces the torsional strain on DNA by breaking, detorting and reconnecting single strands of DNA. Irinotecan's action on topoisomerase I allows single strand breaks to accumulate, ultimately leading to cell cycle arrest and cell death.

Oxaliplatin was introduced to the global market in the late 1990s. It is a platinum-based compound that cross-links DNA, preventing its replication and transcription. The 5-FU, leucovorin, and oxaliplatin combination, FOLFOX, is highly effective in the metastatic setting, but its long-term use is limited by a cumulative dose-dependent side effect of peripheral sensory neuropathy.

Novel biologic agents have been recently introduced into clinical use and are monoclonal antibodies to proteins key to tumor growth pathways. Bevacizumab is a fully humanized antibody against vascular endothelial growth factor (VEGF), and results in inhibition of tumor angiogenesis. Cetuximab and panitumumab are antibodies to the human epidermal growth factor receptor (EGFR; also called HER1). EGFR blockade inhibits cell growth and induces apoptosis. Mutations of the KRAS gene, downstream from EGFR, negate the potential effects of EGFR inhibitors, and so only patients with wild-type KRAS benefit from this treatment (Karapetis et al., 2008). These medications are generally well tolerated, although rare but concerning side effects have been documented (Table 1B). As all of these agents are new to clinical use, their side effect profiles are likely to be refined over time.

Agent	Fluorouracil	Irinotecan	Oxaliplatin
Common Side Effects	Nausea/Vomiting Diarrhea Stomatitis Hand-foot syndrome Bone marrow suppression Hyperbilirubinemia	Nausea/Vomiting Diarrhea Abdominal pain Bone marrow suppression Hair loss Asthenia	Nausea/Vomiting Diarrhea Peripheral sensory neuropathy Stomatitis Bone marrow suppression
Rare Side Effects	Cardiac complications Liver fibrosis/failure	Colitis/ ileitis/ bowel perforation Thromboembolic events Liver impairment, including SOS	Thromboembolic events Liver impairment, including CASH

Table 1A. Side effects of cytotoxic agents used in metastatic colorectal cancer.

An overview of the side effect profiles of each of these drugs is given in Table 1. Of particular interest is the potential of chemotherapy to induce specific liver toxicity in the setting of future liver surgery, discussed further below.

Agent	Bevacizumab	Cetuximab	Panitumumab
Common Side Effects	Hypertension Bleeding Abdominal pain Asthenia Nausea/Vomiting Diarrhea/constipation	Rash Infusion/hypersensitivity reactions Headache Abdominal pain Nausea/vomiting Diarrhea/constipation Bone marrow suppression	Rash Infusion/hypersensitivity reactions Abdominal pain Nausea/vomiting Diarrhea/constipation Asthenia Peripheral edema
Rare Side Effects	GI perforation GI fistula Delayed wound healing Congestive heart failure Thromboembolism	Respiratory complications Cardiopulmonary Arrest	Respiratory complications

Table 1B. Side effects of biologic agents used in metastatic colorectal cancer.

4. Rationale for neoadjuvant chemotherapy

Neoadjuvant chemotherapy could be considered in instances where the CRLM are resectable, or when CRLM are not technically resectable. The rationale for giving upfront chemotherapy for each of these circumstances differs, which bears some discussion.

4.1 Unresectable colorectal liver metastasis

The utility of using chemotherapy to downstage CRLM which are unresectable to a resectable status was first described by Bismuth et al (1996). Since then, in the setting of unresectable CRLM, unless some adjunctive approach such as PVE or two-stage hepatectomy is considered, all patients with unresectable CRLM should be considered for chemotherapy. After detailed imaging, chemotherapy is administered for 2 - 6 cycles, and then repeat detailed imaging is performed to evaluate for response. Patients with a response significant enough to make them candidates for resection are then reconsidered for surgery. Patients whose liver lesions do not respond or progress on chemotherapy continue on palliative-intent chemotherapy, with consideration for second-line and/or clinical trial agents.

This approach has several benefits. Firstly, it defines a group of responders whose tumor biology is more favorable, and in whom aggressive resection is most likely to be of benefit. Secondly, it provides an *in vivo* measurement of the effectiveness of the given chemotherapy regimen for a given patient. Depending on the response, decisions can then be made about continuing with the same agents or switching regimens - either as adjunctive therapy following surgery, or as palliative-intent chemotherapy when surgery is not possible.

4.2 Resectable colorectal liver metastasis

In patients with initially resectable CRLM, the decision to administer upfront chemotherapy is much more complicated. A neoadjuvant chemotherapy approach has some advantages. First, it allows the delivery of systemic treatment early in the patient's treatment course. Occult or micrometastatic disease is treated before it becomes clinically visible, when the burden of disease is low. Neoadjuvant therapy further allows the patient to receive chemotherapy during optimal health, as undoubtedly some surgical patients will experience morbidity that will delay or preclude the administration of cytotoxic drugs. Secondly, neoadjuvant chemotherapy allows the clinician to assess tumor biology. Response to chemotherapy can be measured on serial imaging. Progression of disease, whether in or outside the liver, indicates resistance to the chemotherapy regimen used and thus provides the opportunity to select an alternative combination that may be more effective. Progression of disease while on chemotherapy is an independent predictor of worse survival and liver surgery may not be beneficial in this population (Adam et al., 2004b). Thus, this information further aids in selection of appropriate liver surgery patients.

There are also some disadvantages that accompany neoadjuvant chemotherapy for CRLM. First, current chemotherapy regimens have the potential for liver damage. This risk is mitigated by careful monitoring and by limited durations of pre-operative chemotherapy. Secondly, disease progression on chemotherapy may preclude some patients who were initial surgical candidates from liver resection. This has been a rare event in trials of neodjuvant chemotherapy, and likely portends a worse overall prognosis (Nordlinger et al., 2008; Bathe et al., 2009). Thus, it may actually spare patients from surgery if they are unlikely to achieve a survival benefit. Finally, up-front chemotherapy may cause some tumors to disappear completely, making subsequent decision-making more difficult. These challenges are discussed in more detail in Section 5.

5. Clinical trials

5.1 The role of neoadjuvant chemotherapy in unresectable liver-only metastases

Chemotherapy has long been used as the sole treatment modality for patients with CRLM, with the goal of palliation and the prolongation of life by a few months. With the finding that hepatectomy can lead to long-term survival in 30 - 40% of patients, this goal changed. In initially unresectable patients, chemotherapy is now used with the aim of downstaging lesions to the point of resectability. If this is not achievable, then the goal shifts towards more traditional palliative-intent treatment.

Clinical trials in the setting of liver-only metastases have thus begun to focus on determining the optimal chemotherapy regimen, in terms of maximizing response and resection rates, and also in terms of minimizing perioperative morbidity associated with the effects of intensive preoperative chemotherapy. In early cohort and phase II studies of unresectable patients, treatment with 5-FU, leucovorin and oxaliplatin and/or irinotecan (FOLFOX/FOLFIRI) led to a measurable response rate of 59 - 72% and achievement of margin-negative resections in 12-38% of patients (Giachetti et al., 1999; Adam et al., 2004a; Masi et al., 2009). In patients undergoing resection after downstaging, median survival from the start of chemotherapy was 37 - 48 months, compared to 14 - 15 months in those who did not respond sufficiently to allow resection and/or were not candidates for resection following chemotherapy. These results were obtained with the administration of, on average, 10 - 12 cycles of chemotherapy over a 5 - 6 month period. No perioperative deaths were reported in these studies, although Masi et al. (2009) reported a perioperative morbidity rate of 27% including 8% transient liver failure.

Two phase II trials have evaluated tumor response and secondary resection rates with the addition of biologic agents to FOLFOX/FOLFIRI chemotherapy. In initially unresectable patients, Wong et al. (2011) reports an objective response rate of 40% and a margin-negative resection rate of 10% after administration of capecitabine, oxaliplatin, and bevacizumab (CAPOX+B). With only 12 months of follow-up reported, median survival times have not been reached in this study. Of note, patients in this study received a median of only 4 cycles of preoperative CAPOX+B and 2 patients who achieved a complete response did not undergo resection. Bevacizumab was stopped, on average, 10 weeks prior to hepatectomy but a 4% rate of grade 2 or 3 intestinal perforation was reported. Overall, the perioperative morbidity rate was 28%, with no liver failure events reported.

In the CELIM trial (Folprecht et al., 2011), patients with unresectable CRLM were randomized to cetuximab plus either FOLFOX or FOLFIRI. The objective response rate was 62%, with a 70% response rate in the subset of patients who were *K-ras* wildtype - a known predictor of responsiveness to cetuximab. The overall margin-negative resection rate was 34% and patients received a median of 8 treatment cycles over a 5-month period prior to surgery. Survival data have not yet been published. Perioperative mortality was 4% and major morbidities occurred in 35%.

The addition of bevacizumab has not been conclusively shown to improve response rate or resectability rate, either in the phase II trial reviewed here or, as a secondary end-point in phase III trials (Saltz et al., 2008). On the other hand, the response rates reported in the CELIM trial are quite compelling reasons to consider cetuximab-containing regimens when attempting to downstage unresectable liver metastases, particularly in *K-ras* wildtype patients.

With modern chemotherapeutic regimens, usually incorporating oxaliplatin or irinotecan and biologic agents, responses to chemotherapy are well over 50% (Folprecht et al., 2010; Gruenberger, 2008a, 2008b). Downstaging of initially unresectable disease to resectable disease occurs in 13 - 40% of patients with liver-only metastases who have received systemic chemotherapy (Table 2 and Table 3). Higher rates of conversion to resectability are generally reported in surgical series (Table 3). The wide range of incidences of conversion of unresectable liver metastases to a resectable status is partly a function of the variations in definitions of resectability among surgeons and other oncologic specialties. This phenomenon was well illustrated in the series by Folprecht et al. (2010).

Reference	Agents	N	RR (%)	Liver Resection (%)
Levi et al., 1999	5-FU, LV, Oxaliplatin	90	66	34
De Gramont et al., 2000	5-FU, LV, Oxaliplatin	210	54	7
Giacchetti et al., 2000	5-FU, LV, Oxaliplatin	100	53	32
Scheithauer et al., 2003	Capecitabine, Oxaliplatin	89	48	9
Teufel et al., 2004	5-FU, LV, Irinotecan	35	31	9
Tournigand et al., 2004	FOLFIRI → FOLFOX FOLFOX → FOLFIRI	109 111	56 54	9 22
Sorbye et al., 2004	5-FU, LV, Oxaliplatin	82	62	11
Bajetta et al., 2004	Capecitabine, Irinotecan	140	46	6
Cassidy et al., 2004	Capecitabine, Oxaliplatin	96	55	5
Kohne et al., 2005	5-FU, LV, Irinotecan	214	62	7
Falcone et al., 2007	FOLFIRI FOLFOXIRI	122 122	41 66	6 15
Tabernero et al., 2007	FOLFOX, Cetuximab	43	72	23

Table 2. Incidence of successful hepatic metastasectomy in first-line chemotherapy trials.

Overall, these experiences have served to make response and resection rates important end points in trials of new chemotherapeutic agents for CRLM. Downstaging unresectable liver-only disease followed by surgery is accompanied by reasonable perioperative complication rates and has become the accepted standard.

Reference	Agents	N	Liver Resection (%)
Adam et al., 2001	Mostly oxaliplatin-based	701	13.5
Rivoire et al., 2002	5-FU, LV, Oxaliplatin	131	44
Moehler et al., 2003	5-FU, LV, Irinotecan	46	6.5
Pozzo et al., 2004	5-FU, LV, Irinotecan	40	32.5
Delaunoit et al., 2005	92% oxaliplatin-based	795	3.3
Masi et al., 2006	FOLFOXIRI	74	26
Folprecht et al., 2010	FOLFIRI + cetuximab FOLFOX + cetuximab	55 56	38 40

Table 3. Rates of successful liver resection in surgical series where neoadjuvant chemotherapy was used to downstage tumour bulk.

5.2 The role of neoadjuvant chemotherapy in resectable colorectal liver metastases

There are few clinical trials of neodjuvant chemotherapy in the upfront resectable setting. The EORTC 40983 trial provides the only level I evidence for its use (Nordlinger et al., 2008). This trial enrolled 364 patients with up to four colorectal liver metastases to receive perioperative chemotherapy and liver resection versus surgery alone. The chemotherapy consisted of 12 cycles of FOLFOX4, with half given pre-operatively and half post-operatively. In the chemotherapy arm, 80 percent of patients completed the preoperative schedule and 70% completed the entire regimen. At the time of surgery, 3% had a complete response, 40% a partial response, and 38% stable disease. Only 8 patients had progression that precluded surgery. Ultimately, 3 year progression-free survival went from 28.1 months in the surgery arm to 35.4 months in the multimodality arm, for a hazard ratio of 0.79. Final analysis of overall survival is still pending.

A similar trend has been seen in nonrandomized trials. Bathe et al. (2009) published a phase II trial of 5-FU, leucovorin, and irinotecan as pre-operative chemotherapy for patients with resectable liver metastases. The study enrolled 35 patients, of whom 76 percent had responsive or stable disease during chemotherapy. Thirty-one patients went to surgery, with 30 patients having R0 resection. Post-operative chemotherapy was also delivered to 22 patients. Median disease-free survival (DFS) was 23 months and 2 year DFS was 47 percent. The study was halted early due to a high rate of thromboembolic complications. Meanwhile, Watkins et al. (2010) employed a strategy of neoadjuvant capecitabine and oxaliplatin in a heterogeneous group of patients with stage IV colorectal cancer, among them 32 patients with resectable liver only disease. Liver resection was ultimately performed in 19 patients. Median overall survival in the entire group was 52.9 months.

Reddy et al. (2009) published a multi-institutional study of patients undergoing surgery for initially resectable, synchronous colorectal liver metastasis. A variety of treatment regimens were used, including pre-operative chemotherapy, post-operative chemotherapy, pre- and post-operative treatment, and no chemotherapy. This study found post-operative treatment for six months or longer was associated with improved overall survival in the synchronous liver metastases setting. The heterogeneity of the treatment regimens in terms of timing relative to surgery, duration of therapy, and drugs used makes this analysis difficult to interpret.

A summary of randomized and observational studies of neoadjuvant chemotherapy was recently published (Chua et al., 2010). With a heterogeneous group of chemotherapy protocols and patients, they estimated an objective response rate of 64% (range 44 - 100%) and a median overall survival of 46 months (range 20-67 months).

Alternative approaches to neoadjuvant chemotherapy are available. Portier et al. (1996) studied chemotherapy in the adjuvant setting with positive results. They randomized 173 patients to surgery alone versus surgery with adjuvant 5-FU/leucovorin for six months. The 5 year disease-free survival was 26.7% for the surgery alone arm and 33.5% for the combined treatment. Hepatic artery infusional chemotherapy has been advocated by some groups as well. Kemeny et al. (1999) randomized 156 patients undergoing liver resection to post-operative systemic 5-FU based chemotherapy versus 5-FU-based hepatic artery infusional chemotherapy along with systemic chemotherapy. The median survival was 59.3 months in the systemic arm and 72.2 months in the combined arm. Two other trials have found similar results (Lygidakis et al., 2001; Kemeny et al., 2002). Despite promising results, this technique has not gained popularity. The technical difficulty and expertise needed to perform the procedure safely has limited its use to a few highly specialized cancer centres, and would pose difficulty in expanding its use to the extraordinary numbers of patients with colorectal cancer.

6. Special problems related to neoadjuvant chemotherapy for colorectal liver metastases

6.1 Hepatotoxicity

As the administration of neoadjuvant chemotherapy has become more popular, reports have emerged that clearly demonstrate associated hepatotoxicity, which may adversely affect operative outcomes. The type of hepatic injury depends on the agents administered, while the degree of hepatotoxicity is related to duration of therapy, as well as the chemotherapeutic agents used.

Steatosis was one of the first lesions observed in association with chemotherapy. In a phase II clinical trial where irinotecan-based chemotherapy was administered prior to surgery, we observed that 66% of patients had hepatic steatosis (Bathe et al., 2009). Others have observed lower rates of steatosis, ranging from 9 - 30% (Vauthey et al., 2006). This large range may be due to differences in definitions or severity of steatosis, as well as to population-specific factors such as incidence of diabetes and obesity. Vauthey et al. (2006) reported that no specific chemotherapy regimen was particularly associated with steatosis. However, steatohepatitis, which involves a monomorphic and neutrophilic inflammatory response in addition to steatosis, occurs in a minority of individuals, and it is particularly associated with exposure to irinotecan containing regimens—20.2% vs. 4.2% with no chemotherapy (Vauthey et al., 2006).

Vascular changes including hepatic sinusoidal dilatation, peliosis, hemorrhagic centrilobular necrosis and regenerative nodular hyperplasia have also been observed. These lesions are particularly common in individuals who have received oxaliplatin-based regimens (Aloia et al., 2006b; Kandutsch et al., 2008; Karoui et al., 2006; Vauthey et al., 2006). Sinusoidal congestion and dilatation is present in 18 -23% of individuals who have had oxaliplatin (Aloia et al., 2006b; Vauthey et al., 2006; Wicherts et al., 2011a). Regenerative nodules appear in individuals who have had a prolonged exposure to chemotherapy, and they appear to represent an end-stage vascular injury (Aloia et al., 2006b; Wicherts et al., 2011a).

The effects of each of these lesions on liver function and clinical outcomes following liver resection vary. Steatosis has been associated with an increase in postoperative morbidity although mortality rates do not appear to be adversely affected (Belghiti et al., 1998; Kooby et al., 2003). Steatohepatitis is clearly associated with increased mortality. In the series described by Vauthey and colleagues, steatohepatitis was associated with a 90-day mortality rate of 14.7%, whereas the mortality was only 1.6% in individuals without steatohepatitis (2006). The impact of sinusoidal dilatation and other vascular injuries from chemotherapy on operative outcomes is not clear. In a number of series, sinusoidal dilatation was not associated with increased morbidity and mortality following liver resection (Kishi et al., 2010; Nordlinger et al., 2008; Kandutsch et al., 2008; Vauthey et al., 2006). However, the more severe vascular lesions, such as hemorrhagic centrilobular necrosis and regenerative nodular hyperplasia, may be associated with increased transfusion requirements and liver dysfunction (Aloia et al., 2006b; Wicherts et al., 2011a). The influence of chemotherapy on operative morbidity is proportional to the duration of neoadjuvant chemotherapy (Aloia et al., 2006b; Karoui et al., 2006; Kishi et al., 2010). This has led to a general recommendation to limit the degree of exposure to chemotherapy in the preoperative phase to a period of two to three months, if possible. In addition, lower morbidity rates have been reported when liver resection is performed more than 4 weeks after stopping chemotherapy (Welsh et al., 2007).

There is evidence that some of the biological agents modify the degree of hepatic injury induced by cytotoxic agents. In one report, the prevalence of sinusoidal injury and fibrosis was lower in patients who received cetuximab, and the prevalence of steatohepatitis was lower in patients who received bevacizumab (Pessaux et al., 2010). The addition of bevacizumab or cetuximab to neoadjuvant chemotherapy did not appear to increase the morbidity rates after hepatectomy, and was not associated with any additional histopathologic evidence of hepatic injury. In individuals exposed to 5-FU and oxaliplatin, bevacizumab appears to diminish the incidence and severity of sinusoidal dilatation (Klinger et al., 2009; Ribero et al., 2007). Bevacizumab does not appear to adversely affect postoperative liver function (Wicherts et al., 2011b), but the effects of cetuximab on liver function require further study.

6.2 Thromboembolic complications

Any systemic therapy regimen that increases the risk for thromboembolic complications should be viewed with caution when administered in the preoperative setting. Thromboembolic events that occur preoperatively may delay surgery, and patients on anticoagulants will have an increased risk of bleeding from liver resection.

In our own experience, individuals who had irinotecan-based neoadjuvant chemotherapy had a particularly high risk of thromboembolic complications. Significant thromboembolic events have previously been reported with irinotecan and bolus 5-FU/leucovorin (Pan et al., 2005; Rothenberg et al., 2001). Another study utilizing a similar chemotherapy regimen prior to liver resection did not demonstrate such a high thromboembolic event rate (Pozzo et al., 2004). Therefore it is difficult to determine whether the chemotherapy itself represents a risk factor for thromboembolic complications. A number of contributory risk factors are also present in this patient population in addition to the underlying malignancy. In particular, the insertion of indwelling central venous catheters can be associated with increased risk of thromboembolic complications (Seddighzadeh, Shetty, & Goldhaber, 2007). Given the spurious nature of reports on thromboembolic complications in irinotecan-containing neoadjuvant chemotherapy regimens, it is premature to completely dismiss their role in the management of colorectal liver metastases.

Bevacizumab is also associated with a risk of thromboembolic complications including arterial thrombosis (Kozloff et al., 2010; Schutz et al., 2010). Therefore, caution should be utilized when using bevacizumab containing regimens in the preoperative setting. Having said this, a number of series have been reported in which preoperative bevacizumab was not associated with a particularly high rate of thromboembolic complications, and surgery done more than 8 weeks after the last dose of bevacizumab was considered safe (Gruenberger et al., 2008b; Wicherts et al., 2011b).

6.3 Planning the liver resection following a significant response to chemotherapy

In this chapter we have already shown that unresectable tumors can be downstaged with chemotherapy to a point where they are rendered resectable. However, the question remains whether it is oncologically appropriate to remove less leiver in the case of liver metastases that have shrunk with chemotherapy. A liver-sparing approach would be adequate if the metastasis shrank in a concentric fashion. However, if intratumoral cell death from chemotherapy had a more random distribution, then doing a liver-sparing resection may result in leaving islands of viable tumor in the space previously occupied by the tumor.

Our group studied the histologic patterns of response to chemotherapy to define whether lesions actually shrank in a centripetal fashion (Ng et al, 2008). Our detailed histopathologic analysis demonstrated that tumor did indeed shrink centripedally. However, there were also regional differences in the degree of chemotherapy-induced cell death and fibrosis, resulting in the appearance of islands of viable tumor outside of the confines of the main tumor. Fortunately, these islands of viable tumor always resided close to the gross residual tumor. These observations provided support to the practice of removing only the residual tumor (and possibly preserving liver parenchyma), although a margin of > 1 cm might be desirable to avoid leaving behind more peripheral islands of viable tumor.

6.4 Management of a complete response to chemotherapy

Management of patients who have sustained a complete response to chemotherapy is also controversial. A series of 15 patients with complete radiographic response to chemotherapy was reported by Elias et al. (2004). All were submitted to surgery. In four patients, the lesions could be found at laparotomy, and were therefore resected. In the other 11 patients, the site of liver metastases could not be found at the time of laparotomy and were therefore left in situ. Three of these lesions eventually recurred within a median follow-up of 31.3 months. Benoist and colleagues reported another series of 66 patients with complete disappearance of metastases on CT. Thirty-one patients were observed. Within a year, 23 of these lesions reappeared on CT scan. Of the patients who went for surgery, 20 had macroscopically visible tumor at surgery, 15 had invisible metastases that were resected, and viable tumor cells were seen in 12 of the final pathologic specimens (Benoist et al., 2006). These observations suggest that, in the majority of individuals who have experienced a radiographic complete response to chemotherapy, residual tumor is present. Therefore, there is a rationale to remove all segments of liver in which tumor had resided prior to chemotherapy. Alternatively, patients can be treated expectantly with extremely close follow-up, and ablative treatments can be administered as soon as tumor recurs.

6.5 Response as a prognostic marker

One rationale for neoadjuvant chemotherapy is that it is utilized as a means of selecting patients for resection. In particular, if extrahepatic disease appears during preoperative chemotherapy, then it is not likely that the patient will benefit from hepatic metastasectomy.

Clinical management is not as well defined in patients who experience disease progression while on chemotherapy yet who still have resectable disease confined to the liver. Most data suggest that progression on chemotherapy is associated with a worse prognosis. A large retrospective series reported by Adam and coworkers demonstrated that patients who progressed on chemotherapy prior to liver resection had a 5-year overall survival and disease-free survival of only 8% and 3%, respectively (Adam et al., 2004). Similarly, Gruenberger's group reported a median recurrence-free survival of 24.7 months in patients who had a response to chemotherapy, 8.2 months in patients who had stable disease, and only 3.0 months in patients who had progressive disease (Gruenberger et al., 2008a). Others have also demonstrated the prognostic value of response to chemotherapy (Chan et al., 2010; Small et al., 2009). These observations have prompted reflection on whether individuals who have progressed on chemotherapy should be considered candidates for liver resection. On the other hand, some have observed that response to chemotherapy is not prognostic in certain circumstances, such as in synchronous metastases (Gallagher et al., 2009). Moreover, it is not clear whether resection could still provide some clinical advantage in those patients with progression. More research is required to determine the best treatment algorithm for patients who have progressed on chemotherapy yet still have technically resectable disease.

6.6 The need for a working multidisciplinary tumor conference

If neoadjuvant chemotherapy is to be considered in the management of colorectal liver metastases, then a coordinated and well-functioning multidisciplinary group is essential. It begins with review of imaging by a radiologist with specialty in the area. In consultation with the surgical team, a decision on resectability should be made from initial imaging. This stratifies the patient into: unresectable/pallative treatment; unresectable but suitable for chemotherapy in an attempt at conversion to resectable status; and resectable at presentation. With this information, the medical oncologist is given clear goals for treatment and an appropriate systemic regimen is chosen. It is important that the medical oncologist understands the concerns of the surgeon with respect to the potential hepatotoxicity of any chemotherapy, and the need to limit the course of treatment to only that which is necessary in the neoadjuvant setting. Administration of drugs such as bevacizumab in the perioperative period is also concerning and further highlights the need to coordinate the timing of chemotherapy and surgery. The surgeon should have a role in ongoing monitoring of patients undergoing a "conversion to resectable" approach in order to decide when the patient has reached a resectable state. The role of an experienced liver surgeon, as well as medical oncologist and others, in the delivery of care cannot be overemphasized. This approach to care has been endorsed by the National Comprehensive Cancer Network and others (NCCN, 2011; Vickers et al., 2010).

7. Future considerations

The administration of chemotherapy prior to resection of liver metastases is gaining popularity. There are a number advantages to this approach but there are also some disadvantages, as we have outlined in this article. Trials will be required, trials will be required that compare outcomes related to preoperative or perioperative chemotherapy versus postoperative chemotherapy. The design of these trials will be particularly important and will require some forethought. For example, there are some agents, such as bevacizumab and irinotecan, that are unlikely to be successful in an adjuvant setting given results from adjuvant trials in the non-metastatic setting (Saltz et al., 2007; Allegra et al., 2011). More research is required to understand the underlying cause of hepatotoxicity associated with certain chemotherapy agents. Understanding the mechanisms of hepatotoxicity may aid in developing strategies to reduce it, and ultimately enhance the safety of liver resection following chemotherapy. As biological or targeted therapies become more frequently utilized, it may be that current criteria for measuring response (Response Evaluation Criteria In Solid Tumors; RECIST) are insufficient to determine whether there is a benefit to any chemotherapy. This is due to the phenomenon that many of these agents induce more of a cytostatic rather than cytocidal response. Therefore, new methods of determining biological response (including the use of biomarkers and metabolic measures such as PET) will have to be investigated when gauging response. Eventually biomarkers will be developed to predict the likelihood of response to a particular chemotherapy and the identification of such biomarkers would result in truly personalized cancer care. Furthermore, prognostic biomarkers would help to select patients who would most likely benefit from surgery. Ultimately a combination of predictive and prognostic biomarkers would be very useful for this field and will constitute an important part of decision-making in the future.

8. References

Abdalla, E.K., Adam, R., Bilchik, A.J., Jaeck, D., Vauthey, J.N., & Mahvi, D. (2006). Improving resectability of hepatic colorectal metastases: expert consensus statement. *Annals of Surgical Oncology,* Vol. 13, No. 10 (October 2006), pp.1271-80, ISSN 1534-4681.

Abdalla, E. K., Vauthey, J.-N., Ellis, L. M., Ellis, V., Pollock, R., Broglio, K.R., Hess, K. & Curley, S.A. (2004). Recurrence and outcomes following hepatic resection, radiofrequency ablation, and combined resection/ablation for colorectal liver metastases. *Annals of Surgery* Vol. 239, No. 6 (June 2004), pp.818-827, ISSN 0003-4932.

Adam, R., Avisar, E., Ariche, A., Giachetti, S., Azoulay, D., Castaing, D., Kunstlinger, F., Levi, F. & Bismuth, F. (2001). Five-year survival following hepatic resection after neoadjuvant therapy for nonresectable colorectal. *Annals of Surgical Oncology,* Vol. 8, No. 4(January 2001), pp. 347-353, ISSN 1534-4681.

Adam, R., Delvart, V., Pascal, G., Valeanu, A., Castaing, D., Azoulay, D., Giacchetti, S., Paule, B., Kunstlinger, F., Ghemard, O., Levi, F., Bismuth, H. (2004a). Rescue surgery for unresectable colorectal liver metastases downstaged by chemotherapy – A model to predict survival. *Annals of Surgery,* Vol.240, No. 2 (August 2004), pp.242-256, ISSN 0003-4932.

Adam, R., Pascal, G., Castaing, D., Azoulay, D., Delvart, V., Paule, B., Levi, F. & Bismuth, H. (2004). Tumor progression while on chemotherapy: a contraindication to liver resection for multiple colorectal metastases? *Annals of Surgery,* Vol. 240, No. 6 (December 2004b), pp. 1052-1064, ISSN 0003-4932.

Adam, R., de Haas, R.J., Wicherts, D., Vibert, E., Salloum, C., Azoulay, D. & Castaing, D. (2011). Concomitant extrahepatic disease in patients with colorectal liver metastases: when is there a place for surgery? *Annals of Surgery,* Vol. 253, No. 2 (February 2011), pp.349-359, ISSN 0003-4932.

Allegra, C.J., Yothers, G., O'Connell, M.J., Sharif, S., Petrelli, N.J., Colangelo, L.H., Atkins, J.N., Seay, T.E., Fehrenbacher, L., Goldberg, R.M., O'Reilly, S., Chu L., Azar, C.A., Lopa, S. & Wolmark, N. (2011). Phase III trial assessing bevacizumab in stages II and III carcinoma of the colon: Results of NASBP protocol C-08. *Journal of Clinical Oncology,* Vol. 29, No. 1 (January 2011), pp. 11-16, ISSN 1527-7755.

Aloia, T.A., Vauthey, J.N., Loyer, E.M., Ribero, D., Pawlik, T.M., Wei, S.H., Curley, S.A., Zorzia, D. & Abdalla, E.K. (2006a). Solitary colorectal liver metastasis: resection determines outcome. *Archives of Surgery,* Vol. 141, No. 5 (May 2006), pp.460-466, ISSN 0004-0010.

Aloia, T., Sebagh, M., Plasse, M., Karam, V., Levi, F., Giacchetti, S., et al. (2006b). Liver histology and surgical outcomes after preoperative chemotherapy with fluorouracil plus oxaliplatin in colorectal cancer liver metastases. *Journal of Clinical Oncology,* Vol. 24, No. 31(November 2006), pp. 4983-4990, ISSN 1527-7755.

Bathe, O.F., Ernst, S., Sutherland, F.R., Dixon, E., Butts, C., Bigam, D., Holland, D., Porter, GA., Koppel, J. & Dowden, S. (2009). A phase II experience with neodjuvant irinotecan (CPT-11), 5-fluorouracil (5-FU) and leucovorin (LV) for colorectal liver metastases. *BMC Cancer,* Vol. 9 (May 2009), pp. 156, ISSN 1471-2407.

Behrns, K.E., Tsiotos, G.G., DeSouza, N.F., Krishna, M.K., Ludwig, J., Nagorney, D.M. (1998). Hepatic steatosis as a potential risk factor for major hepatic resection. *Journal of Gastrointestinal Surgery,* Vol 2, No. 3 (May-June 1998), pp. 292-8, ISSN 1873-4626.

Bajetta, E., Di Bartolomeo, M., Mariani, L., Cassata, A., Artale, S., Frustaci, S., Pinotti, G., Bonetti, A., Carreca, I., Biasco, G., Bonaglia, L., Marini, G., Iannelli, A., Cortinovis, D., Ferrario, E., Beretta, E., Lambiase, A. & Buzzoni, R. (2004). Randomized multicenter Phase II trial of two different schedules of irinotecan combined with capecitabine as first-line treatment in metastatic colorectal carcinoma. *Cancer,* Vol. 100, No. 2 (January 2004), pp. 279-287, ISSN 1097-0142.

Benoist, S., Brouquet, A., Penna, C., Julié, C., El Hajjam, M., Chagnon, S., Mitry, E., Rougier, P. & Nordlinger, B. (2006). Complete response of colorectal liver metastases after chemotherapy: Does it mean cure? *Journal of Clinical Oncology,* Vol., 24, No. 24 (August 2006), pp. 3939-3945, ISSN 1527-7755.

Bismuth, H., Adam, R., Levi, F., Farabos, C., Waechter, F., Castaing, D., Majno, P., & Engerran, L. (1996). Resection of nonresectable liver metastases from colorectal cancer after neoadjuvant chemotherapy. *Annals of Surgery,* Vol. 224, No. 4 (October 1996), pp. 509-522, ISSN 0003-4932.

Brouquet, A., Mortenson, M.M., Vauthey, J.N., Rodriguez-Bigas, M.A., Overman, M.J., Chang, G.J., Kopetz, S., Garrett, C., Curley, S.A. & Abdalla, E.K. (2010). Surgical strategies for synchronous colorectal liver metastases in 156 consecutive patients: classic, combined or reverse strategy? *Journal of the American College of Surgeons,* Vol. 210, No. 6 (June 2010), pp.934-41, ISSN 1879-1190.

Carpizo, D.R., & D'Angelica, M. (2009). Liver resection for metastatic colorectal cancer in the presence of extrahepatic disease. *The Lancet Oncology,* Vol. 10, No. 8(August 2009), pp.801-809, ISSN 1474-5488.

Cassidy, J., Tabernero, J., Twelves, C., Brunet, R., Butts, C., Conroy, T., Debraud, F., Figer, A., Grossmann, J., Sawada, N., Schoffski, P., Sobrero, A., Van Cutsem, E. & Diaz-

Rubio, E. (2004). XELOX (capecitabine plus oxaliplatin): active first-line therapy for patients with metastatic colorectal cancer. *Journal of Clinical Oncology*, Vol. 22, No. 11 (June 2004), pp. 2084-2091, ISSN 1527-7755.

Cellini, C., Hunt, S.R., Fleshman, J.W., Birnbaum, E.H., Bierhals, A.J., & Mutch, M.G. (2010). Stage IV rectal cancer with liver metastases: is there a benefit to resection of the primary tumor? *World Journal of Surgery*, Vol. 34, No. 5 (May 2010), pp.1102-1108, ISSN 1432-2323.

Chan, G., Hassanain, M., Chaudhury, P., Vrochides, D., Neville, A., Cesari, M., Kavan, P., Marcus, V. & Metrakos P. (2010). Pathological response grade of colorectal liver metastases treated with neoadjuvant chemotherapy. *HPB (Oxford)*, Vol. 12, No. 4 (May 2010), pp. 277-284, ISSN:1477-2574.

Charnsangavej, C., Clary, B., Fong, Y., Grothey, A., Pawlik, T.M., & Choti, M.A. (2006). Selection of patients for resection of hepatic colorectal metastases: expert consensus statement. *Annals of Surgical Oncology*, Vol.13, No.10 (October 2006), pp.1261-1268, ISSN 1534-4681.

Choti, M.A., Sitzmann, J.V., Tiburi, M.F., Sumetchotimetha, W., Rangsin, R., Schulick, R D., Lillemoe, K.D., Yeo, C.J. & Cameron, J.L. (2002). Trends in long-term survival following liver resection for hepatic colorectal metastases. *Annals of Surgery* Vol. 235, No. 6 (June 2002), pp.759-766, ISSN 0003-4932.

Chua, T.C., Saxena, A., Liauw, W., Kokandi, A. & Morris, D.L. (2010). Systematic review of randomized and nonrandomized trials of the clinical response and outcomes of neoadjuvant systemic chemotherapy for resectable colorectal liver metastases. *Annals of Surgical Oncology*, Vol. 17, No. 2 (February 2010), pp. 492-501, ISSN 1534-4681.

Chun, Y.S., Vauthey, J.N., Ribero, D., Donadon, M., Mullen, J.T., Eng, C., Madoff, D.C., Chang, D.Z., Ho, L., Kopetz, S., Wei, S.H., Curley, S.A. & Abdalla, E.K. (2007). Systemic chemotherapy and two-stage hepatectomy for extensive bilateral colorectal liver metastases: perioperative safety and survival. *Journal of Gastrointestinal Surgery*, Vol.11, No.11 (November 2007), pp.1498-1504, ISSN 1873-4626.

Compton, C., Hawk, E., Grochow, L., et al. (2008). Chapter 81 - Colon Cancer, In: *Abeloff's Clinical Oncology, 4th ed.* Abeloff, M.D., Armitage, J.O., Niederhuber, J.E., Kastan, M.B., & McKenna, W.G. pp. 1477-1525. Elsevier, ISBN 978-0-443-06694-8, Philadelphia.

Cook, A.D., Single, R., & McCahill, L.E. (2005). Surgical resection of primary tumors in patients who present with stage IV colorectal cancer: an analysis of surveillance, epidemiology, and end results data, 1988 to 2000. *Annals of Surgical Oncology*, Vol.12, No.8 (August 2005), pp.637-645, ISSN 1534-4681.

Cummings, L.C., Payes, J.D., & Cooper, G.S. (2007). Survival after hepatic resection in metastatic colorectal cancer: a population-based study. *Cancer*, Vol. 109, No. 4 (February 2007), pp.718-726, ISSN 1097-0142.

Delaunoit, T., Alberts, S.R., Sargent, D.J., Green, E., Goldberg, R.M., Krook, J., Fuchs, C., Ramanathan, R.K., Williamson, S.K., Morton, R.F. & Findlay, B.P. (2005). Chemotherapy permits resection of metastatic colorectal cancer: Experience from Intergroup N9741. *Annals of Oncology*, Vol. 16, No. 3 (March 2005), pp. 425-429, ISSN 1569-8041.

De Gramont, A., Figer, A., Seymour, M., Homerin, M., Hmissi, A., Cassidy, J., Boni, C., Cortes-Funes, H., Cervantes, A., Freyer, G., Papamichael, D., Le Bail, N., Louvet, C.,

Hendler, D., de Braud, F., Wilson, C., Morvan ,F. & Bonetti A. (2000). Leucovorin and fluorouracil with or without oxaliplatin as first-line treatment in advanced colorectal cancer. *Journal of Clinical Oncology,* Vol. 18, No. 16 (August 2000), pp. 2938-2947, ISSN 1527-7755.

Douillard, J. Y., Siena, S., Cassidy, J., Tabernero, J., Burkes, R., Barugel, M., Humblet, Y., Bodoky, G., Cunningham, D., Jassem, J., Rivera, F., Kocákova, I., Ruff, P., Błasińska-Morawiec, M., Šmakal, M., Canon, J.L., Rother, M., Oliner, K.S., Wolf, M. & Gansert J. (2010). Randomized, phase III trial of panitumumab with infusional fluorouracil, leucovorin, and oxaliplatin (FOLFOX4) versus FOLFOX4 alone as first-line treatment in patients with previously untreated metastatic colorectal cancer: the PRIME study. *Journal of Clinical Oncology,* Vol. 28, No. 31 (November 2010), pp.4697-4705, ISSN 1527-7755.

Elias, D., Youssef, O., Sideris, L., Dromain, C., Baton, O., Boige, V., & Ducreux, M. (2004). Evolution of missing colorectal liver metastases following inductive chemotherapy and hepatectomy. *Journal of Surgical Oncology, Vol. 86,* No. 1 (April 2004), pp. 4-9, ISSN 1096-9098.

Falcone, A., Ricci, S., Brunetti, I., Pfanner, E., Allegrini, G., Barbara, C., Crino, L., Benedetti, G., Evangelista, W., Fanchini, L., Cortesi, E., Picone, V., Vitello, S., Chiara, S., Granetto, C., Porcile, G., Fioretto, L., Orlandini, C., Andreuccetti, M. & Masi, G. (2007). Phase III trial of infusional fluorouracil, leucovorin, oxaliplatin, and irinotecan (FOLFOXIRI) compared with infusional fluorouracil, leucovorin, and irinotecan (FOLFIRI) as first-line treatment for metastatic colorectal cancer: the Gruppo Oncologico Nord Ovest. *Journal of Clinical Oncology,* Vol. 25, No. 13 (May 2007), pp. 1670-1676, ISSN 1527-7755.

Fernandez, F.G., Drebin, J.A., Linehan, D.C., Dehdashti, F., Siegel, B.A., & Strasberg, S.M. (2004). Five-year survival after resection of hepatic metastases from colorectal cancer in patients screened by positron emission tomography with F-18 fluorodeoxyglucose (FDG-PET). *Annals of Surgery,* Vol. 240, No. 3 (Spetmber 2004), pp.438-450, ISSN 0003-4932.

Figueras, J., Valls, C., Rafecas, A., Fabregat, J., Ramos, E., & Jaurrieta, E. (2001). Resection rate and effect of postoperative chemotherapy on survival after surgery for colorectal liver metastases. *British Journal of Surgery,* Vol. 88, No. 7 (July 2001), pp. 980-985, ISSN 0007-1323.

Figueras, J., Torras, J., Valls, C., Llado, L., Ramos, E., Marti-Ragué, J., Serrano, T. & Fabregat, J. (2007). Surgical resection of colorectal liver metastases in patients with expanded indications: a single-center experience with 501 patients. *Diseases of the Colon and Rectum,* Vol. 50, No. 4 (April 2007), pp.478-488, ISSN 0012-3706.

Folprecht, G., Gruenberger, T., Bechstein, W.O., Raab, H.R., Lordick, F., Hartmann, J.T., Lang, H., Frilling, A., Stoehlmacher, J. & Weitz, J. (2010). Tumour response and secondary resectability of colorectal liver metastases following neoadjuvant chemotherapy with cetuximab: the CELIM randomised phase 2 trial. *The Lancet Oncology,* Vol. 11, No. 1 (January 2010), pp.38-47, ISSN 1474-5488.

Fong, Y., Cohen, A. M., Fortner, J. G., Enker, W. E., Turnbull, A. D., Coit, D. G., Marrero, A.M., Prasad, M., Blumgart, L.H. & Brennan, M.F. (1997). Liver resection for colorectal metastases. *Journal of Clinical Oncology,* Vol. 15, No. 3 (March 1997), pp.938-946, ISSN 1527-7755.

Gallagher, D. J., Zheng, J., Capanu, M., Haviland, D., Paty, P., Dematteo, R. P., D'Angelica, M., Fong, Y., Jarnagin, W.R., Allen, P.J. & Kemeny, N. (2009). Response to neoadjuvant chemotherapy does not predict overall survival for patients with synchronous colorectal hepatic metastases. *Annals of Surgical Oncology,* Vol. 16, No. 7 (July 2009), pp. 1844-1851, ISSN 1534-4681.

Giacchetti, S., Itzhaki, M., Gruia, G., Adam, R., Zidani, R., Kunstlinger, F., Brienza, S., Alafaci, E., Bertheault-Cvitkovic, F., Jasmin, C., Reynes, M., Bismuth, H., Misset, J.L. & Levi, F. (1999). Long-term survival of patients with unresectable colorectal cancer liver metastases following infusional chemotherapy with 5-fluorouracil, leucovorin, oxaliplatin and surgery. *Annals of Oncology,* Vol. 10, No. 6 (June 1999), pp. 663-669, ISSN 1569-8041.

Giacchetti, S., Perpoint, B., Zidani, R., Le Bail, N., Faggiuolo, R., Focan, C., Chollet, P., Llory, J.F., Letourneau, Y., Coudert, B., Bertheaut-Cvitkovic, F., Larregain-Fournier, D., Le Rol, A., Walter, S., Adam, R., Misset, J.L. & Levi, F. (2000). Phase III multicenter randomized trial of oxaliplatin added to chronomodulated fluorouracil-leucovorin as first-line treatment of metastatic colorectal cancer. Journal of Clinical Oncology, Vol. 18, No. 1 (January 2000), pp. 136-147, ISSN 1527-7755.

Gruenberger, B., Scheithauer, W., Punzengruber, R., Zielinski, C., Tamandl, D., & Gruenberger, T. (2008a). Importance of response to neoadjuvant chemotherapy in potentially curable colorectal cancer liver metastases. *BMC Cancer,* Vol. 8 (April 2008), pp. 120, ISSN 1471-2407.

Gruenberger, B., Tamandl, D., Schueller, J., Scheithauer, W., Zielinski, C., Herbst, F. & Gruenberger, T.. (2008b). Bevacizumab, capecitabine, and oxaliplatin as neoadjuvant therapy for patients with potentially curable metastatic colorectal cancer. *Journal of Clinical Oncology,* Vol. 26, No. 11 (April 2008), pp. 1830-1835, ISSN 1527-7755.

de Haas, R.J., Adam, R., Wicherts, D.A., Azoulay, D., Bismuth, H., Vibert, E., Salloum, C., Perdigao, F., Benkabbou, A. & Castaing, D. (2010). Comparison of simultaneous or delayed liver surgery for limited synchronous colorectal metastases. *British Journal of Surgery,* Vol. 97, No. 8 (August 2010), pp.1279-1289, ISSN 0007-1323.

Kandutsch, S., Klinger, M., Hacker, S., Wrba, F., Gruenberger, B., & Gruenberger, T. (2008). Patterns of hepatotoxicity after chemotherapy for colorectal cancer liver metastases. *European Journal of Surgical Oncology, Vol. 34,* No. 11 (November 2008), pp. 1231-1236, ISSN 0748-7983.

Karapetis, C. S., Khambata-Ford, S., Jonker, D. J., O'Callaghan, C. J., Tu, D., Tebbutt, N. C., Simes, R.J., Chalchal, H., Shapiro, J.D., Robitaille, S., Price, T.J., Shepherd, L., Au, H.J., Langer, C., Moore, M.J. & Zalcberg, J.R. (2008). K-ras mutations and benefit from cetuximab in advanced colorectal cancer. *New England Journal of Medicine,* Vol. 359, No. 17 (October 2008), pp. 1757-1765, ISSN 0028-4793.

Karoui, M., Penna, C., Amin-Hashem, M., Mitry, E., Benoist, S., Franc, B., Rougier, P. & Nordlinger, B. (2006). Influence of preoperative chemotherapy on the risk of major hepatectomy for colorectal liver metastases. *Annals of Surg, Vol. 243,* No. 1 (January 2006), pp. 1-7, ISSN 0003-4932.

Kemeny, N., Huang, Y., Cohen, A.M., Shi, W., Conti, J.A., Brennan, M.F., Bertino, J.R., Turnbull, A.D., Sullivan, D., Stockman, J., Blumgart, L.H. & Fong, Y. (1999). Hepatic arterial infusion of chemotherapy after resection of hepatic metastases from colorectal cancer. *New England Journal of Medicine,* Vol. 341, No. 27 (December 1999), pp. 2039 - 2048, ISSN 0028-4793.

Kemeny, M.M., Adak, S., Gray, B., Macdonald, J.S., Smith, T., Lipsitz, S., Sigurdson, E.R., O'Dwyer, P.J. & Benson, A.B.3rd. (2002). Combined-modality treatment for resectable metastatic colorectal carcinoma to the liver: Surgical resection of hepatic metastases in combination with continuous infusion of chemotherapy—An intergroup study. *Journal of Clinical Oncology,* Vol. 20, No. 6 (March 2002), pp.1499 - 1505, ISSN 1527-7755.

Kishi, Y., Zorzi, D., Contreras, C. M., Maru, D. M., Kopetz, S., Ribero, D., Motta, M., Ravarino, N., Risio, M., Curley, S.A., Abdalla, E.K., Capussotti, L. & Vauthey, J.N. (2010). Extended preoperative chemotherapy does not improve pathologic response and increases postoperative liver insufficiency after hepatic resection for colorectal liver metastases. *Annals of Surgical Oncology,* Vol. 17, No. 11 (November 2010), pp. 2870-2876, ISSN 1534-4681.

Klinger, M., Eipeldauer, S., Hacker, S., Herberger, B., Tamandl, D., Dorfmeister, M., Koelblinger, C., Gruenberger, B. & Gruenberger, T. (2009). Bevacizumab protects against sinusoidal obstruction syndrome and does not increase response rate in neoadjuvant XELOX/FOLFOX therapy of colorectal cancer liver metastases. *European Journal of Surgical Oncology,* Vol. 35, No. 5 (May 2009), pp. 515-520, ISSN 0748-7983.

Kohne, C.H., van Cutsem, E., Wils, J., Bokemeyer, C., El-Serafi, M., Lutz, M.P., Lorenz, M., Reichardt, P., Ruckle-Lanz, H., Frickhofen, N., Fuchs, R., Mergenthaler, H.G., Langenbuch, T., Vanhoefer, U., Rougier, P., Voigtmann, R., Muller, L., Genicot, B., Anak, O. & Nordlinger, B. (2005). Phase III study of weekly high-dose infusional fluorouracil plus folinic acid with or without irinotecan in patients with metastatic colorectal cancer: European Organisation for Research and Treatment of Cancer Gastrointestinal Group Study 40986. *Journal of Clinical Oncology,* Vol. 23, No. 22 (August 2005), pp. 4856-4865, ISSN 1527-7755.

Kooby, D., Fong, Y., Suriawinata, A., Gonen, M., Allen, P., Klimstra, D., DeMatteo, R.P., D'Angelica, M., Blumgart, L.H. & Jarnagin, W.R. (2003). Impact of steatosis on perioperative outcome following hepatic resection. *Journal of Gastrointestinal Surgery, Vol. 7,* No. 8 (December 2003), pp. 1034-1044, ISSN 1873-4626.

Kozloff, M. F., Berlin, J., Flynn, P. J., Kabbinavar, F., Ashby, M., Dong, W., Sing, A.P. & Grothey, A. (2010). Clinical outcomes in elderly patients with metastatic colorectal cancer receiving bevacizumab and chemotherapy: results from the BRiTE observational cohort study. *Oncology,* Vol. 78, No. 5-6 (November 2010), pp. 329-339, ISSN 0030-2414.

Levi, F., Zidani, R., Brienza, S., Dogliotti, L., Perpoint, B., Rotarski, M., Letourneau, Y., Llory, J.F., Chollet, P., Le Rol, A. & Focan, C. (1999). A multicenter evaluation of intensified, ambulatory, chronomodulated chemotherapy with oxaliplatin, 5-fluorouracil, and leucovorin as initial treatment of patients with metastatic colorectal carcinoma. International Organization for Cancer Chronotherapy. *Cancer,* Vol. 85, No. 12 (June 1999), pp. 2532-2540, ISSN 1097-0142.

Lyass, S., Zamir, G., Matot, I., Goitein, D., Eid, A., & Jurim, O. (2001). Combined colon and hepatic resection for synchronous colorectal liver metastases. *Journal of Surgical Oncology,* Vol. 78, No. 1 (September 2001), pp.17-21, ISSN 1096-9098.

Lygidakis, N.J., Sgourakis, G., Vlachos, L., Raptis, S., Safioleas, M., Boura, P., Kountouras, J. & Alamani, M. (2001). Metastatic liver disease of colorectal origin: The value of locoregional immunochemotherapy combined with systemic chemotherapy following liver resection. Results of a prospective randomized study. *Hepatogastroenterology,* Vol. 48, No. 48 (November/December 2001), pp. 1685–1691, ISSN 0172-6390.

Martin, R.C.G., Augenstein, V., Reuter, N.P., Scoggins, C.R., & McMasters, K.M. (2009). Simultaneous versus staged resection for synchronous colorectal cancer liver metastases. *Journal of the American College of Surgeons,* Vol. 208, No. 5 (May 2009), pp.842-850, ISSN 1879-1190.

Masi, G., Cupini, S., Marcucci, L., Cerri, E., Loupakis, F., Allegrini, G., Brunetti, I.M., Pfanner, E., Viti, M., Goletti, O., Filipponi, F. & Falcone, A. (2006). Treatment with 5-fluorouracil/folinic acid, oxaliplatin, and irinotecan enables surgical resection of metastases in patients with initially unresectable metastatic colorectal cancer. *Annals of Surgical Oncology,* Vol. 13, No. 1 (January 2006), pp. 58-65, ISSN 1534-4681.

Masi, G., Loupakis, F., Pollina, L., Vasile, E., Cupini, S., Ricci, S., Brunetti, I.M., Ferraldeschi, R., Naso, G., Filiponni, F., Pietrabissa, A., Goletti, O., Baldi, G., Fornaro, L, Andreuccetti, M. & Falcone, A. (2009). Long-term outcome of initially unresectable metastatic colorectal cancer patients treated with 5-fluorouracil/leucovorin, oxaliplatin, and irinotecan (FOLFOXIRI) followed by radical surgery of metastases. *Annals of Surgery,* Vol. 249, No. 3 (Marhc 2009), pp.420-425, ISSN 0003-4932.

Moehler, M., Hoffmann, T., Zanke, C., Hohl, H., Burg, H., Ehscheid, P., Schwindt, P., Adami, B., Schroeder, M., Klein, O., Baldus, M., Galle, P.R. & Heike, M. (2003). Safety and efficacy of outpatient treatment with CPT-11 plus bolus folinic acid/5-fluorouracil as first-line chemotherapy for metastatic colorectal cancer. *Anticancer Drugs,* Vol. 14, No. 1 (January 2003), pp. 79-85, ISSN 1473-5741.

National Comprehensive Cancer Network (2011). Colon Cancer. In: *NCCN Clinical Practice Guidelines in Oncology.* Accessed April 6, 2011. Available from: http://www.nccn.org.

Ng, J.K., Urbanski, S.J., Mangat, N., McKay, A., Sutherland, F.R., Dixon, E., Dowden, S., Ernst, S., Bathe, O.F. (2008). Colorectal liver metastasis contract centripetally, with a response to chemotherapy: A histomorphologic study. *Cancer,* Vol. 115, No. 2 (January 2008), pp. 362-71, ISSN 1097-0142.

Nikfarjam, M., Shereef, S., Kimchi, E.T., Gusani, N.J., Jiang, Y., Avella, D.M., Mahraj, R.P. & Staveley-O'Carroll, K.F. (2009). Survival outcomes of patients with colorectal liver metastases following hepatic resection or ablation in the era of effective chemotherapy. *Annals of Surgical Oncology,* Vol. 16, No. 7 (July 2009), pp.1860-1867, ISSN 1534-4681.

Nordlinger, B., Sorbye, H., Glimelius, B., Poston, G.J., Schlag, P.M., Rougier, P., Bechstein, W.O., Primrose, J.N., Walpole, E.T., Finch-Jones, M., Jaeck, D., Mirza, D., Parks, R.W., Collette, L., Praet, M., Bethe, U., Van Cutsem, E., Scheithauer, W. & Gruenberger, T. (2008). Perioperative chemotherapy with FOLFOX4 and surgery versus surgery alone for respectable liver metastasis from colorectal cancer (EORTC Intergroup trial 40983): a randomised control trial. *Lancet,* Vol. 371, No. 9617 (March 2008), pp. 1007-1015, ISSN 0140-6736.

Nordlinger, B., Van Cutsem, E., Gruenberger, T., Glimelius, B., Poston, G., Rougier, P., Sobrero, A., Ychou, M. (2009). Combination of surgery and chemotherapy and the role of targeted agents in the treatment of patients with colorectal liver metastases: Recommendations from an expert panel. *Annals of Oncology,* Vol. 20, No. 6 (June 2009), pp.985-992, ISSN 1569-8041.

Pan, C. X., Loehrer, P., Seitz, D., Helft, P., Juliar, B., Ansari, R., Pletcher, W., Vinson, J., Cheng, L. & Sweeney, C. (2005). A phase II trial of irinotecan, 5-fluorouracil and leucovorin combined with celecoxib and glutamine as first-line therapy for advanced colorectal cancer. *Oncology,* Vol. 69, No. 1 (August 2005), pp. 63-70, ISSN 0030-2414.

Pawlik, T. M., Scoggins, C. R., Zorzi, D., Abdalla, E. K., Andres, A., Eng, C., Curley, S.A., Loyer, E.M., Muratore, A., Mentha, G., Capussotti, L. & Vauthey, J.N. (2005). Effect of surgical margin status on survival and site of recurrence after hepatic resection for colorectal metastases. *Annals of Surgery,* Vol. 241, No. 5 (May 2005), pp.715-724, ISSN 0003-4932.

Pessaux, P., Panaro, F., Casnedi, S., Zeca, I., Marzano, E., Bachellier, P., Jaeck, D. & Chenard, M.P. (2010). Targeted molecular therapies (cetuximab and bevacizumab) do not induce additional hepatotoxicity: preliminary results of a case-control study. *European Journal of Surgical Oncology, Vol. 36,* No. 6 (June 2010), pp. 575-582, ISSN 0748-7983.

Portier, G., Elias, D., Bouche, O., Rougier, P., Bosset, J.F., Saric, J., Belghiti, J., Piedbois, P., Guimbaud, R., Nordlinger, B., Bugat, R., Lazorthes, F. & Bedenne, L. (2006). Multicenter randomized trial of adjuvant fluoruracil and folinic acid compared with surgery alone after resection of colorectal liver metastasis: FFCD ACHBTH AURC 9002 trial. *Journal of Clinical Oncology,* Vol. 24, No.10, (November 2006), pp. 4976-4982, ISSN 1527-7755.

Pozzo, C., Basso, M., Cassano, A., Quirino, M., Schinzari, G., Trigila, N., Vellone, M., Giuliante, F., Nuzzo, G. & Barone, C. (2004). Neoadjuvant treatment of unresectable liver disease with irinotecan and 5-fluorouracil plus folinic acid in colorectal cancer patients. *Annals of Oncology,* Vol. 15, No. 6 (June 2004), pp. 933-939, ISSN 1569-8041.

Reddy, S.K., Zorzi, D., Lum, Y.W., Barbas, A.S., Pawlik, T.M., Ribero, D., Abdalla, E.K., Choti, M.A., Kemp, C., Vauthey, J.N., Morse, M.A., White, R.R., Clary, B.M. (2009). Timing of multimodality therapy for resectable synchronous colorectal liver metastases: a retrospective multi-institutional analysis. *Annals of Surgical Oncology,* Vol 16, No. 7 (July 2009), pp. 1809-1819, ISSN 1534-4681.

Rennes University Hospital. (2009). Evaluation of 2 Resection Strategies of Synchronous Colorectal Cancer Metastases (METASYNC) - NCT00264979. US National Institute of Health. Accessed: April 11, 2001. Available from http://clinicaltrials.gov/ct2/show/NCT00264979?term=hepatic+synchronous&rank=1

Ribero, D., Wang, H., Donadon, M., Zorzi, D., Thomas, M. B., Eng, C., Chang, D.Z., Curley, S.A., Abdalla, E.K., Ellis, L.M. & Vauthey, J.N. (2007). Bevacizumab improves pathologic response and protects against hepatic injury in patients treated with oxaliplatin-based chemotherapy for colorectal liver metastases. *Cancer, Vol. 110,* No. 12 (December 2007), pp. 2761-2767, ISSN: 1097-0142.

Rivoire, M., De Cian, F., Meeus, P., Negrier, S., Sebban, H. & Kaemmerlen, P. (2002). Combination of neoadjuvant chemotherapy with cryotherapy and surgical resection for the treatment of unresectable liver metastases from colorectal carcinoma. *Cancer,* Vol. 95, No. 11 (December 2002), pp. 2283-2292, ISSN 1097-0142.

Robertson, D.J., Stukel, T.A., Gottlieb, D.J., Sutherland, J.M., & Fisher, E.S. (2009). Survival after hepatic resection of colorectal cancer metastases: a national experience. *Cancer,* Vol. 115, No. 4 (February 2009), pp. 752-759, ISSN 1097-0142.

Rothenberg, M.L., Meropol, N J., Poplin, E.A., Van Cutsem, E., & Wadler, S. (2001). Mortality associated with irinotecan plus bolus fluorouracil/leucovorin: summary findings of an independent panel. *Journal of Clinical Oncology, Vol. 19,* No. 18 (Septmber 2001), pp. 3801-3807, ISSN 1527-7755.

Ruo, L., Gougoutas, C., Paty, P.B., Guillem, J.G., Cohen, A.M. & Wong, W.D. (2003). Elective bowel resection for incurable stage IV colorectal cancer: Prognostic variables for asymptomatic patients. *Journal of the American College of Surgeons,* Vol. 196, No. 5 (May 2003), pp.722-728, ISSN 1879-1190.

Saltz, L. B., Clarke, S., Díaz-Rubio, E., Scheithauer, W., Figer, A., Wong, R., Koski, S., Lichinitser, M., Yang, T.-S., Rivera, F., Couture, F., Sirzen, F. & Cassidy, J. (2008). Bevacizumab in combination with oxaliplatin-based chemotherapy as first-line therapy in metastatic colorectal cancer: a randomized phase III study. *Journal of Clinical Oncology,* Vol. 26, No. 12 (May 2008), pp. 2013-2019, ISSN 1527-7755.

Saltz, L.B., Niedzwiecki, D., Hollis, D., Goldberg, R.M., Hantel, A., Thomas, J.P., Fields, A.L., & Mayer, R.J. (2007). Irinotecan fluorouracil plus leucovorin is not superior to fluorouracil plus leucovorin alone as adjuvant treatment for stage III colon cancer: Results of CALGB 89803. *Journal of Clinical Oncology,* Vol. 25, No. 23 (August 2007), pp. 3456-3461, ISSN 1527-7755.

Scheele, J. & Altendorf-Hofmann. A. (1999). Resection of colorectal liver metastases. *Langenbeck's Archives of Surgery,* Vol. 384, No. 4 (August 1999), pp.313-327, ISSN 1435-2443.

Scheithauer W, Kornek GV, Raderer M, Schüll B, Schmid K, Kovats E, Schneeweiss B, Lang F, Lenauer A, Depisch D. (2003). Randomized multicenter phase II trial of two different schedules of capecitabine plus oxaliplatin as first-line treatment in advanced colorectal cancer. *Journal of Clinical Oncology,* Vol. 21, No. 7 (April 2003), pp. 1307-1312, ISSN 1527-7755.

Scheer, M.G.W., Sloots, C.E.J., van der Wilt, G.J., & Ruers, T.J.M. (2008). Management of patients with asymptomatic colorectal cancer and synchronous irresectable metastases. *Annals of Oncology,* Vol. 19, No. 11 (November 2008), pp.1829-1835, ISSN 1569-8041.

Schutz, F.A., Je, Y., Azzi, G.R., Nguyen, P.L., & Choueiri, T.K. (2011). Bevacizumab increases the risk of arterial ischemia: a large study in cancer patients with a focus on different subgroup outcomes. *Annals of Oncology, Vol.* 22, No. 6 (June 2011), pp. 1404-1412, ISSN 1569-8041.

Seddighzadeh, A., Shetty, R., & Goldhaber, S. Z. (2007). Venous thromboembolism in patients with active cancer. *Thrombosis and Haemostasis,* Vol. 98, No. 3 (Septmber 2007), pp. 656-661, ISSN 0340-6245.

Small, R. M., Lubezky, N., Shmueli, E., Figer, A., Aderka, D., Nakache, R., Klausner, J.M. & Ben-Haim, M. (2009). Response to chemotherapy predicts survival following resection of hepatic colo-rectal metastases in patients treated with neoadjuvant therapy. *Journal of Surgical Oncology,* Vol. 99, No. 2 (February 2009), pp. 93-98, ISSN 1096-9098.

Sorbye, H., Glimelius, B., Berglund, A., Fokstuen, T., Tveit, K.M., Braendengen, M., Ogreid, D. & Dahl, O. (2004). Multicenter phase II study of Nordic fluorouracil and folinic acid bolus schedule combined with oxaliplatin as first-line treatment of metastatic colorectal cancer. *Journal of Clinical Oncology,* Vol 22., No. 1 (January 2004), pp. 31-38, ISSN 1527-7755.

Tabernero, J., Van Cutsem, E., Diaz-Rubio, E., Cervantes, A., Humblet, Y., Andre, T., Van Laethem, J.L., Soulie, P., Casado, E., Verslype, C., Valera, J.S., Tortora, G., Ciardiello, F., Kisker, O. & de Gramont, A. (2007). Phase II trial of cetuximab in combination with fluorouracil, leucovorin, and oxaliplatin in the first-line treatment of metastatic colorectal cancer. *Journal of Clinical Oncology,* Vol. 25, No. 33 (November 2007), pp. 5225-5235, ISSN 1527-7755.

Tournigand, C., Andre, T., Achille, E., Lledo, G., Flesh, M., Mery-Mignard, D., Quinaux, E., Couteau, C., Buyse, M., Ganem, G., Landi, B., Colin, P., Louvet, C. & de Gramont, A. (2004). FOLFIRI followed by FOLFOX6 or the reverse sequence in advanced colorectal cancer: a randomized GERCOR study. *Journal of Clinical Oncology,* Vol. 22, No. 2 (January 2004), pp. 229-237, ISSN 1527-7755.

Teufel, A., Steinmann, S., Siebler, J., Zanke, C., Hohl, H., Adami, B., Schroeder, M., Klein, O., Höhler, T., Galle, PR., Heike, M. & Moehler, M. (2004). Irinotecan plus folinic acid/continuous 5-fluorouracil as simplified bimonthly FOLFIRI regimen for first-line therapy of metastatic colorectal cancer. *BMC Cancer,* Vol. 4 (July 2004), pp. 38, ISSN 1471-2407.

Vauthey, J. N., Pawlik, T. M., Ribero, D., Wu, T. T., Zorzi, D., Hoff, P. M., Xiong, H.Q., Eng, C., Lauwers, G.Y., Mino-Kenudson, M., Risio, M., Muratore, A., Capussotti, L., Curley, S.A. & Abdalla, E.K. (2006). Chemotherapy regimen predicts steatohepatitis and an increase in 90-day mortality after surgery for hepatic colorectal metastases. *Journal of Clinical Oncology,* Vol. 24, No. 13 (May 2006), pp. 2065-2072, ISSN 1527-7755.

Vickers, M., Samson, B., Colwell, B., Cripps, C., Jalink, D., El-Sayed, S., Chen, E., Porter, G., Goel, R., Villeneuve ,J., Sundaresan, S., Asselah, J., Biagi, J., Jonker, D., Dawson, L., Letourneau, R., Rother, M., Maroun, J., Thirlwell, M., Hussein, M., Tehfe, M., Perrin, N., Michaud, N., Hammad, N., Champion, P., Rajan, R., Burkes, R., Barrette, S., Welch, S., Yarom, N. & Asmis T.. (2010). Eastern Canadian Colorectal Cancer Consensus Conference: setting the limits of resectable disease. *Current Oncology,* Vol. 17, No. 3 (June 2010), pp. 70-77, ISSN 1718-7729.

Wang, X., Hershman, D.L., Abrams, J.A., Feingold, D., Grann, V.R., Jacobson, J.S. & Neugat, A.I. (2007). Predictors of survival after hepatic resection among patients with colorectal liver metastasis. *British Journal of Cancer,* Vol. 97, No. 12 (December 2007), pp.1606-1612, ISSN 0007-0920.

Watkins, D.J., Chau, I., Cunningham, D., Mudan, S.S., Karanjia, N., Brown, G., Ashley, S. & Norman, A.R. (2010). Defining patient outcomes in stage IV colorectal cancer: A prospective study with baseline stratification according to disease respectability status. *British Journal of Cancer,* Vol. 102, No. 2 (January 2010), pp. 255-61, ISSN 0007-0920.

Welsh, F.K., Tilney, H.S., Tekkis, P.P., John, T.G., & Rees, M. (2007). Safe liver resection following chemotherapy for colorectal metastases is a matter of timing. *British Journal of Cancer,* Vol. 96, No. 7 (April 2007), pp. 1037-1042, ISSN 0007-0920.

Wicherts, D. A., de Haas, R. J., Sebagh, M., Ciacio, O., Levi, F., Paule, B., Giacchetti, S., Guettier, C., Azoulay, D., Castaing, D. & Adam, R. (2011a). Regenerative nodular hyperplasia of the liver related to chemotherapy: impact on outcome of liver surgery for colorectal metastases. *Annals of Surgical Oncology,* Vol. 18, No. 3 (March 2011), pp. 659-669, ISSN 1534-4681.

Wicherts, D. A., de Haas, R. J., Sebagh, M., Saenz Corrales, E., Gorden, D. L., Levi, F., Paule, B., Azoulay, D., Castaing, D. & Adam, R. (2011b). Impact of bevacizumab on functional recovery and histology of the liver after resection of colorectal metastases. *British Journal of Surgery,* Vol. 98, No. 3 (March 2011), pp. 399-407, ISSN 0007-1323.

Wicherts, D.A., Miller, R., de Haas, R.J., Bitsakou, G., Vibert, E., Veilhan, L.-A., Azoulay, D., Bismuth, H., Castaing, D. & Adam, R. (2008). Long-term results of two-stage hepatectomy for irresectable colorectal cancer liver metastases. *Annals of Surgery,* Vol. 248, No. 6 (Decmber 2008), pp.994-1005, ISSN 0003-4932.

Wong, R., Cunningham, D., Barbachano, Y., Saffery, C., Valle, J., Hickish, T., Mudan, S., Brown, G., Khan, A., Wotherspoon, A., Strimpakos, A.S., Thomas, J., Compton, S., Chua, Y.J. & Chua, I. (2011). A multicentre study of capecitabine, oxaliplatin plus bevacizumab as perioperative treatment of patients with poor-risk colorectal liver-only metastases not selected for upfront resection. *Annals of Oncology* Epub (Feb 2011): doi: 10.1093/annonc/mdq714. ISSN 1569-8041.

Yang, A.D., Brouquet, A., & Vauthey, J.-N. (2010). Extending limits of resection for metastatic colorectal cancer: risk benefit ratio. *Journal of Surgical Oncology,* Vol. 102, No. 8 (December 2010), pp.996-1001, ISSN 0748-7983.

12

Chemotherapy in the Combined Modality Treatment of Penile Carcinoma

Jennifer Wang and Lance C. Pagliaro
The University of Texas MD Anderson Cancer Center
USA

1. Introduction

Penile carcinoma is a rare malignancy accounting for 0.4% to 0.6% of all cancers in men in the United States and Europe (Perksy, 1977). Penile cancers usually originate from the epithelium of the inner prepuce and glans with squamous cell histology accounting for >95% of cancers; melanoma and basal cell carcinoma account for another 3% (Cubilla, 2009). There is a predictable pattern of spread with the first site of metastasis occurring at the regional femoral and iliac nodes (Wood, 2010). The lymphatics of the prepuce connect to the lymphatics from the skin of the shaft, and the lymphatics of the glans and corporal bodies join together in the superficial inguinal nodes. The superficial lymph nodes drain into the deep inguinal nodes, which in turn, drain into the pelvic nodes (internal and external iliac nodes and obturator nodes). This lymphatic system is illustrated in Figure 1. Penile lymphatic drainage occurs bilaterally through crossover drainage at multiple levels. Direct metastasis to the deep inguinal lymph nodes can uncommonly occur, but metastasis directly to the pelvic lymph nodes is rare. Histologic subtypes appear to possess different risks of developing metastatic lymph nodes with sarcomatoid tumors having the highest risk of around 90% (Cubilla, 2009).

Once a diagnosis of penile cancer is determined, treatment is based on stage of disease. The most recent seventh edition of the TNM staging system for penile carcinoma as designated by the American Joint Committee on Cancer is presented in Tables 1 and 2 (Edge et al., 2010).

The Netherlands Cancer Institute evaluated the prognostic value of the TNM staging classification. The current inconsistencies between staging and prognosis include different clinical 5 year disease-specific survival for tumors invading corpus spongiosum and corpora cavernosa and no significant differences in the 5-year disease-specific survival between T2 and T3 tumors or N1 and N2 disease (Leijte et al., 2007). A revision of the current T2 TNM staging system to take this prognostic difference into consideration has been proposed.

2. Treatment overview

2.1 Local disease

Treatment, as with other malignancies, is stratified based on staging. For local control, surgical amputation is the oncologic gold standard for definitive treatment with local recurrence rates ranging from 0-8% (McDougal et al., 1986). Penile tumors with favorable histology with Tis, Ta, grade 1 tumors, and certain grade 2 tumors are at lower risk for metastases. The goal in these patients is for organ-sparing treatment. These treatment

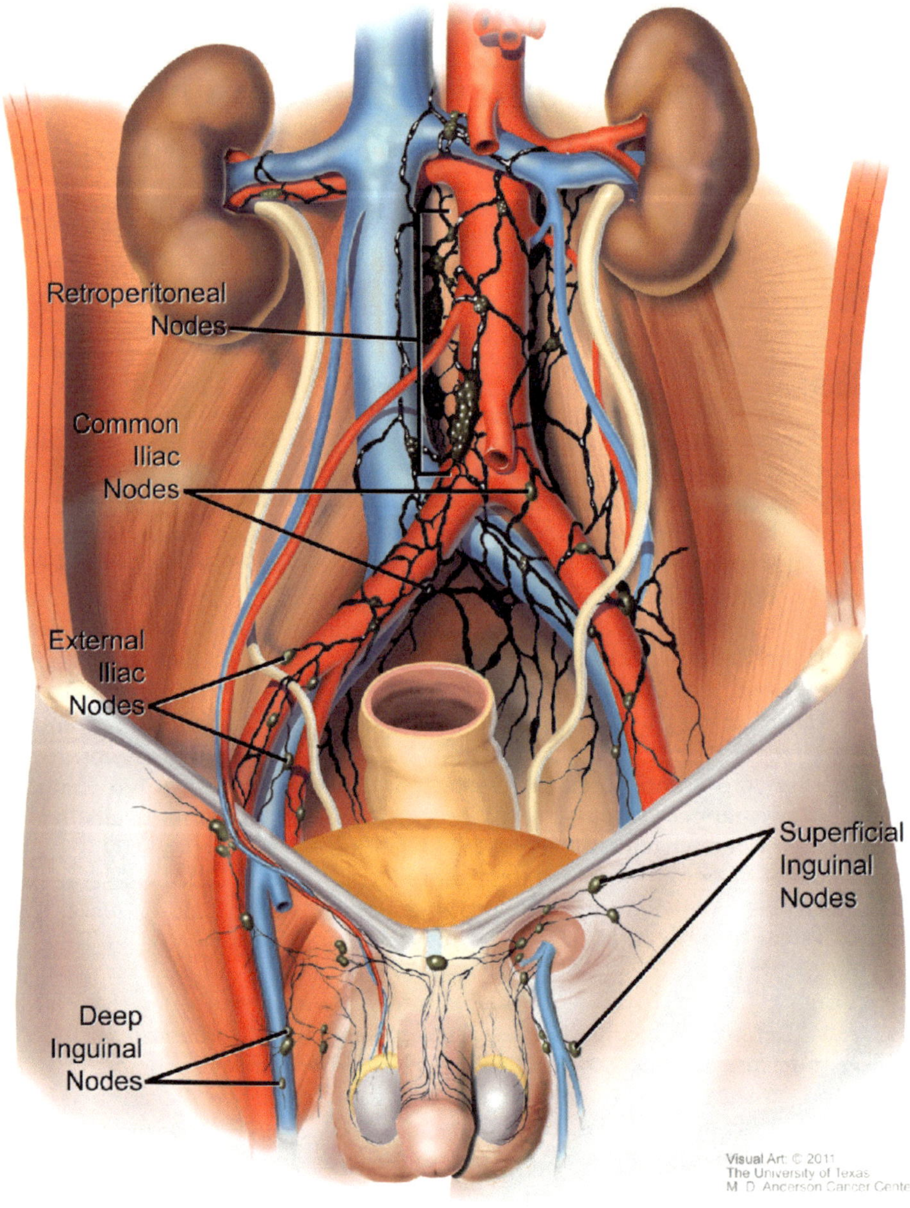

Fig. 1. Lymphatic drainage of the penis (Medical Graphics and Photography, UT M.D. Anderson Cancer Center, 2011).

options include topical therapy, radiotherapy, Mohs surgery, laser ablation, and partial penectomy. Surgery, radiation, and laser therapy have not been compared in a randomized fashion, and in general, the treatment of choice depends on factors such as tumor size, location, and center experience without noted significant differences in local recurrence rates amongst these options (Pagliaro & Crook, 2009; Pizzocaro et al., 2009). Ablative surgery with partial penectomy does have a lower risk of local recurrence compared to more conservative measures. Proximal tumors or more advanced stages require total penectomy. Appropriate treatment is essential and requires a balance between avoiding overtreatment with ensuring appropriate removal of all cancerous tissues (Leijte et al., 2007).

Primary Tumor (T)	
TX	Primary tumor cannot be assessed
T0	No evidence of primary tumor
Tis	Carcinoma in situ
Ta	Noninvasive verrucous carcinoma
T1a	Tumor invades subepithelial connective tissue without lymph vascular invasion and is not poorly differentiated (i.e., grade 3–4)
T1b	Tumor invades subepithelial connective tissue and exhibits lymph vascular invasion or is poorly differentiated
T2	Tumor invades corpus spongiosum or cavernosum
T3	Tumor invades urethra
T4	Tumor invades other adjacent structures
Regional Lymph Nodes (N)	
Clinical Stage Definition	
cNX	Regional lymph nodes cannot be assessed
cN0	No palpable or visibly enlarged inguinal lymph nodes
cN1	Palpable mobile unilateral inguinal lymph node
cN2	Palpable mobile multiple or bilateral inguinal lymph nodes
cN3	Palpable fixed inguinal nodal mass or pelvic lymphadenopathy unilateral or bilateral
Pathologic Stage Definition	
pNX	Regional lymph nodes cannot be assessed
pN0	No regional lymph node metastasis
pN1	Metastasis in a single inguinal lymph node
pN2	Metastasis in multiple or bilateral inguinal lymph nodes
pN3	Extranodal extension of lymph node metastasis or pelvic lymph nodes(s) unilateral or bilateral
Distant Metastasis (M)	
M0	No distant metastasis
M1	Distant metastasis*

*Lymph node metastasis outside the true pelvis in addition to visceral or bone sites.

Table 1. Definitions of TNM (AJCC, 2010) Used with the permission of the American Joint Committee on Cancer (AJCC), Chicago, Illinois. The original source for this material is the AJCC Cancer Staging Manual, Seventh Edition (2010) published by Springer Science and Business Media LLC, www.springer.com.

Stage 0	Tis	N0	M0
	Ta	N0	M0
Stage I	T1a	N0	M0
Stage II	T1b	N0	M0
	T2	N0	M0
	T3	N0	M0
Stage IIIa	T1-3	N1	M0
Stage IIIb	T1-3	N2	M0
Stage IV	T4	Any N	M0
	Any T	N3	M0
	Any T	Any N	M1

Table 2. Stage Grouping for Penile Cancer (AJCC, 2010) Used with the permission of the American Joint Committee on Cancer (AJCC), Chicago, Illinois. The original source for this material is the AJCC Cancer Staging Manual, Seventh Edition (2010) published by Springer Science and Business Media LLC, www.springer.com.

2.2 Nodal disease

Metastatic disease in the inguinal region is the most important prognostic factor for survival in penile squamous cell carcinoma. The presence of palpable inguinal lymph nodes is not a definitive indicator of metastatic disease as it may also be secondary to inflammation in as many as 50% of cases at the time of initial diagnosis (Pizzocaro et al., 2009). Likewise, occult metastatic disease can escape detection, and multiple studies have shown an incidence of lymph node metastases in up to 40% of patients who are clinically node negative (Delacroix & Pettaway, 2010). Utilization of imaging with ultrasound, CT, and MRI may identify distortion of lymph node architecture; however, they are also not completely reliable in differentiating between causes (Heyns, 2010b).

Clinical features that suggest advanced regional disease include size of inguinal lymph nodes greater than 4 cm, bilateral and multiple enlarged nodes, overlying skin changes, and enlarged pelvic lymph nodes (Delacroix & Pettaway, 2010). Pathologically, the most important prognostic factors for lymph node spread include tumor grade, lymphovascular invasion, perineural invasion, pathological subtype, tumor depth or thickness, anatomic site, size, and growth pattern, with the first three factors being the most predictive (Cubilla, 2009; Pagliaro, 2011; Pagliaro & Crook, 2009).

The optimal management in patients without inguinal adenopathy consists of a variety of approaches to the lymph nodes including surveillance, fine needle aspiration cytology, dynamic sentinel lymph node biopsy, and different variations of lymphadenectomies (Graafland, 2010; Heyns, 2010a). Lymphadenectomies are divided into early versus delayed, with early lymphadenectomy defined as within 6 weeks after treatment of the primary tumor and delayed defined as therapeutic after the development of palpable nodes during follow-up. Johnson and Lo compared early versus late therapeutic inguinal lymph node dissection and reported a 3-year survival rate of 71% versus 57% and a 5-year survival rate of 50% versus 30% favoring the early group (Johnson & Lo, 1984). This benefit is likely due to the incidence of clinically occult metastatic disease and suggests that surgery with microscopic disease rather than bulky nodal disease leads to fewer post-operative complications and results in improved overall survival. However, lymphadenectomy does also come with significant morbidities and an associated mortality of 3%, high costs for the approximately 80% of clinically node negative patients who will be free of lymph node involvement (Pagliaro & Crook, 2009; Heyns, 2010a).

The survival in patients with established lymph node metastases after surgical dissection is variable from 20-60%, a range that correlates with the extent of metastatic disease (Heyns, 2010a; Pagliaro, 2011). Metastatic enlargement of the regional nodes can lead to morbidity with skin necrosis and chronic infection; death, which usually occurs within two years if left untreated, can occur from hemorrhage, sepsis, and failure to thrive. However, unlike many other malignancies, regional nodal metastatic disease can be cured with lymphadenectomy alone in appropriately selected patients (Delacroix & Pettaway, 2010).

2.3 Prognostic factors for combined modality consideration

Overall, the pathologic features that are associated with long term survival after attempted curative lymphadenectomy include the following: two or fewer lymph nodes involved, unilateral involvement, no extranodal extension, and absence of pelvic nodal metastases (Pagliaro, 2011). Once bilateral or pelvic lymph nodes are involved (stage N2 or N3 disease), the 5-year overall and disease-free survival rates drop to only 10-20% and are even more dismal with the presence of extranodal extension (Pizzocaro, 1996).

When lymph nodes are initially fixed, chemotherapy is a rational upfront strategy since surgery would be difficult. In the absence of distant metastases, select patients may be candidates for neoadjuvant therapy in the hopes of downstaging to operable disease with curative intent (Leijte, 2007).

3. Combined modality management

3.1 Chemotherapy response rates

Neoadjuvant chemotherapy for solid tumors requires that there be chemotherapeutic drugs or combinations that exceed a certain threshold of efficacy. Historically, the treatments were first found to have high response rates in the setting of advanced metastatic disease, then tested in the adjuvant or neoadjuvant setting. For the treatment of advanced metastatic penile cancer, various combinations were studied and most had only modest response rates. The activity of combination cisplatin and 5-fluorouracil was first reported by Hussain et al in 1990 where 5 advanced penile squamous cell carcinoma patients were treated with sequential cisplatin and 5-fluorouracil, all five achieved partial response, and one even improved to resectable disease (Hussain et al., 1990). Double agent cisplatin and irinotecan was studied in the phase II EORTC 30992 trial that evaluated 26 patients with T3, T4, N1, N2, N3 or M1 disease. Of these 26 patients, 7 were treated in the neoadjuvant setting. They had 8 total responses, 2 CRs and 6 PRs with 3 of the patients receiving neoadjuvant chemotherapy proceeding to lymphadenectomy having pathologically negative lymph nodes. The overall response rate was 30.8% (Theodore et al., 2008).

The most studied triple-drug regimen is cisplatin, methotrexate, and bleomycin. Dexeus et al initially described this regimen with a response in 10 of 14 patients, including 2 CRs (Dexeus et al., 1991). Additional studies by Haas, Hakenberg, Corral, and Leijte found responses, but at the expense of significant hematological and pulmonary toxicities (Protzel

& Hakenberg, 2009). Newer regimens have better toxicity profiles and higher response rates. Bleomycin is no longer recommended for the treatment of penile cancer.

3.2 Neoadjuvant chemotherapy

The literature regarding neoadjuvant chemotherapy for penile cancer is limited with the first prospective series just recently published (Pagliaro et al., 2010). There have been seven retrospective studies assessing the role of neoadjuvant chemotherapy in cases of fixed inguinal lymph nodes (Protzel & Hakenberg, 2009). Pizzocaro et al were able to achieve partial responses with neoadjuvant chemotherapy in 9 of 16 patients (56%) followed by lymphadenectomy with the best results achieved with a cisplatin/5-fluorouracil combination (Pizzocaro et al., 1996). Leijte et al studied 20 patients with initially unresectable penile cancer who received neoadjuvant chemotherapy at the Netherlands Cancer Institute between 1972 and 2005. Several regimens were sequentially used throughout that time period including: single agent bleomycin until 1985, then bleomycin, vincristine, and methotrexate until 1999, then cisplatin and 5-fluorouracil until 2001, and cisplatin, bleomycin, and methotrexate since 2001, with one patient treated with cisplatin and irinotecan in a clinical trial. Twelve patients had a clinical response to chemotherapy (2 complete, 10 partial), and 8 of the 9 patients who went on to resection with curative intent were clinically disease-free at median follow-up time of 20 months (Leijte et al., 2007). There was a significant difference in overall survival in those who responded to chemotherapy (56% overall survival at 5 years) compared to the nonresponders with stable or progressive disease through treatment (0% overall survival at 5 years) due to recurrence after consolidative surgery as shown in Figure 2 (Leijte et al., 2007).

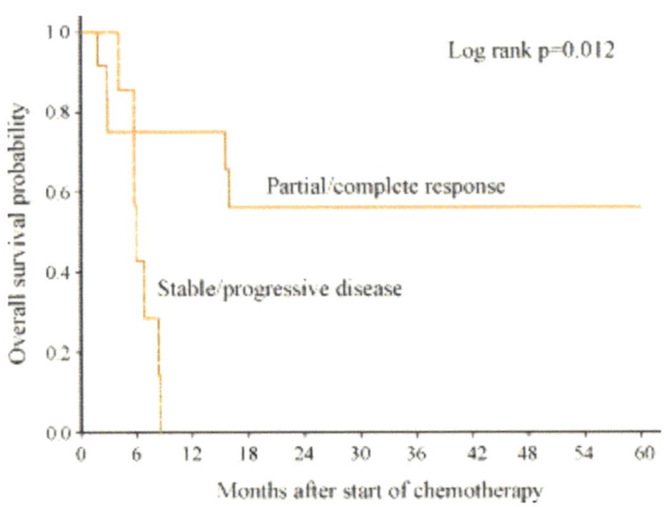

Fig. 2. Overall survival of patients grouped according to response to neoadjuvant chemotherapy (Reproduced from Leijte et al, 2007, with permission).

In another retrospective study, Bermejo et al reviewed 10 patients with advanced penile carcinoma treated from 1985 to 2000 who had received consolidation surgery after having stable, partial, or complete responses on various chemotherapy regimens. After receiving induction regimens consisting of paclitaxel/ifosfamide/cisplatin, bleomycin/methotrexate/ cisplatin, and paclitaxel/carboplatin, the authors found that 4 patients achieved CR, 1 achieved PR, and 5 had stable disease after chemotherapy with responses tending to occur quickly during treatment, often after the first or second cycles. After surgical consolidative lymphadenectomy, pathology revealed that 3 patients had no evidence of metastatic disease in the lymph nodes, with all 3 of these patients having had received paclitaxel, ifosfamide, and cisplatin as their neoadjuvant regimen (Bermejo, 2007). Culkin and Beer's literature review of cisplatin-based neoadjuvant chemotherapy found a clinical response in 69% with 23% of patients having no disease in follow-up after surgery. In summary, these authors found that neoadjuvant chemotherapy could render patients disease-free, and in combination with surgical consolidation, could lead to prolonged survival of patients with advanced penile cancer with low toxicity in regards to surgical complications (Culkin & Beer, 2003).

The design of the first prospective study of neoadjuvant chemotherapy for metastatic penile cancer was based on data related to efficacy of paclitaxel, ifosfamide, and cisplatin in head and neck squamous cell carcinoma (Pagliaro et al., 2010). Thirty patients with clinical stage N2 or N3 disease without evidence of distant metastases were enrolled into a phase II trial of which twenty-three (76.7%) completed four courses of neoadjuvant chemotherapy. N2 and N3 disease was defined by the 1987 to 2002 TNM staging system as palpable, mobile, multiple or bilateral inguinal lymph nodes (N2) or fixed inguinal nodal mass or pelvic lymphadenopathy, unilateral or bilateral (N3). The four cycles were on 21 to 28-day durations depending on count recovery, and paclitaxel was dosed at 175mg/m^2 over 3 hours on day 1, ifosfamide 1200mg/m^2 IV over 2 hours on days 1-3, and cisplatin 25mg/m^2 IV over 2 hours on days 1-3. Twenty-two patients went on to subsequent surgery with bilateral inguinal lymph node dissection and either unilateral or bilateral pelvic lymph node dissection. Three patients (13.6% of those who completed the treatment) had no tumor remaining in the surgical specimen, and 11 patients (36.7% of those enrolled) survived without recurrence, with median follow-up of 34 months at the time of publication (Figure 3A). A total of 3 CRs and 12 PRs were achieved for an overall response rate of 50%.

Figure 3A-B shows an estimated median time to progression of 8.1 months, ranging from 5.4 months to greater than 50 months and an overall survival of 17.1 months, ranging from 10.3 months to greater than 60 months. Univariate analysis showed significantly worse time to tumor progression and overall survival among the patients who did not have an objective response to chemotherapy (Figure 3C-D), had bilateral residual tumor at resection, or had extranodal extension detected after chemotherapy (Pagliaro et al, 2010).

This study determined the outcomes of a specific multimodality approach with neoadjuvant chemotherapy and surgical consolidation; however, it was not randomized and thus was not designed to demonstrate superiority over surgery. However, from the previously published series of penile carcinoma with stage TX, N2-3, M0 disease that document the progression-free and overall survival, as previously mentioned, long-term, disease-free survival was seldom achieved with surgery alone. Based on other series, the estimated long-term survival for patients with pelvic lymph node metastases and/or extranodal extension was only 10-15% with surgery alone. Importantly, there also were no chemotherapy-related deaths or increased surgical morbidity or mortality following this neoadjuvant regimen as compared to the effective, yet toxic, bleomycin, methotrexate, cisplatin regimen.

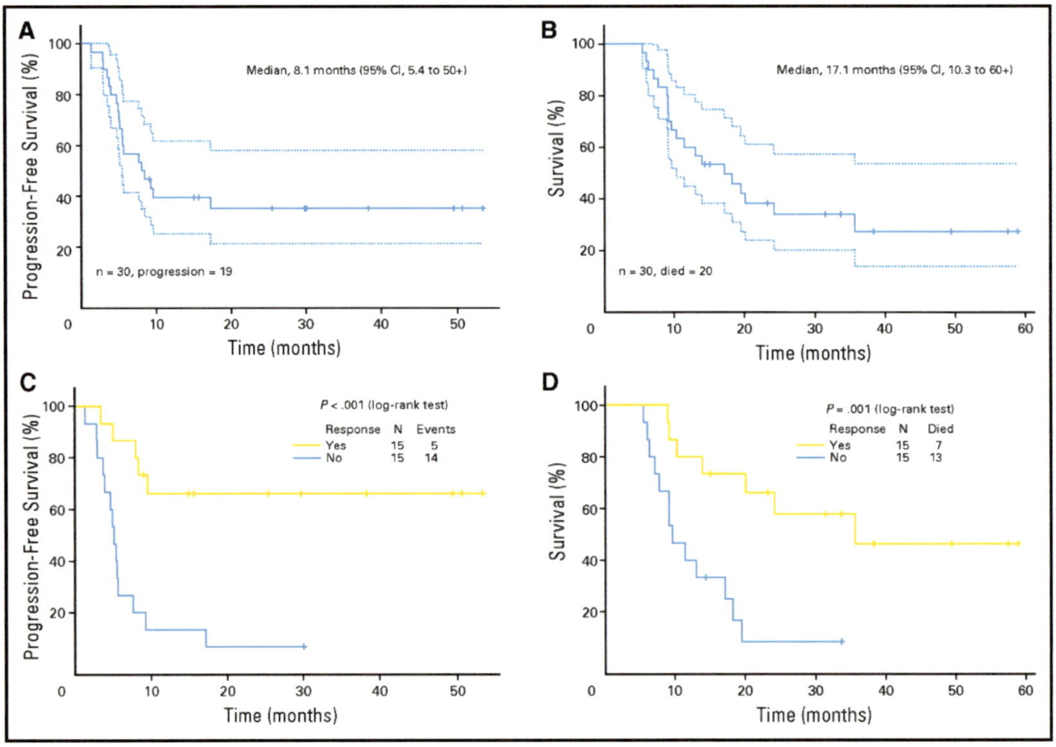

Fig. 3. Overall and progression-free survival for patients treated with neoadjuvant paclitaxel, ifosfamide, and cisplatin chemotherapy (Reproduced from Pagliaro et al, 2010, with permission).

In a special commentary by Pettaway et al, the authors recommend that neoadjuvant chemotherapy should be considered with N1 disease with mobile mass greater than 4 cm, N2-N3 disease, or recurrent regional disease after therapeutic lymph node dissection (Pettaway et al., 2010). This algorithm is demonstrated in Figure 4.

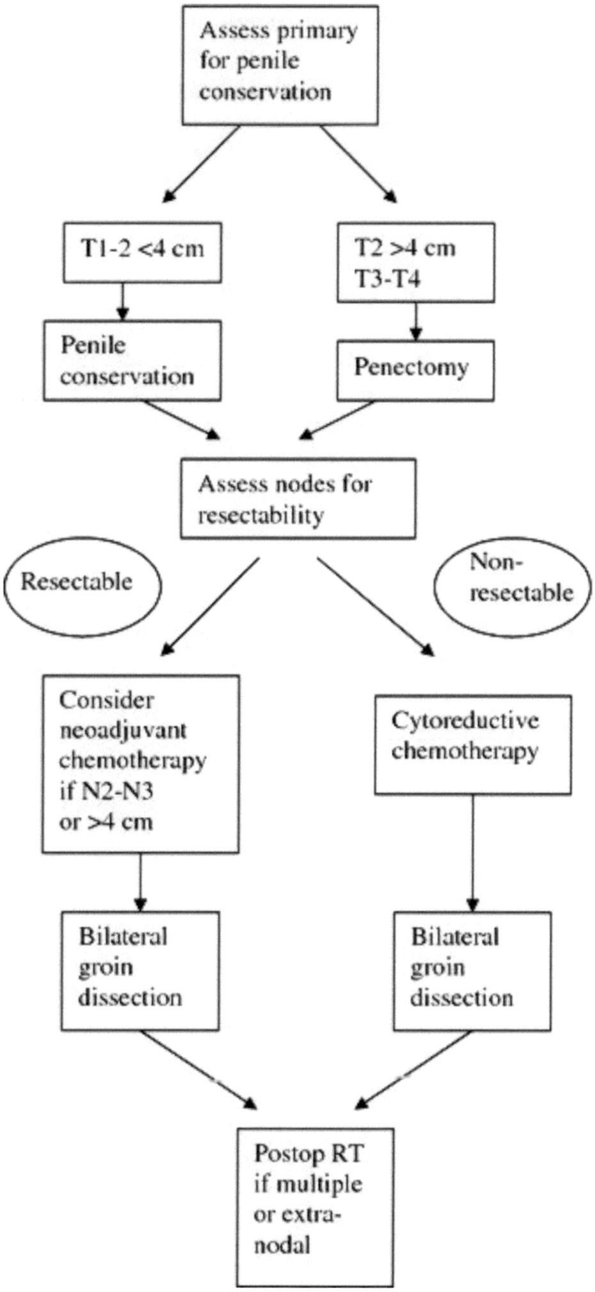

Fig. 4. Algorithm for management of bulky lymph node metastases (Reproduced from Pagliaro and Crook 2009, with permission).

3.3 Post-chemotherapy surgery

Surgical techniques include radical inguinal lymphadenectomy, the gold standard for inguinal metastasis where all lymph nodes in the superficial and deep compartments of the inguino-femoral region are removed, and pelvic lymphadenectomy when indicated depending on degree of inguinal disease (Pettaway et al., 2010). Chemotherapy has not yet been assessed in a neoadjuvant setting for an aim of organ-sparing surgery. There are also no data in regards to using radiation as consolidation treatment in metastatic penile cancer at this time though it is a promising thought given its utility in other squamous cell carcinomas (NCCN, 2010).

3.4 Adjuvant chemotherapy

Little literature exists regarding adjuvant chemotherapy. In a Pizzocaro et al study of 12 patients who received adjuvant vincristine, bleomycin, and methotrexate, only 1 developed progression with a mean remission time of 42 months (Pizzocaro & Piva, 1988). In another Pizzocaro study, the 5-year survival was 82% after adjuvant chemotherapy compared to only 37% in historical controls without adjuvant treatment (Pizzocaro et al., 1996). In Hakenberg's study, mean duration of remission with adjuvant cisplatin, bleomycin, and methotrexate was only 26 months with 1 treatment-associated death (Hakenberg et al., 2006).

3.5 The role of radiotherapy

Radiation in the neoadjuvant setting has not been studied in detail. A retrospective series in India looked at 77 patients over a 20 year period who had palpable pathological node positive disease at least 4 cm in size. Thirty-four of these patients received 40 Gy/4 weeks of radiation followed by consolidative surgery. The irradiated patients had less extranodal extension (9% versus 33%) with a 70% 5 year disease-free survival. However, there was high morbidity with this approach with local complication rate of 100% with skin necrosis or infection (Ravi et al., 1994).

4. Conclusion

Squamous cell carcinoma of the penis is an uncommon disease, which essentially precludes randomized clinical studies. The prognosis for metastatic penile carcinoma is known to be very poor with either surgery or chemotherapy alone. Evidence from a recent prospective study (Pagliaro et al, 2010) showed promising results with a multimodal approach with the paclitaxel, ifosfamide, and cisplatin chemotherapy regimen before surgery for curative intent in metastatic disease. This disease truly necessitates a multidisciplinary approach in prognostication and management of these patients to improve survival while reducing morbidity or mortality of unnecessary procedures. Not only are members of medical oncology and urology involved, but wound care and plastic surgery specialists have important roles. This now represents a reasonable standard of care for the treatment of regional metastatic disease.

Future directions should include additional studies to promote the further understanding of the utility of neoadjuvant chemotherapy in lower stage disease that may lead to improved organ-sparing, predictive factors for chemotherapy response, possible addition of biologic agents, role of radiation, and measures to decrease the morbidity of surgery. Squamous cell carcinoma of the penis is now becoming a multidisciplinary disease with many exciting opportunities on the horizon.

5. References

Bermejo, C., Busby, J. E., Spiess, P. E., Heller, L., Pagliaro, L. C. & Pettaway, C. A. (2007) Neoadjuvant chemotherapy followed by aggressive surgical consolidation for metastatic penile squamous cell carcinoma, *J Urol. 177*, 1335-8.

Cubilla, A. L. (2009) The role of pathologic prognostic factors in squamous cell carcinoma of the penis, *World J Urol. 27*, 169-77.

Culkin, D. & Beer, T. M. (2003) Advanced penile carcinoma, *J Urol. 170*, 359-365.

Delacroix, S. E., Jr. & Pettaway, C. A. (2010) Therapeutic strategies for advanced penile carcinoma, *Curr Opin Support Palliat Care. 4*, 285-92.

Dexeus, F. H., Logothetis, C. J., Sella, A., Amato, R., Kilbourn, R., Fitz, K. & Striegel, A. (1991) Combination chemotherapy with methotrexate, bleomycin and cisplatin for advanced squamous cell carcinoma of the male genital tract, *J Urol. 146*, 1284-

Edge, S. B., Byrd D. R., Carducci, M. A., Compton, C. C., eds. (2010) AJCC Cancer Staging Manual. 7th ed. New York: Springer.

Graffland, N. M., Lam, W., Leitje, J. A., Yap, T., Gallee, M. P., Corbishley, C., van Werkhoven, E., Watkin, N. & Horenblas, S. (2010) Prognostic Factors for Occult Inguinal Lymph Node Involvement in Penile Carcinoma and Assessment of the High-Risk EAU Subgroup: A Two-Institution Analysis of 342 Clinically Node-Negative Patients, *Eur Urol. 58*, 742-7.

Hakenberg, O. W., Nippgen, J. B., Froehner, M., Zastrow, S. & Wirth, M. P. (2006) Cisplatin, methotrexate and bleomycin for treating advanced penile carcinoma, *BJU Int. 98*, 1225-7.

Heyns, C. F., Fleshner, N., Sangar, V., Schlenker, B., Yuvaraja, T. B. & van Poppel, H. (2010) Management of the lymph nodes in penile cancer, *Urology. 76*, S43-57.

Heyns, C. F., Mendoza-Valdes, A. & Pompeo, A. C. (2010) Diagnosis and staging of penile cancer, *Urology. 76*, S15-23.

Hussein, A. M., Benedetto, P. & Sridhar, K. S. (1990) Chemotherapy with cisplatin and 5-fluorouracil for penile and urethral squamous cell carcinomas, *Cancer. 65*, 433-8.

Johnson, D. E. & Lo, R. K. (1984) Management of regional lymph nodes in penile carcinoma. Five-year results following therapeutic groin dissections, *Urology. 24*, 308-11.

Leijte, J. A., Gallee, M., Antonini, N., & Horenblas, S. (2006) Evaluation of current (2002) TNM classification of penile carcinoma, *J Urol. 180*,933-938.

Leijte, J. A., Kerst, J. M., Bais, E., Antonini, N. & Horenblas, S. (2007) Neoadjuvant chemotherapy in advanced penile carcinoma, *Eur Urol. 52*, 488-94.

McDougal, W. S., Kirchner, F. K., Jr., Edwards, R. H. & Killion, L. T. (1986) Treatment of carcinoma of the penis: the case for primary lymphadenectomy, *J Urol. 136*, 38-41.

Neto, A. S., Tobias-Machado, M., Ficarra, V., Wroclawski, M. L., Amarante, R. D., Pompeo, A. C. & Giglio, A. D. (2011) Dynamic Sentinel Node Biopsy for Inguinal Lymph Node Staging in Patients with Penile Cancer: A Systematic Review and Cumulative Analysis of the Literature, *Ann Surg Oncol.*

NCCN Clinical Practice Guidelines in Oncology: National Comprehensive Cancer Network (2010).

Pagliaro, L. C. & Crook, J. (2009) Multimodality therapy in penile cancer: when and which treatments?, *World J Urol. 27*, 221-5.

Pagliaro, L. Penile Cancer, in Kantarjian, H. M., Wolff, R. A. & Koller, C. A. eds. (2011) MD Anderson Manual of Medical Oncology, 2nd ed. New York: McGraw-Hill.

Pagliaro, L. C., Williams, D. L., Daliani, D., Williams, M. B., Osai, W., Kincaid, M., Wen, S., Thall, P. F. & Pettaway, C. A. (2010) Neoadjuvant paclitaxel, ifosfamide, and cisplatin chemotherapy for metastatic penile cancer: a phase II study, *J Clin Oncol. 28*, 3851-7.

Persky, L. (1977) Epidemiology of cancer of the penis. Recent results, *Cancer Research*, 97-109.

Pettaway, C. A., Pagliaro, L., Theodore, C. & Haas, G. (2010) Treatment of visceral, unresectable, or bulky/unresectable regional metastases of penile cancer, *Urology. 76*, S58-65.

Pizzocaro, G., Algaba, F., Horenblas, S., Solsona, E., Tana, S., Van Der Poel, H. & Watkin, N. A. (2009) EAU penile cancer guidelines 2009, *Eur Urol. 57*, 1002-12.

Pizzocaro, G. & Piva, L. (1988) Adjuvant and neoadjuvant vincristine, bleomycin, and methotrexate for inguinal metastases from squamous cell carcinoma of the penis, *Acta Oncol. 27*, 823-4.

Pizzocaro, G., Piva, L. & Nicolai, N. (1996) Treatment of lymphatic metastasis of squamous cell carcinoma of the penis: experience at the National Tumor Institute of Milan, *Arch Ital Urol Androl. 68*, 169-72.

Protzel, C. & Hakenberg, O. W. (2009) Chemotherapy in patients with penile carcinoma, *Urol Int. 82*, 1-7.

Ravi, R., Chaturvedi, H. K. & Sastry, D. V. (1994) Role of radiation therapy in the treatment of carcinoma of the penis, *Br J Urol. 74*, 646-51.

Theodore, C., Skoneczna, I., Bodrogi, I., Leahy, M., Kerst, J. M., Collette, L., Ven, K., Marreaud, S. & Oliver, R. D. (2008) A phase II multicentre study of irinotecan (CPT 11) in combination with cisplatin (CDDP) in metastatic or locally advanced penile carcinoma (EORTC PROTOCOL 30992), *Ann Oncol. 19*, 1304-7.

Wood, H. M. & Angermeier, K. W. (2010) Anatomic considerations of the penis, lymphatic drainage, and biopsy of the sentinel node, *Urol Clin North Am. 37*, 327-34.

Neoadjuvant Chemotherapy for Soft Tissue Sarcoma of the Extremity or Trunk, Gastrointestinal Stromal Tumors, and Retroperitoneal Sarcoma

Lloyd Mack and Walley Temple
University of Calgary
Canada

1. Introduction

Soft tissue sarcomas (STS) are a heterogeneous group of tumors (Table 1) that account for approximately 1% of all adult cancer (Clark et al., 2005). There are more than 50 subtypes that are stratified by their histological appearance, presence or absence of characteristic gene translocations, or sensitivity to chemotherapy. They can be found in nearly any site in the body, but upper and lower extremity soft tissue sarcomas make up approximately 60% of all cases (Zagars et al., 2003). Soft tissue sarcomas of the trunk make up another 10% with retroperitoneal tumors comprising approximately 15% (Stoeckle et al., 2001). Gastrointestinal stromal tumors are the most common mesenchymal tumor of the gastrointestinal tract (Miettinen M & Lasota, J 2006). They can occur anywhere along the gastrointestinal tract but are most commonly found in the stomach (60%) or small intestine (30%). Other sites are quite rare including rectum (3%), colon (1-2%), and esophagus (<1%).

Histology	Subtype
Malignant fibrous histiocytoma	
Liposarcoma	Well-differentiated, myxoid, round cell, pleomorphic
Leiomyosarcoma	
Synovial	Monophasic, biphasic
Fibrosarcoma	
Rhabdomyosarcoma	Embryonal, alveolar, pleomorphic
Malignant peripheral nerve sheath tumor	
Angiosarcoma	Hemangiopericytoma, lymphangiosarcoma
Undifferentiated/ unclassified	
Rare/ miscellaneous	Alveolar soft parts, clear cell, epithelioid, malignant mesenchymal, malignant granular cell, mixed mesodermal, endometrial stromal

Table 1. Common Histologies and Subtypes of Soft Tissue Sarcoma

The incidence rate for soft tissue sarcoma is approximately 6/ 100000/ year (Ferrari et al., 2011). Soft tissue sarcomas make up a small fraction of the overall cancer burden. However, it occurs in all ages including young adults so there is a disproportionately high economic impact in a working population. Approximately 3300 to 6000 gastrointestinal stromal tumors are diagnosed annually in the United States with an estimated incidence of 0.68/ 100000/ year (Tran et al., 2005). The true incidence may be higher depending on the proportion of gastrointestinal tumors being tested for c-kit or platelet-derived growth factor receptor alpha (PDGFRA).
The heterogeneity of these tumors presents a challenge in the diagnosis and treatment of soft tissue sarcomas and their relative infrequency limits the ability to conduct meaningful clinical trials. This chapter will focus on neoadjuvant chemotherapy for adult soft tissue sarcomas primarily of the extremity and trunk. Separate sections on retroperitoneal sarcomas and gastrointestinal stromal tumors (GIST) will focus on their unique biology and potential neoadjuvant treatment strategies.

2. Initial assessment

All patients with a suspected soft tissue sarcoma are assessed with a full history concentrating on presenting symptoms such as mass, pain, and neurovascular deficits as well as constitutional symptoms. For suspected STS of the retroperitoneum or for primary GIST, attention is directed to complaints associated with an abdominal mass, early satiety, back pain and the development of lymphedema or leg discomfort as well as symptoms of gastrointestinal hemorrhage and bowel or urinary obstruction. Physical examination includes the chest to rule out obvious findings of metastatic disease such as pleural effusion, abdomen for organomegaly or mass, and evaluation of the involved extremity and draining lymph node basins. For the extremity, assessment of tumor size, determination of whether a mass is mobile and superficial versus fixed and deep to muscular fascia, and an appropriate neurovascular assessment including documentation of limb function is required.
Initial imaging includes plain radiographs of the affected area, chest x-ray and cross-sectional imaging of the mass with either computer tomography (CT) scan or magnetic resonance imaging (MRI). MRI usually gives the most information regarding invasion of important neurovascular structures in STS of the extremity or trunk (Heslin & Smith, 1999). CT is often quite comparable and can assess potential periosteal or bony invasion, although uncommon. CT scan of the chest, abdomen and pelvis is appropriate for the initial evaluation of retroperitoneal tumors and GISTs.
Image or surgeon directed core biopsy obtaining multiple samples generally makes the diagnosis of STS in >90% of cases (Hoeber et al., 2001; Welker et al., 2000). In cases where core biopsy is non-diagnostic, an incisional biopsy is needed and should be performed by an experienced soft tissue oncology surgeon. The incision is made longitudinally on the limb directly over the palpable mass so the biopsy tract or incision can be removed at the time of definitive surgery. Small (≤3 cm), superficial soft tissue masses can be removed by excisional biopsy, again using a longitudinal incision with minimal skin flaps, careful hemostasis, and a complete yet minimal margin. GISTs are usually biopsied via an endoscopic approach when in the stomach, duodenum or rectum; or by percutaneous approach or surgery if inaccessible via endoscopy. Retroperitoneal sarcomas are more commonly being diagnosed with image directed core biopsy, especially in centers where a neoadjuvant approach to treatment is considered.

Pathologic assessment is performed by a pathologist experienced in the diagnosis and grading of STS including microscopic evaluation, immunohistochemistry, and cytogenetic and molecular pathologic evaluation as appropriate (Coindre et al., 1988). This may include fluorescent in situ hybridization (FISH) or RT-PCR assessing for recurrent chromosomal translocations which may be present in up to one third of sarcomas. For GIST, c-Kit (CD117 (KIT)) immunohistochemistry staining is positive in 95% of cases (Fletcher et al., 2002). Analysis for known mutations of KIT and PDGF genes may be used in morphologically typical GIST that are CD117 negative. Mitotic count is prognostic and should be expressed as the number of mitoses per 50 high-power fields. Further, mutational analysis has predictive value for sensitivity to molecular targeted therapy.

Staging recommendations include CT chest for extremity or trunk STS and CT chest, abdomen, and pelvis for retroperitoneal sarcoma and GIST subtypes. CT abdomen and pelvis is also employed for some subtypes of STS including myxoid liposarcoma which has a more variable metastatic pattern. Sentinel lymph node biopsy is considered in uncommon histological subtypes of extremity soft tissue sarcoma including clear cell, epitheliod, or angiosarcoma where lymph node metastases are more common (Maduekwe et al., 2009).

3. Local treatment

3.1 Local treatment for soft tissue sarcoma of the extremity or trunk

Level I evidence confirms equivalent outcomes with limb-sparing surgery and adjuvant irradiation compared to amputation or wide excision alone (Pisters et al., 1994; Rosenberg et al., 1982; Yang et al., 1998). The ideal specific combinations of surgery, radiotherapy and possible chemotherapy remain controversial. Multidisciplinary discussions and planning is vital; final treatment recommendations often depend more on location of the tumor and local expertise than overall evidence.

Most centers follow treatment protocols using either pre-operative or post-operative irradiation and limb-sparing, function-preserving surgery for STS. The optimum timing of radiation therapy was evaluated in a randomized control trial that showed no overall differences in local control, disease-free survival or overall survival between treatment arms (O'Sullivan et al., 2002). Wound complications were higher (35% v 17%; p=0.01) in the group treated with pre-operative radiation, and were most significant in the lower limb. Those treated with postoperative radiation had better function at 6 weeks post surgery but no significant differences at later time points (Davis et al., 2002). However, there was more late radiation morbidity from fibrosis in the postoperative radiation arm. Significant fibrosis was associated with more joint stiffness and edema adversely affecting patient function (Davis et al., 2005).

Soft tissue sarcomas superficial to muscular fascia or atypical lipomas/ well-differentiated liposarcomas are more often treated with limb-sparing surgery alone with clear microscopic margins (Kooby et al., 2004; Pisters et al., 2007). However, combination of limb sparing surgery and irradiation in some fashion is the standard of care for the majority of soft tissue sarcomas of the extremity or trunk.

3.2 Identification of high-risk soft tissue sarcoma

Important factors predictive of a higher local recurrence for STS include positive margins following resection, presentation with locally recurrent disease, and high grade pathology (Eilber et al., 2003; Pisters et al., 1996). Prognostic factors predictive of systemic recurrence and death include older age at diagnosis (> 60 years), increasing tumor size (>5, 5 to 10, or > 10 cm), higher tumor grade, depth (deep to muscular fascia) and site (head and neck, abdominal, retroperitoneal and trunk worse than extremity) (Coindre et al., 2001; Kattan et al., 2002; Pisters et al., 1996). In a large series of 1225 patients treated with limb-sparing surgery and radiation for localized STS, the risk of local or distant relapse was highest in the first few years, with approximately two thirds of recurrences by 2 years and more than 90% by 5 years (Zagars et al., 2003). Unfortunately, approximately 50% of those with high risk STS die of their disease. Hence, it is in these high risk sub-groups that the role of chemotherapy is usually explored.

4. Effective chemotherapeutic agents

Doxorubicin is the most active agent in metastatic STS excluding GISTs with response rates from 20-30%(Edmonson et al., 1993; Eriksson 2010). Ifosfamide is the second most commonly used agent with response rates of 15-30%. Combination chemotherapy of doxorubicin and ifosfamide or cyclofosfamide appears to have an increased tumor response in the metastatic setting but the toxicity is similarly increased (Eriksson 2010). A randomized trial is currently enrolling comparing doxorubicin alone versus doxorubicin plus ifosfamide in the metastatic setting (Verschraegen et al., 2010). At present, either doxorubicin or ifosfamide or the combination is considered first line for metastatic soft tissue sarcoma. Similarly, doxorubicin or ifosfamide or the combination is the most common agents used in the adjuvant setting.

Other potential agents for treatment of soft tissue sarcomas in the metastatic setting include dacarbazine or its oral analogue temozolomide (often in the multidrug combination of MAID - mesna, doxorubicin, ifosfamide and dacarbazine), gemcitabine, taxanes such as paclitaxel, the combination of gemcitabine and docetaxel, vinca alkaloids such as vinorelbine, trabectedin , as well as etoposide. Although these agents have been used as second or third line in the metastatic setting, use in the adjuvant setting is uncommon.

4.1 Adjuvant chemotherapy for soft tissue sarcoma of the extremity and trunk

The use of adjuvant chemotherapy in soft tissue sarcoma is controversial. Some randomized trials have suggested chemotherapy improves disease-free and overall survival while many have not (Frustaci et al. 2001). Issues with the study of adjuvant chemotherapy in STS include the lack of a highly effective agent, the heterogeneity of tumors within the grouping STS, the rareness of the disease, and the potential dilution of effect in clinical trials by inclusion of all patients regardless of risk, including those unlikely to benefit.

The largest meta-analysis of doxorubicin-based chemotherapy assessed individual patient data from 14 trials and did show an improvement in disease-free survival but no improvement in overall survival (Tierney et al., 1997). However, subset analysis notes an absolute 7% improvement in disease-free survival and an absolute 4% improvement in overall survival for the subgroup of patients with STS of the trunk or extremity with tumors greater than 5 cm and high grade (grades 2 or 3 out of 3). Other subtypes of STS by location, size, or grade showed no differences in disease-free or local survival. The same meta-analysis notes insufficient evidence to make recommendations for adjuvant chemotherapy for retroperitoneal sarcomas. Further, it was felt there are insufficient data to determine whether single-agent doxorubicin or combination chemotherapy should be recommended. An updated meta-analysis with four additional trials including the use of ifosfamide in the adjuvant studies found the hazard ratios of local, distant and overall survival were 0.73 (95% CI 0.56-0.95), 0.65 (95% CI 0.53-0.80), and 0.67 (95% CI 0.56-0.82) respectively in favor of adjuvant chemotherapy (Pervaiz et al., 2008).

5. Neoadjuvant therapies for soft tissue sarcoma of the extremity and trunk

Early administration of chemotherapy in STS can theoretically treat micro-metastatic disease, decrease the rate of distant metastatic disease and improve overall survival. Early non-randomized trials suggest a higher response rate for primary tumors compared to chemotherapy given in the setting of distant metastases (Rouessse et al., 1987). Therefore, preoperative chemotherapy may have a role in downstaging primary tumors to improve resectability. Finally, response to chemotherapy in vivo could affect choices of postoperative adjuvant chemotherapy.

5.1 Neoadjuvant systemic chemotherapy

One randomized trial has assessed neoadjuvant systemic chemotherapy for STS. The small (134 patients) multicenter trial by Gortzak et al. (2001) assessed preoperative chemotherapy with doxorubicin and ifosfamide vs. no preoperative therapy in patients aged 15-75 with high risk STS. High risk was defined as tumors ≥ 8 cm of any grade, or grade II/III tumors < 8 cm, or grade II/III locally recurrent tumors or grade II/III tumors with inadequate surgery performed in the previous 6 weeks which required further surgery. Preoperative chemotherapy consisted of three cycles of doxorubicin (q 3 weeks -50mg/m2 bolus) and ifosfamide (5 g/m2) by 24-hour infusion. Surgery occurred within 3 weeks of completion of chemotherapy. Surgery was planned at randomization in both arms and could include amputation, compartmental resection, wide or marginal excision. Postoperative radiation could be used if marginal surgery, for microscopically positive margins with no possibility of further surgery with limb salvage, or in cases of surgery for local recurrence. Although 150 were initially entered into the trial, 134 were eligible with randomization of 67 to each arm. The response rate was 28% in the chemotherapy arm (8% complete, 20% partial); no different than the usual response in the setting of metastatic disease. Side effects from chemotherapy arm included alopecia, nausea and emesis (95%), and leukocytopenia (32%). There was an 8% grade IV leukocytopenia rate and one grade V complication (death) from febrile neutropenia. Surgical outcomes included 88% limb salvage and 12% amputation rate. At median follow-up of 7.3 years, 5 year disease-free survival was 52% and 56% in the surgery alone and chemotherapy arms respectively (p=0.35). Overall 5-year survival was 64 and 65% respectively (p=0.22). A priori sample size calculations estimated 269 patients were required to detect a 15% increase in 5-year survival. Although closed prior to its planned accrual, it was felt the study results made it unlikely that a major survival benefit would be achieved with preoperative systemic doxorubicin and ifosfamide. The authors note preoperative chemotherapy was feasible and did not compromise subsequent surgery, radiation treatments or wound healing.

A retrospective analysis by Meric et al. (2000) had similar findings with regards to surgical complications. They compared 204 patients having surgery first to 105 who had preoperative chemotherapy with various regimes including combinations or single agent doxorubicin, ifosfamide, dacarbazine, cyclophosphamide, or mesna. Generally, those in the neoadjuvant chemotherapy group had large tumors (12 vs. 8 cm), a higher proportion of high grade tumors (90 vs. 64%) and were younger (age 47 vs. 55 years of age). The incidence of surgical complications was similar (34 vs. 41% for extremity; 29 vs 34% for retroperitoneal/ visceral) with the majority of complications being wound infections or other wound complications. The main predictors of wound complications were preoperative radiation, autologous flap coverage, and those with lower extremity tumors, rather than the use of neoadjuvant chemotherapy.

A two center retrospective analysis by Grobmyer et al. ((2004) assessed preoperative systemic chemotherapy with doxorubicin, ifosfamide and mesna followed by surgery (74 patients) versus surgery alone (282 patients) for the time period 1990-2001. Inclusion criteria included high-grade, deep, >5cm extremity soft tissue sarcomas. Overall, there was a younger median age in the group treated with neoadjuvant chemotherapy (50 years vs. 62 years) and more of the synovial sarcoma histological subtype. Size was similar but slightly larger in the neoadjuvant group (median 12 cm vs. 10 cm). With potential imbalances that may favor the surgery alone arm, the unadjusted hazard ratio for the effect of neoadjuvant chemotherapy on disease-specific survival was 0.75 (95% CI:0.45-1.2). Following multivariate analysis including factors size, histology and age, the HR for the effect of neoadjuvant chemotherapy on disease-specific survival was 0.52 (95%CI:0.30-0.92). Three year disease-specific survival for tumors greater than 10 cm was 83 %(72-95) vs. 62% (53-71) for those treated with neoadjuvant chemotherapy vs. surgery alone respectively. The authors felt the study suggests an association between neoadjuvant chemotherapy and disease-specific survival but caution the retrospective nature of the study had distinct limitations.

At present, there is no convincing evidence for the routine use of systemic dose neoadjuvant chemotherapy alone in the treatment of soft tissue sarcoma of the extremity. However, neoadjuvant protocols continue to be developed. The overall challenge with neoadjuvant systemic chemotherapy has been the lack of a highly effective agent.

5.2 Neoadjuvant chemoradiation

A number of primarily single center trials assess the approach of neoadjuvant chemoradiation in the treatment of STS. Advantages of combining chemotherapy and radiation include the potential of using a lower dose of radiation and possibly avoiding side effects such as wound complications associated with high dose preoperative radiation. Downstaging can occur and resection margins may be less radical, especially near critical neurovascular structures. Although the literature often suggests neoadjuvant chemotherapy given with radiation may still theoretically treat micro-metastatic disease, it is important to recognize that the chemotherapy dose is often significantly reduced, in which case it is being used primarily as a radiosensitizer. Generally trials can be divided into those with neoadjuvant chemoradiation usually with chemotherapy as a radiosensitizer versus trials with systemic neoadjuvant chemotherapy with radiation interdigitated between cycles.

Based on a prior pilot study, an important phase II trial by the Radiation Therapy Oncology Group assessed systemic dose preoperative chemotherapy interdigitated with preoperative radiation therapy followed by 3 cycles of postoperative chemotherapy (Delaney et al., 1996; Kraybill et al., 2006). Sixty-six patients were enrolled with 64 analyzed. Preoperative chemotherapy consisted of 3 cycles of mesna, doxorubicin, ifosfamide and dacarbazine (MAID) with 44 Gy of preoperative radiation; twenty-two Gy was given in 11 daily fractions between cycle 1 and 2 as well as cycle 2 and 3. Seventy-nine percent completed preoperative chemotherapy and 59% completed all chemotherapy. Three patients died from grade 5 toxicity (hematologic/ infectious) and 83% had grade 4 toxicities with the majority being hematologic. There was a 22% partial response rate based on radiology and 27% had no viable tumor at pathologic review. Sixty-one patients came to surgery with 58 R0 resections including 5 amputations. The 3-year rate of local regional failure was 10.1%. Three year disease-free, distant disease-free, and overall survival was 56.6%, 64.5%, and 75.1% respectively. The three-year survival rates were promising compared to the literature dealing primarily with large, high grade tumors. The trial authors conclude that an aggressive neoadjuvant regime can be delivered in a cancer cooperative group. However, the substantial toxicity of the treatment precludes its use outside of clinical trials. It is suggested the future of this regime may be a modified version with possible targeted therapies and reduced doses of cytotoxic agents.

The most recent publication of neoadjuvant chemoradiation where full dose chemotherapy is used involves 25 patients with intermediate or high-grade soft tissue sarcomas with 3 cycles of pre and postoperative epirubicin and ifosfamide with 28 Gy of irradiation given in 8 fractions during cycle 2 of chemotherapy (Ryan et al., 2008). Sixteen patients completed the entire treatment but 21 had grade 4 toxicity which was generally hematologic such as febrile neutropenia and anemias. Postoperative wound complications occurred in 20%. Forty percent of resected specimens showed >95% pathologic necrosis. The 2-year overall and disease-free survival rates were 84 and 62%. Although the high pathologic response rate was encouraging, the relatively high rate of major toxicity limited the use of this protocol.

Overall, full dose systemic chemotherapy with interdigitated radiation has not been successful in convincingly improving disease-free or overall survival for patients with high-risk tumors. Although higher response rates have been reported, these generally have trended with higher toxicity.

A phase I trial of concurrent preoperative doxorubicin and radiation used full-dose radiation (50Gy) with varying doses of 4-day continuous doxorubicin (Pisters et al., 2004). This is the only reported trial of truly concurrent chemoradiation. The maximum tolerated dose of continuous-infusion doxorubicin was 17.5mg/m2/week. Among 22 patients treated with this dose and full-dose radiation, 50% had a greater than 90% tumor necrosis rate including 2 patients with a complete pathologic response. Six patients (23%) experienced major wound complications requiring hospital admission; two patients required re-operation.

An early neoadjuvant chemoradiation regime where chemotherapy was used as a radiosensitizer was developed and popularized by Eilber et al. (2003) at the University of Calfornia, Los Angeles (UCLA). An initial protocol combined intra-arterial doxorubicin and sequential hypofractionated radiation (35 Gy in 3.5 Gy fractions) followed by limb-sparing surgery. In a small series, all patients avoided amputation and the local recurrence rate was 3%; the best local control rate in the literature. However, postoperative wound complications were considerable with 23% of patients requiring re-operation. Following further experimentation of the protocol, the most widely published regime included 28 Gy in 3.5 daily fractions. Further, intra-arterial chemotherapy was changed to being given intravenously. Eilber et al. (2001) noted that a pathologic complete response following neoadjuvant chemoradiation was associated with improved local recurrence as well as overall survival.

Further modification of the Eilber protocol occurred at the University of Calgary (Mack et al., 2005). This protocol uses 3 consecutive days of systemic doxorubicin with sequential 10 fractions of 3 Gy preoperative irradiation; total dose 30 Gy. The largest report of this protocol assessed 75 consecutive patients with a 3% 5 year local recurrence rate and a 63% 5

year overall survival. The major wound complication rate of 4% was much lower than other preoperative full-dose radiation protocols. Although local recurrence rates are quite favorable, overall survival data appears unchanged compared to the literature. Wanebo et al. (1995) also reported on 66 patients treated with preoperative doxorubicin and 3-4600 cGY of radiation. In this tricentre study, the 5-year local recurrence rate was 2% and 5 year overall survival was 59%. Other series have been published using various modifications of the Eilber protocol or neoadjuvant chemoradiation strategies with similarly low local recurrence rates (Goodnight et al., 1985; Levine et al., 1993; Pisters et al., 2002).
Therefore, the role of using chemotherapy as a radiosensitizer has promise in terms of local control but not in terms of distant disease control or overall survival. Thus far, this approach has been explored primarily in single centers and has not been studied in a comparative trial.

5.3 Neoadjuvant chemotherapy and regional hyperthermia

Another modification of neoadjuvant chemotherapy is the combination of chemotherapy or radiation with hyperthermia; the tumor is heated to improve the effects of the chemotherapy or radiation. The theory of using hyperthermia is that heat kills cells via thermal toxicity, increases drug efficacy, and induces a tumoricidal immune response.
In a phase III trial of 341 patients with large, high-grade sarcomas (extremity or trunk), patients were randomized to neoadjuvant etoposide, ifosfamide and doxorubicin plus or minus concurrent hyperthermia (Issels et al., 2010). Treatment response was 12.7% in the neoadjuvant chemotherapy arm and 28.8% in the neoadjuvant chemotherapy with hyperthermia arm. The majority of patients (90%) went on to surgery with 6.7% and 8.9% having an amputation in the combination arm and chemotherapy arm respectively. However, only about two thirds had a definitive surgical resection with approximately one third not having a definitive surgery as felt to be impossible. The reasons for unresectability were not explicitly described. The R0 resection rate was quite low at 51% and 41.6% in the combination and chemotherapy alone arms respectively. Approximately two thirds of patients had adjuvant radiation. Local control was improved in the hyperthermia arm (HR 0.58, 95% Cl 0.41-0.83;p=0.003) compared to the chemotherapy alone group. Further, overall survival was better in the combined arm (HR 0.66; 95% CI 0.45-0.98, p=0.038).
Although there have been other phase II trials of this combination treatment, few centers have adopted the approach (Schlemmer et al., 2010). At present, the potential benefits of this new intervention are restricted to patients with very high-risk soft tissue sarcomas in the context of a clinical trial.

5.4 Isolated limb infusion or perfusion

Isolated limb perfusion (ILP) uses high-dose regional chemotherapy where the blood supply to the limb is isolated from the rest of the body by an extracorporeal circulation. It involves a complex and invasive technique by clamping and cannulating the major artery and vein after heparinization of the patient, connection to an oxygenated high-flow extracorporeal circuit, ligation of collateral vessels, and the application of a tourniquet at the root of the limb to occlude superficial veins (Hoekstra 2008). Isolated limb infusion (ILI) is a modified, more minimally invasive technique via percutaneously placed catheters (Kroom & Thompson 2009). Further, ILI is low flow and performed under hypoxic conditions. The intent is still to provide regional chemotherapy but without the potential morbidity of a surgical procedure.

Most commonly, agents used for soft tissue sarcoma of the extremity include tumor necrosis factor-alpha (TNF-α), melphalan, doxorubicin, cisplatin, carboplatin and actinomycin-D (Hoekstra 2008; Kroon & Thompson 2009). TNF-α is only available in Europe. The use of either procedure is limited to large soft tissue tumors initially felt to be unresectable without amputation. It is sometimes used in a palliative fashion in those with large unresectable and symptomatic tumors in the setting of small volume metastatic disease. Although relatively toxic to local tissues, it also has quite high response rates and may allow limb salvage in 70-90% in the short-term and as high as 60% at 5 to 10 years (Di Filippo et al., 2009; Grunhagen et al., 2005; Moncrieff et al., 2008). Complete and partial response rates range from 0-70% and 0-74% respectively (Hoekstra 2008). A randomized trial found no differences in response with varying doses of TNF-α but systemic toxicity did correlate with higher drug dosage (Bonvalot et al., 2005).

6. Retroperitoneal sarcoma

6.1 Local treatment for retroperitoneal sarcomas

Unlike extremity/ trunk STS where surgery and radiation is accepted as the standard of care, the most appropriate treatment of retroperitoneal sarcoma is less clear. En bloc resection of the retroperitoneal STS plus adjacent organs to obtain a negative margin is the most common treatment (Lewis et al., 1998). Unfortunately, as many as 20-60% of tumors are deemed unresectable at presentation or gross residual disease remains after a resection attempt (Catton et al., 1994; Lewis et al., 1998; Sindelar et al., 1993) In this group, there is no survival benefit to partial or incomplete gross resection (Lewis et al., 1998). Even when completely resected, about 25% of cases have microscopically positive margins; potentially higher depending on the intensity of the pathologic evaluation. In a large series, 19% and 41% local recurrence rates at 2 and 5 years respectively were described for those having a complete resection (Lewis et al., 1998). Local recurrence without the development of systemic disease is the leading cause of death in retroperitoneal sarcomas.

Some centers are commonly using preoperative irradiation in an effort to improve upon local control and possibly overall survival for retroperitoneal sarcoma. Theoretical advantages of preoperative irradiation include the gross tumor volume is more clearly demarcated since still in situ, radiosensitive viscera are displaced by the tumor outside of the radiation field, the biologically effective dose is lower preoperatively as the tumor is still well oxygenated, a higher dose can be delivered to the tumor since there are fewer surgical adhesions (less scar), and the tumor is treated preoperatively prior to potential contamination by surgery (Raut & Pisters 2006). Two prospective protocols from the MD Anderson Cancer Center and the University of Toronto employed pre-operative irradiation (45-50 Gy) followed by surgery (Pawlik et al., 2006). At median follow-up of 40 months, combined results showed 5-year local recurrence free, disease free and overall survival rates of 60%, 46%, and 61% respectively. Using 45 Gy of pre-operative irradiation but with the use of surgically placed intra-abdominal spacers to displace small intestine and allow maximal irradiation to the tumor margin, White et al. (2007) describe an 80% 5 year local control rate in a series of 23 patients.

Unfortunately, a phase III trial randomizing between preoperative external beam irradiation (45-50.4 Gy) and surgery versus surgery alone was closed due to poor accrual (Raut & Pisters 2006).

6.2 Neoadjuvant chemotherapy and chemoradiation

The high local recurrence rate after surgery alone has led to combined modality approaches to potentially improve local control. As noted, preoperative irradiation protocols are the most commonly explored. However, there have also been a few attempts of neoadjuvant chemotherapy or neoadjuvant chemoradiation protocols. A study of 16 patients with 3 to 5 cycles of preoperative chemotherapy alternating with irradiation therapy led to 11 surgical resections and 4 R0 resections in advanced, large (median 17 cm) retroperitoneal sarcomas (Robertson et al., 1995). Two further studies of concurrent chemoradiation noted feasible complication rates (11% admission rate for toxicity) and a fairly high (26%) complete pathologic response rate (Eilber et al., 1995; Pisters et al., 2003). Finally, a retrospective review of 55 patients having neoadjuvant chemotherapy (plus preoperative radiation in 56%) found no difference in disease-specific or overall survival compared to predicted outcomes (Donahue et al. 2010). However, those with a greater than 95% pathologic necrosis (25% of cohort) had much improved disease-specific survival compared to non-responders.

A phase II trial of preoperative combined modality treatment for intermediate or high-grade retroperitoneal sarcoma with doxorubicin and ifosfamide followed by preoperative irradiation followed by surgery and an intraoperative or postoperative boost was closed due to poor accrual (Raut & Pisters 2006). Concerns regarding the rare incidence of this tumor subtype and institution specific protocols were the most likely reasons for insufficient timely accrual.

7. Gastrointestinal stromal tumors (GISTs)

7.1 Local treatment of gastrointestinal stromal tumors

The mainstay of treatment for GIST is complete surgical excision with negative margins without dissection of clinically negative nodes (Dematteo et al., 2002). Adjuvant irradiation does not have a role for these intra-abdominal tumors.

7.2 Role of imatinib

The prognosis of GISTs is primarily related to mitotic index and tumor size (Table 2) (Fletcher et al., 2002). The risk of relapse is based on these factors as well as site, surgical margins and whether tumor rupture has occurred (Casali & Blay, 2009). Most patients with localized disease and deemed low risk have surgery alone.

For patients with intermediate or high-risk tumors, adjuvant imatinib is considered. Imatinib is a highly active targeted therapy for patients with GIST. The ACOSOG Z9001 trial compared one year of adjuvant imatinib with placebo in patients with complete resection of their primary GIST which was intermediate or high-risk based on size alone (Dematteo et al., 2007). Based on 756 patients and an interim analysis, the relapse free survival at one year was 97% in the imatinib arm compared to 83% in the placebo arm. This was highly significant and the trial was unblinded; those on placebo crossed over to one year of adjuvant imatinib. There was no overall survival benefit at this point in the trial and this may never be demonstrated due to the crossover of patients after the interim analysis. Therefore, the use of adjuvant imatinib in all patients has been questioned until an overall survival benefit can be demonstrated. Fortunately, a European placebo controlled trial continues and is powered to detect overall survival differences (Joensuu et al., 2011).

	Size	Mitotic Count
Very low risk	< 2 cm	<5/ 50 high power fields (HPF)
Low risk	2-5 cm	<5/ 50 HPF
Intermediate risk	< 5 cm 5-10 cm	6-10/ 50 HPF <5/ 50 HPF
High risk	>5 cm >10 cm Any size	>5/ 50 HPF Any mitotic count >10/ 50 HPF

Table 2. Approach for Defining Risk of Aggressive Behavior in GISTs.

Finally, those patients presenting with locally advanced inoperable tumors or with metastatic disease, palliative intent chemotherapy with imatinib is the standard of care (Blanke et al., 2008). Objective response rates of 50-60% occur with only 10-15% of tumors having primary progression. The first-line dose is 400 mg per day; however, those with exon 9 KIT mutations appear to do better with 800 mg daily (Verweij et al., 2004). Further, in cases of tumor progression, imatinib is increased to 800 mg daily. Second-line therapy includes sunitinib and other anti-tyrosine kinase agents or clinical trial (Casali & Blay, 2010). Gastrointestinal stromal tumors are considered refractory to conventional, systemic chemotherapy (Trent et al., 2003).

7.3 Neoadjuvant imatinib in gastrointestinal stromal tumors (GISTs)

Since GISTs have a high response (50-60%) to imantinib in the metastatic setting, neoadjuvant strategies have been explored to attempt to reduce the surgical procedure required or downstage (Blanke et al., 2008 Verweij et al., 2004). Currently, ESMO guidelines recommend neoadjuvant imantinib in patients for whom a complete R0 resection is not feasible and for patients who are candidates for less mutilating surgery (Casali & Blay, 2009). Similarly, NCCN guidelines recommend neoadjuvant imatinib for marginally resectable tumors or resectable tumors with risk of significant morbidity. Finally, Canadian guidelines consider neoadjuvant imatinib if surgery may result in significant morbidity of loss of organ function (Blackstein et al., 2006). Generally, in these scenarios, subsequent surgery is considered 4-12 months later after maximal tumor response (Figure 1).

A phase II trial of neoadjuvant imatinib was reported by Eisenberg et al. (2009) for advanced primary (30 patients) and metastatic/recurrent yet operable (22 patients) gastrointestinal stromal tumors. Imatinib was used for 8-12 weeks prior to surgery at 600 mg per day. Generally, imatinib was tolerated with 21% grade 3 complications, 12% grade 4 and 2% grade five complications. The response rates by RECIST criteria for primary tumors is partial (7%), stable (83%), and unknown (10%). For those with metastatic/ recurrent yet operable tumors the response was partial (4.5%), stable (91%), and progression (4.5%). Postoperative complications were consistent with a surgical patient series with extensive and re-operative surgery. The type of surgery performed included a single or partial organ resection (53%), multi-organ resection (36%), as well as combinations of organs and peritoneal implants (11%). In the advanced primary tumor group, an R0 resection (no residual gross or microscopic disease) was possible in 77%, R1 (no residual gross disease but microscopic residual) in 15% and R2 (gross disease remaining) in 8%. In the metastatic or recurrent yet operable setting, similar rates were 58%, 5%, and 32% respectively for R0, R1, and R2 resections. The two-year progression free survival was 80.5% and 82.7% in the two groups,. The 2-year overall survival was 93.3% and 90.9% in the group with advanced primary versus metastatic or recurrent yet operable disease, respectively. The overall conclusions of this multicenter trial were that neoadjuvant imatinib in the case of locally advanced primary or metastatic GIST was feasible, requires multidisciplinary considerations, and was not associated with increased postoperative complications.

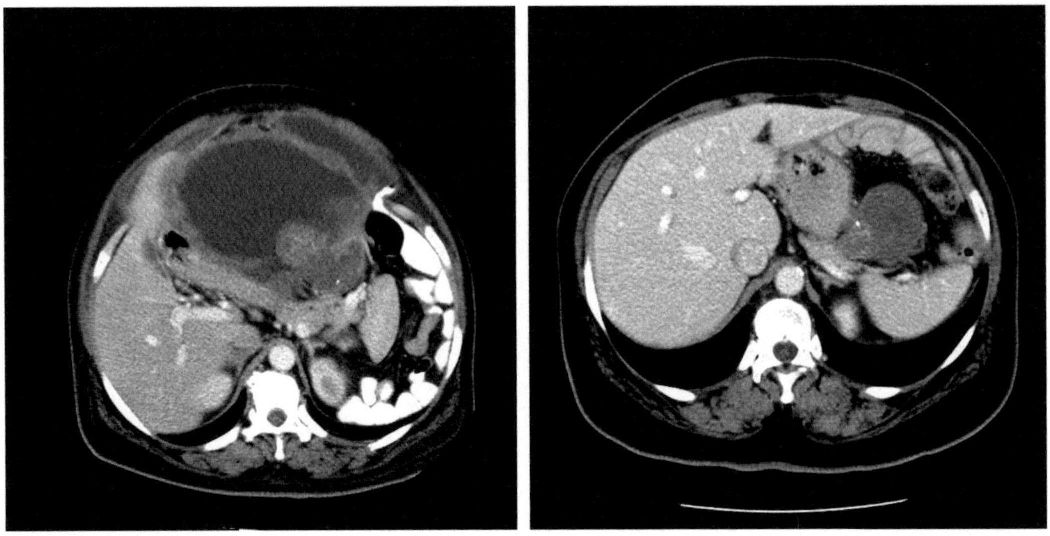

Fig. 1. CT Scans showing Large GIST Before (left) and After (right) Neoadjuvant Imatinib.

8. Future directions

The main difficulties with the use of neoadjuvant therapies for soft tissue sarcoma of the extremity, trunk or retroperitoneum include issues with the lack of a highly effective agent, the heterogeneity of tumors subtypes, the rareness of patients with the disease for participation in clinical trials, and the potential dilution of effect in clinical trials by inclusion of all patients regardless of risk, including those unlikely to benefit. By contrast, patients with gastrointestinal stromal tumors now have a highly effective agent (imatinib) in the metastatic setting with the potential of exploring additional neoadjuvant protocols.

Identification of similar chromosomal translocations and gene microarray technology are playing increasing roles in the diagnosis of soft tissue sarcoma and potential identification of therapeutic targets (Borden et al., 2003; Nielsen et al., 2006). Dynamic positron emission technology (PET) imaging is being used to evaluate treatment responses after initial cycles of neoadjuvant chemotherapy (Dimitrakopoulou-Strauss et al., 2010). Further, there does appear to be a histopathologic correlation of treatment response and PET imaging which may allow early treatment decisions as to continuing or discontinuing neoadjuvant chemotherapy (Benz et al., 2009).

9. Conclusion

Although limb-sparing, function-preserving surgery plus radiation in some fashion is the current standard of care for soft tissue sarcoma of the extremity or trunk, neoadjuvant chemotherapy and chemoradiation strategies continue to be explored and employed especially in large, high-risk tumors. At present, the success of these strategies have been limited primarily due to the lack of an effective agent in soft tissue sarcoma, especially in terms of distant disease free and overall survival rates. The development of new, targeted therapies based on the distinct histologic and biologic differences among subtypes of soft tissue sarcoma is required.

The use of a highly effective agent, imatinib as well as other tyrosine kinase inhibitors in the treatment of gastrointestinal stromal tumors, either neoadjuvantly, adjuvantly, or in the metastatic setting will hopefully correlate with similar development of targeted therapies for soft tissue sarcoma.

10. References

Benz, M.R., Czernin, J., Allen-Auerbach, M.S., Tap, W.D., Dry, S.M., Elashoff, D., Chow, K., Evilevitch, V., Eckardt, J.J., Phelps, M.E., Weber, W.A., & Eilber, F.C. (2009). FDG-PET/CT imaging predicts histopathologic treatment responses after the initial cycle of neoadjuvant chemotherapy in high-grade soft-tissue sarcomas. *Clinical cancer research*, Vol. 15, No. 8, (April 2009), pp. 2856-63, ISSN 1078-0432.

Blanke C.D., Demetri, G.D, von Mehren, M. Heinrich, M.C., Eisenberg, B., Fletcher, J.A., Corless, C.L., Fletcher, C.D., Roberts, P.J., Heinz, D., Wehre, E., Nikolova, Z., & Joensuu, H. (2008). Long-term results from a randomized phase II trial of standard-versus higher-dose imatinib mesylate for patients with unresectable or metastatic gastrointestinal stromal tumours expressing KIT. *Journal of clinical oncology.*, Vol. 26, No. 4, (February 2008), pp. 620-5, ISSN 1527-7755.

Bonvalot, S., Laplanche, A., Lejeune, F., Stoeckle, E., Le Pechoux, C., Vanel, D., Terrier, P., Lumbroso, J., Ricard, M., Antoni, G., Cavalcanti, A., Robert, C., Lassau, N., Blay, J.Y., & Le Cesne, A. (2005). Limb salvage with isolated perfusion for soft tissue sarcoma: could less TNF-alpha be better? *Annals of oncology*, Vol. 16, No. 7, (July 2005), pp. 1061-8, ISSN 1569-8041.

Borden, E.C., Baker, L.H., Bell, R.S., Bramwell, V., Demetri, G.D., Eisenberg, B.L., Fletcher, C.D., Fletcher, J.A., Ladanyi, M., Meltzer, P., O'Sullivan, B., Parkinson, D.R., Pisters, P.W., Saxman, S., Singer, S., Sundaram, M., van Oosterom, A.T., Verweij, J., Waalen, J., Weiss, S.W., & Brennan, M.F. (2003). Soft tissue sarcomas of adults: state of the translational science. *Clinical cancer research*, Vol. 9, No. 3, (June 2003), pp. 1941-56, ISSN 1078-0432.

Casali, P.G. & Blay, J.-Y. (2010). Gastrointestinal stromal tumours: ESMO clinical practice guidelines for diagnosis, treatment and follow-up. *Annals of Oncology,*. Vol. Suppl. 5, (May 2010), pp. v98-102, ISSN 1569-8041.

Catton, C.N., O'Sullivan, B.Kotwall, C. Cummings, B., Hao, Y., & Fornasier, V. (1994). Outcome and prognosis in retroperitoneal soft tissue sarcoma. *International journal of radiation oncology biology physics*, Vol. 29, No. 5, (July 1994), pp. 1005-1010.

Clark, M.A., Fisher, C., Judson, I., & Thomas, J.M. (2005). Soft-tissue sarcomas in adults. *New England journal of medicine*, Vol. 353, pp. 701-11, ISSN 0028-4793.

Coindre, J., Nguyen, B.B., Bonichon, F., de Mascarel, I., & Trojani, M. (1988). Histopathologic grading in spindle cell soft tissue sarcomas. *Cancer*, Vol. 61, No. 11, (June 1988), pp. 2305-9, ISSN 1097-0142.

Coindre, J.M., Terrier, P., Guillou, L., Doussal, V.L., Collin, F., Ranchere, D., Sastre, X., Vilain, M.O., Bonichon, F., & Bui, B.N. (2001). Predictive value of grade for metastasis development in the main histologic types of adult soft tissue sarcomas: a study of 1240 patients from the French Federation of Cancer Centers Sarcoma Group. *Cancer,* Vol. 91, No. 10, (May 2001), pp. 1914-26, ISSN 1097-0142.

Davis, A.M., O'Sullivan, B, Bell, R.S., Turcotte, R., Catton, C.N., Wunder, J.S., Chabot, P., Hammond, A., Benk, V., Isler, M., Freeman, C., Goddard, K., Bezjak, A., Kandel, R.A., Sadura, A., Day, A., James, K., Tu, D., Pater, J., & Zee, B. (2002). Function and health status outcomes in a randomized trial comparing preoperative and postoperative radiotherapy in extremity soft tissue sarcoma. *Journal of clinical oncology,* Vol. 20, No. 22, (November 2002), pp. 4472-7, ISSN 1527-7755.

Davis, A.M., O'Sullivan, B, Turcotte, R., Bell, R., Catton, C., Chabot, P., Wunder, J., Hammond, A., Benk, V., Kandel, R., Goddard, K., Freeman, C., Sadura, A., Zee, B., Day, A., Tu, D., Pater, J., A Canadian Sarcoma Group and NCI Canada Clinical Trials Group Randomized Trial. (2005). Late radiation morbidity following randomization to preoperative versus postoperative radiotherapy in extremity soft tissue sarcoma. *Radiotherapy and oncology,* Vol. 75, No. 1, (April 2005), pp. 48-53, ISSN 0167-8140.

DeLaney, T.F., Spiro, I.J., Suit, H.D., Phil, D., Gebhardt, M.C., Hornicek, F.J., Mankin, H.J., Rosenberg, A.L., Rosenthal, D.E., Miryousefi, F., Ancukiewicz, M., & Harmon, D.C. (2003). Neoadjuvant chemotherapy and radiotherapy for large extremity soft-tissue sarcomas. *International journal of radiation oncology biology and physics,* Vol., 56, No. 4, (July 2003), pp. 1117-27, ISSN 0360-3016.

DeMatteo, R.P., Heinrich, M.C., El-rifai, W.M. & Demetri, G. (2002). Clinical management of gastrointestinal stromal tumors: before and after STI-571. *Human pathology,* Vol. 33, No. 5, (May 2002), pp. 466-77, ISSN 0046-8177.

Di Fiiippo, F., Giacomini, P., Rossi, C.R., Santinami, M., Garinei, R., Anza, M., Deraco, M., Botti, C., Perri, P., Cavaliere, F., Di Angelo, P., Sofra, C., Sperduti, I., Pasqualoni, R., Di Filippo, S., Corrias, F., Armenti, A., & Ferraresi, V. (2009). Hyperthermic isolated perfusion with tumor necrosis factor-alpha and doxorubicin for the treatment of limb-threatening soft tissue sarcoma: the experience of the Italian Society of Integrated Locoregional Treatment in Oncology (SITILO). *In vivo,* Vol. 23, No. 2, (March 2009), pp. 363-7, ISSN 1791-7549.

Dimitrakopoulou-Stauss, A., Strauss, L.G., Egerer, G., Vasamiliette, J., Mechtersheimer, G., Schmitt, T., LEhner, B., Haberkorn, Stroebel, P., & Kasper, B. (2010). Impact of dynamic ^{18}F-FDG PET on the early prediction of therapy outcome in patients with high-risk soft-tissue sarcomas after neoadjuvant chemotherapy: a feasibility study. *Journal of nuclear medicine,* Vol. 51, No. 4, (April 2010), pp. 551-8. ISSN 0161-5505.

Donahue, T.R., Kattan, M.W., Nelson, S.D., Tap, W.D., Eilber, F.R., Eilber, F.C. (2010). Evaluation of neoadjuvant therapy and histopathologic response in primary, high-grade retroperitoneal sarcomas using the sarcoma nomograms. *Cancer,* Vol. 1116, No. 16, (August 2010), pp. 3883-91, ISSN 1097-0142.

Edmonsom, J.H., Ryan, L.M., Blum, R.H., Brooks, J.S., Shiraki, M., Frytak, S., & Parkinson, D.R. (1993). Randomized comparisons of doxorubicin alone versus ifosfamide plus doxorubicin or mitomycin, doxorubicin, and cisplatin against advanced soft tissue sarcoma. *Journal of clinical oncology,* Vol. 11, No. 7, (July 1999), pp. 1269-75, ISSN 1527-7755.

Eilber, F.C., Morton, D.L., Eckardt, J., Grant, T., & Weisenburger, T. (1984). Limb salvage for skeletal and soft tissue sarcomas. *Cancer,* Vol. 53, No. 12, (June 1984), pp. 2579-84, ISSN 1097-0142.

Eilber, F., Eckardt, J., Rosen, G., Forscher, C., Selch, M., & Fu, Y-S. (1995). Preoperative therapy for soft tissue sarcoma. *Hematology/ oncology clinics of North America*, Vol. 9, No. 4, (August 1995), pp. 817-23, ISSN 0889-8588.

Eilber, F.C., Rosen, G., Eckardt, J., Forscher, C., Nelson, S.D., Selch, M., Dorey, F., & Eilber, F.R. (2001). Treatment-induced pathologic necrosis; a predictor of local recurrence and survival in patients receiving neoadjuvant therapy for high-grade extremity soft tissue sarcomas. *Journal of clinical oncology,* Vol. 19, No. 13, (July 2001), pp. 3203-9, ISSN 1527-7755.

Eilber, F.C., Rosen, G., Nelson, S.D., Selch, M., Dorey, F. Eckardt, J., & Eilber, F.R. (2003). High-grade extremity soft tissue sarcomas: factors predictive of local recurrence and its effect on morbidity and mortality. *Annals of surgery.* Vol. 237, No. 2, (February 2003), pp. 218-26, ISSN 0003-4932.

Eisenberg, B.L., Harris, J., Blanke, C., Demetri, G.D., Heinrich, M.C., Watson, J.C., Hoffman, J.P., Okuno, S., Kane, J.M., & von Mehren, M. (2009). Phase II trial of neoadjuvant/ adjuvant imatinib mesylate (IM) for advanced primary and metastatic/ recurrent operable gastrointestinal stromal tumor (GIST) - early results of RTOG 0132. *Journal of surgical oncology.* Vol. 99, No. 1, (January 2009), pp. 42-7, ISSN 1096-9098.

Eriksson, M. (2010). Histology-driven chemotherapy of soft-tissue sarcoma. *Annals of oncology,* Vol. 21, No. Suppl. 7, (October 2010), pp. vii270-76, ISSN 1569-8041.

Ferrari, A., Sultan, I., Huang, T.T., Rodriguez-Galindo, C., Shehadeh, C., Meazza, C., Ness, K.K., Casanova, M., & Spunt, S.L. (2011). Soft tissue sarcoma across the age spectrum: a population-based study from the surveillance epidemiology and end results database. *Pediatric blood & cancer,* Vol. 57, No. 6, (December 2011), pp. 943-9, ISSN 1545-5017.

Fletcher, C.D.M., Berman, J.J., Corless, C., Gorstein, F., Lasota, J., Longley, B.J., Miettinen, M., O'Leary, T.J., Remotti, H. Rubin, B.P., Shmookler, B., Sobin, L.H., & Weiss, S.S. (2002). Diagnosis of gastrointestinal stromal tumors: a consensus approach. *Human pathology.* Vol. 33, No. 5, (May 2002), pp. 459-65, ISSN 0046-8177.

Frustaci, S., Gherlinzoni, F., De Paoli, A., et al. (2001). Adjuvant chemotherapy for adult soft tissue sarcomas of the extremities and girdles: results of the Italian randomized cooperative trial. *Journal of clinical oncology,* Vol. 19, No. 5, (March 2001), pp. 1238-1247, ISSN 1527-7755.

Goodnight, J.E.J., Bargar, W.L., Voegeli, T., & Blaisdell, F.W. (1985). Limb-sparing surgery for extremity sarcomas after preoperative intraarterial doxorubicin and radiation therapy. *American journal of surgery.* Vol.150, No. 1, (July 1985), pp. 109-13, ISSN 0002-9610.

Gortzak, E., Azzarelli, A., Buesa, J. Bramwell, V.H.C., van Coevorden, F., van Geel, A.M., Ezzat, A., Santoro, A., Oosterhuis, J.W., van Glabbeke, M., Kirkpatrick, A., Verweij, J., the E.O.R.T.C. soft tissue bone sarcoma group and the National Institute of Canada clinical trials group/ Canadian sarcoma group. (2001). A randomized phase II study on neo-adjuvant chemotherapy for 'high-risk' adult soft-tissue sarcoma. *European journal of cancer,* Vol. 37, No. 1, (June 2001), pp. 1096-1103, ISSN 0959-8049.

Grobmyer, S.R., Maki, R.G., Demetri, G.D., Mazumdar, M., Riedel, E., Brennan, M.F. & Singer, S. (2004). Neo-adjuvant chemotherapy for primary high-grade extremity soft tissue sarcoma. *Annals of oncology*, Vol. 15, No. 11, (November 2004), pp.1667-72, ISSN 1569-8041.

Grunhagen, D.J., Brunstein, F., Graveland, W.J., van Geel, A.N., de Wilt, J.H., & Eggermont, A.M. (2005). Isolated limb perfusion with tumor necrosis factor and melphalan prevents amputation in patients with multiple sarcomas in arm or leg. *Annals of surgical oncology*, Vol. 12, No. 6, (June 2005), pp. 473-9, ISSN 1534-4681.

Heslin, M.J. & Smith, J.K. (1999). Imaging of soft tissue sarcomas. *Surgical oncology clinics of North America*, Vol. 8, No. 1, (January 1999), pp. 91-107, ISSN 1055 3207.

Hoeber, I., Spillane, A.J., Fisher, C., & Thomas, J.M. (2001). Accuracy of biopsy techniques for limb and limb girdle soft tissue tumors. *Annals of surgical oncology*, Vol., 8, No. 1, pp. 80-7, ISSN 1534-4681.

Hoekstra, H.J. (2008). Extremity perfusion in soft tissue sarcoma. *Surgical oncology clinics of North America*, Vol. 17, No. 4, (October 2008), pp. 805-24, ISSN 1055 3207.

Issels, R.D., Lindner, L.H., Verweij, J., Wust, P., Reichardt, P., Schem, B-C., Abdel-Rahman, S., Daugaard, S., Salat, C., Wendtner, C-M., Vujaskovic, Z., Wessalowski, R., Jauch, K-W., Durr, H.R., Ploner, F., Baur-Melnk, A., Mansmann, U., Hiddemann, W., Blay, J-Y., & Hohenberger, P. (2010). Neo-adjuvant chemotherapy alone or with regional hyperthermia for localized high-risk soft-tissue sarcoma: a randomised phase 3 multicentre study. *Lancet oncology*, Vol. 11, No 6, (June 2010), pp. 561-70, ISSN 1474-5488.

Joensuu, H., Eriksson, M., Hartmann, J., Sudby Hall, K., Schutte, J., Reichardt, A., Schlemmer, E., Wardelmann, G., Ramadori, S., Al-Batran, E., Nilsson, B.E., Monge, O., Kallio, R., Sarlomo-Rikala, M., Bono, P., Leinonen, M., Hohenberger, P. Alvegard, T., & Reichardt, P. (2011). Twelve versus 36 months of adjuvant imatinib (IM) as treatment of operable GIST with a high risk of recurrence: final results of a randomized trial. *Journal of clinical oncology*, Vol. 29, No. 18, (June 2011). ISSN 1527-7755.

Kattan, M.W., Leung, D.H., & Brennan, M.F. (2002). Postoperative nomogram for 12-year sarcoma-specific death. *Journal of clinical oncology*, Vol. 20, No. 3, (February 2002), pp. 791-6, ISSN 1527-7755.

Kraybill, W.G., Harris, J., Spiro, I.J., Ettinger, D.S., DeLaney, T.F., Blum, R.H., Lucas, D.R., Harmon, D.C., Letson, G.D., & Eisenberg , B. (2006). Phase II study of neoadjuvant chemotherapy and radiation therapy in the management of high-risk, high-grade, soft tissue sarcomas of the extremities and body wall: radiation therapy oncology group trial 9514. *Journal of clinical oncology*, Vol. 24, No.4, (February 2006), pp. 619-25, ISSN 1527-7755.

Kraybill, W.G., Harris, J, Spiro, I.J., Ettinger, D.S., Delaney, T.F., Blum, R.H., Licas, D.R., Harmon, D.C., Letson, G.D., & Eisenberg, B. (2010). Long-term results of a phase 2 study of neoadjuvant chemotherapy and radiotherapy in the management of high-risk, high-grade, soft tissue sarcomas of the extremities and body wall. *Cancer*, Vol. 116, No. 19, (November 2010), pp. 4613-21, ISSN 1097-0142.

Kroon, H.M. & Thompson, J.F. (2009). Isolated limb infusion: a review. *Journal of surgical oncology*, Vol. 100, No. 2, (August 2009), pp. 169-77, ISSN1096-9098.

Kooby, D.A., Antonescu, C.R., Brennan, M.F., & Singer, S. (2004). Atypical lipomatous tumor/ well-differentiated liposarcoma of the extremity and trunk wall: importance of histological subtype with treatment recommendations. *Annals of surgical oncology*, Vol. 11, No. 1, (January 2004), pp. 78-84, ISSN 1534-4681.

Levine, E.A., Trippon, M., & DasGupta, T.K. (1993). Preoperative multimodality treatment for soft tissue sarcomas. *Cancer*, Vol. 71, No. 11, (June 1993), pp. 3685-9, ISSN 1097-0142.

Lewis, J.J., Leung, D., Woodruff, J.M., & Brennan, M.F. (1998). Retroperitoneal soft-tissue sarcoma: analysis of 500 patients treated and followed at a single institution. *Annals of surgery*, Vol. 228, No. 3, (September 1998), pp. 355-65, ISSN 0003-4932.

MacDermed, D.M., Miller, L.L., Peabody, T.D., Simon, M.A., Luu, H.H., Haydon, R.C., Montag, A.G., Undevia, S.D., & Connell, P.P. (2010). Primary tumor necrosis predicts distant control in locally advanced soft-tissue sarcomas after preoperative concurrent chemoradiotherapy. International journal of radiation oncology, biology, and physiology, Vol. 76, No. 4, (March 2010), pp. 1147-53, ISSN 0360-3016.

Mack, L.A., Crowe, P.J., Yang, J.L., Schachar, N.S., Morris, D.G., Kurien, E.C., Temple, C.L.F., Lindsay, R.L., Magi, E., DeHaas, W.G., & Temple, W.J. (2004). Preoperative chemoradiotherapy (modified Eilber protocol) provides maximum local control and minimal morbidity in patients with soft tissue sarcoma. *Annals of surgical oncology*, Vol. 12, No. 8, (August 2004), pp. 646-53, ISSN 1534-4681

Maduekwe, U.N., Hornicek, F.J., Springield, D.S., Raskin, K.A., Harmon, D. C., Choy, E. Rosenberg, A.E., Nielsen, G.P., DeLaney, T.F., Chen, Y.L., Ott, M.J., & Yoon, S.S. (2009). Role of sentinel node biopsy in the staging of synovial, epithelioid, and clear cell sarcomas. *Annals of surgical oncology*, Vol. 16, No. 5, (Mary 2009), pp. 1356-63, ISSN 1534-4681.

Meric, F., Milas, M., Hunt, K.K., Hess, K.R., Pisters, P.W.T., Hildebrandt, G., Patel, S.R., Benjamin, R.S., Plager, C., Papadopolous, N.E.J., Burgess, M.A., Pollock, R.E., & Feig, B.W. (2000). Impact of neoadjuvant chemotherapy on postoperative morbidity in soft tissue sarcomas. *Journal of clinical oncology*, Vol. 18, No. 19, (October 2000), pp. 3378-83, ISSN 1527-7755.

Miettinen , M. & Lasota, J. (2006). Gastrointestinal stromal tumors: pathology and prognosis at different sites. *Seminars in diagnostic pathology*, Vol. 23, No. 2, (May 2006), pp. 70-83, ISSN 0740-2570.

Moncrieff, M.D., Kroon, H.M., Kam, P.C., Stalley, P.D., Scolyer, R.A., & Thompson, J.F. (2008). Isolated limb infusion for advanced soft tissue sarcoma of the extremity. *Annals of surgical oncology*, Vol. 15, No. 10, (October 2008), pp. 2749-56, ISSN 1534-4681.

Nielsen, T.O. & West, R.B. (2010). Translating gene expression into clinical care: sarcomas as a paradigm. *Journal of clinical oncology*, Vol. 28, No.10, (April 2010), pp. 1796-805, ISSN 1527-7755.

O'Sullivan, B., Davis, A.M., Turcotte, R., Catton, C.N., Wunder, J., Kandel, R., Goddard, K., Sadura, A., Pater, J., & Zee, B. (2002). Preoperative versus postoperative radiotherapy in soft-tissue sarcoma of the limbs: a randomised trial. *Lancet*, Vol. 359, No. 9325, (June 2002), pp. 2235-41, ISSN 0140-6736.

Pawlik, T.M., Pisters, P.W.T., Mikula, L., Feig, B.W., Hunt, K.K., Cormier, J.N., Ballo, M.T., Catton, C.N., Jones, J.J., O'Sullivan, B., Pollock, R.E., & Swallow, C.J. (2006). Long-term results of two prospective trials of preoperative external beam radiotherapy for localized intermediate- or high-grade retroperitoneal soft tissue sarcoma. *Annals of surgical oncology*, Vol. 13., No. 4, (February 2006), pp. 508-17, ISSN 1534-4681.

Pervaiz, N., Colterjohn, N., Farrokhyar, F., Tozer, R., Figueredo, A., & Ghert, M. (2008). A systematic meta-analysis of randomized controlled trials of adjuvant chemotherapy for localized resectable soft-tissue sarcoma. *Cancer*, Vol. 113, No. 3, (August 2008), pp. 573-81, ISSN 1097-0142.

Pisters, P.W., Harrison, L.B., Woodruff, J.M. Gaynor, J.J., & Brennan, M.F. (1994). A prospective randomized trial of adjuvant brachytherapy in the management of low-grade soft tissue sarcomas of the extremity and superficial trunk. *Journal of clinical oncology*, Vol. 12, No. 6, (June 1994), pp. 1150-5, ISSN 1527-7755.

Pisters, P.W.T., Leung, D.H.Y., Woodruff, J., Shi, W., & Brennan, M.F. (1996). Analysis of prognostic factors in 1,041 patients with localized soft tissue sarcoma of the extremities. *Journal of clinical oncology*, Vol. 14, No. 5, (May 1996), pp. 1679-89, ISSN 1527-7755.

Pisters, P.W.T., Ballo, M.T., & Patel, S.R. (2002). Preoperative chemoradiation treatment strategies for localized sarcoma. *Annals of surgical oncology*, Vol. 9, No. 6, (July 2002), pp. 535-42. ISSN 1534-4681.

Pisters, P.W., Ballo, M.T., Fenstermacher, M.J., Feig, B.W., Hunt, K.K., Raymond, K.A., Burgess, M.A., Zagars, G.K., Pollock, R.E., Benjamin, R.S., & Patel, S.R. (2003). Phase I trial of preoperative concurrent doxorubicin and radiation therapy, surgical resection, and intraoperative electron-beam radiation therapy for patients with localized retroperitoneal sarcoma. *Journal of clinical oncology*, Vol. 21, No. 16, (August 2003), pp. 3092-7, ISSN1527-7755.

Pisters, P.W.T., Patel, S.R., Prieto, V.G., Thall, P.F., Lewis, V.O., Feig, B.W., Hunt, K.K., Yasko, A.W., Lin, P.P. Jacobson, M.G., Burgess, M.A., Pollock, R.E., Zagars, G.K., Benjamin, R.S., & Ballo, M.T. (2004). Phase I trial of preoperative doxorubicin-based concurrent chemoradiation and surgical resection for localized extremity and body wall soft tissue sarcomas. *Journal of clinical oncology*, Vol. 22, No 16, (August 2004), pp. 3375-3380, ISSN1527-7755.

Pisters, P.W., Pollock, R.E., Lewis, V.O., Yasko, A.W., Cormier, J.N., Respondek, P.M., Feig, B.W., Hunt, K.K., Lin, P.P., Zagars, G., Wei, C., & Ballo, M.T. (2007). Long-term results of prospective trial of surgery alone with selective use of radiation for patients with T1 extremity and trunk soft tissue sarcomas. *Annals of surgery*, Vol. 246, No. 4, (October 2007), pp. 675-81, ISSN 0003-4932.

Raut, C.P., Pisters, P.W.T. (2006). Retroperitoneal sarcomas: combined-modality treatment approaches. *Journal of surgical oncology*, Vol. 94, No. 1, (July 2006), pp.81-7, ISSN 1096-9098.

Robertson, J.M., Sondak, V.K., Weiss, S.A., Sussman, J.J., Chang, A.E., & Lawrence, T.S. (1995). Preoperative radiation therapy and iododeoxyuridine for large retroperitoneal sarcomas. *International journal of radiation oncology biology physics*, Vol. 31, No. 1, (January 1995), pp. 87-92, ISSN 0360-3016.

Rosenberg, S.A., Tepper, j, Glatstein, E. Costa, J., Baker, A., Brennan, M., DeMoss, E.V., Seipp, c., Sindelar, W.F., Sugarbaker, P., & Wesley, R. (1982). The treatment of soft-tissue sarcomas of the extremities: prospective randomized evaluations of (1) limb-sparing surgery plus radiation therapy compared with amputation and (2) the role of adjuvant chemotherapy. *Annals of surgery*, Vol. 196, No. 3, (September 1982), pp. 305-15, ISSN 0003-4932.

Rouesse, J.G., Friedman, S., Sevin, D.M., le Chevalier, T., Spielmann, M.L., Contesso, G., Sarrazin, D.M., & Genin, J.R. (1987). Preoperative induction chemotherapy in the treatment of locally advanced soft tissue sarcomas. *Cancer*, Vol. 60, No. 3, (August 1987), pp. 296-300, ISSN 1097-0142.

Ryan, C.W., Montag, A.G., Hosenpud, J.R., Samuels, B., Hayden, J.B., Hung, A.Y., Mansoor, A., Peabody, T.D., Mundt, A.J., & Undevia, S. (2008). Histologic response of dose-intense chemotherapy with preoperative hypofractionated radiotherapy for patients with high-risk soft tissue sarcomas. *Cancer*, Vol. 112, No. 11, (June 2008), pp. 2432-9, ISSN 1097-0142.

Schlemmer, M., Wendtner, C.M., Lindner, L., Abdel-rahman, S., Hiddemann, W., & Issels, R.D. (2010). Thermochemotherapy in patients with extremity high-risk soft tissue sarcoma (HR-STS). *International journal of hyperthermia*, Vol. 26, No. 2, (March 2010), pp. 127-135, ISSN 1464-5157.

Sindelar, W.F., Kinsella, T.J., Chen, P.W., DeLaney, T.F., Tepper, J.E., Rosenberg, S.A., & Glatstein, E. (1993). Intraoperative radiotherapy in retroperitoneal sarcomas. *Archives of surgery*, Vol. 28, No. 4, (April 1993), pp. 402-10, ISSN 0004-0010.

Stoeckle E, Coidre, J.B., Bonvalor, S., Kantor, G., Terrier, P., Bonichon, F., Nguyen Bui, B., & French Federation of Cancer Center Sarcoma Group. (2001). Prognostic factors in retroperitoneal sarcoma: a multivariate analysis of a series of 165 patients of the French Cancer Center Federation Sarcoma Group. *Cancer*, Vol. 92, No. 2, pp. 359-68, ISSN 1097-0142.

Tierney, J.F., Stewart, L.A., & Parmar, M.K.B. (1997). Adjuvant chemotherapy for localized resectable soft-tissue sarcoma of adults: meta-analysis of individual data. *Lancet*, Vol. 350, No. 9092, (December 1997), pp. 1647-54, ISSN 0140-6736.

Tran, T., Davila, J.A., & El-Serag, H.B. (2005). The epidemiology of malignant gastrointestinal stromal tumors: an analysis of 1,458 cases from 1992 to 2000. *American journal of gastroenterology*, Vol. 100, No. 1, (January 2005), pp. 162-8, ISSN 0002-9270.

Trent, J.C., Beach, J., Burgess, M.A., Papadopolous, N., Chen, L.L., Benjamin, R.S., & Patel, S.R. (2003). A two-arm phase II study of temozolomide in patients with advanced gastrointestinal stromal tumors and other soft tissue sarcomas. *Cancer*, Vol. 98, No. 12, (December 2003), pp. 2693-99, ISSN 1097-0142.

Verweij, J., Casali, P.G., Zalcberg, J., LeCesne, A., Reichardt, P., Blay, J.Y., Issels, R., van Oosterom, A., Hogendoom, P.C., Van Glabbeke, M., Bertulli, R., & Judson, I. (2004) Progression-free survival in gastrointestinal stromal tumors with high-dose imatinib: randomized trial. *Lancet*, Vol. 364, No. 9440, pp. 1127-34, ISSN 0140-6736.

Verschraegen, C.F., Chawla, S.P., Mita, M.M., Ryan, C.W., Blakely, L., Keedy, V.L., Santoro, A., Buck, J.Y., Maki, J.J., & Lewis, J.J. (2010). A phase II, randomized, controlled trial of palifosfamide plus doxorubicin versus doxorubicin in patients with soft tissue sarcoma (PICASSO). *Journal of clinical oncology*, Vol. 28, No. 15s, (May 2010), pp. 15s, ISSN 1527-7755.

Wanebo, H.J., Temple, W.J., Popp, M.B., Constable, W., Aron, B., & Cunningham, S.L. (1995). Preoperative regional therapy for extremity sarcoma. A tricenter update. *Cancer*, Vol. 75, No. 9, (May 1995), pp. 2299-2306, ISSN 1097-0142.

Welker, J.A., Henshaw, R.M., Jelinek, J., Shmookler, B.M., & Malawer, M.M. (2000). The percutaneous needle biopsy is safe and recommended in the diagnosis of musculoskeletal masses. *Cancer,* Vol. 89, No. 12, (December 2000), pp. 2677-86, ISSN 1097-0142.

White, J.S., Biberdort, D., DiFrancesco, L.M., Kurien, E., & Temple, W.J. (2007). Use of tissue expanders and pre-operative external beam radiotherapy in the treatment of retroperitoneal sarcoma. *Annals of surgical oncology,* Vol. 14, No. 2, (February 2007), pp. 583-90, ISSN 1534-4681.

Yang, J.C., Chang, A.E., Baker, A.R., Sindelar, W.F., Danforth, D.N., Topalian, S.L., DeLaney, T., Glatstein, E., Steinberg, S.M., Merino, M.J., & Rosenberg, S.A. (1998). Randomized prospective study of the benefit of adjuvant radiation therapy in the treatment of soft tissue sarcomas of the extremity. *Journal of clinical oncology,* Vol. 16, No. 1, (January 1998), pp. 197-203, ISSN 1527-7755.

Zagars, G.K., Ballo, M.T., Pisters, P.W.T., Pollock, R.E., Benjamin, R.S. & Evans, H.L. (2003). Prognostic factors for patients with localized soft-tissue sarcoma treated with conservation surgery and radiation therapy: an analysis of 1225 patients. *Cancer,* Vol. 97, No. 10, (May 2003), pp. 2530-43, ISSN 1097-0142.

14

Effects of Neoadjuvant Chemotherapy in High-Grade Non-Metastatic Osteosarcoma of Extremities

Milan Samardziski[1], Vesna Janevska[2], Beti Zafirova-Ivanovska[3], Violeta Vasilevska[4] and Slavica Kraleva[5]

[1]*University Clinic for Orthopaedic Surgery, Skopje*
[2]*Institute for Pathology, Skopje*
[3]*Institute for Epidemiology and Biostatistics, Skopje*
[4]*University Surgical Clinic "St. Naum Ohridski", Skopje*
[5]*Institute for Radiology and Oncology, Skopje*
Macedonia

1. Introduction

Osteosarcoma is a very rare malignant bone tumor with an incidence of 4-6 cases in 1,000,000 inhabitants and appears mostly in the young and active population aged 10- 30 years (Price & Jeffree, 1977). Amputations and disarticulations as dominant treatment for malignant bone tumors in the beginning of 20th century are rarely and very selectively used today. Before 1970, amputation was the primary treatment for high-grade osteosarcoma and 80% of patients died of lung metastatic disease. Despite aggressive and radical surgery, 5-year survival was low (10-20%) (Rosen et al., 1976). Introducing new sophisticated diagnostic methods (CT and MRI) gave the possibility of precise anatomic definition of the tumors and the borders of infiltration into the surrounding tissues. Better planning of the biopsy and the definite operative procedure, and fostering better patient selection for specific treatment strategies, can decrease the risk of tumor spread into the surrounding tissue and lower the risk of distant metastases. After 1980, improvement of chemotherapeutic protocols with neoadjuvant chemotherapy, better preoperative planning and modern reconstructive options after resection of osteosarcoma led to better survival rates of patients with limb-sparing procedures (Bacci et al., 1993, Bruland & Phil, 1999).

Currently, 80 - 85% of the patients with osteosarcoma on the extremities can be safely treated with wide resection and limb preservation (Di Caprio et al., 2003). A multidisciplinary approach to diagnosis and treatment, combination chemotherapy and a number of options for reconstruction after osteosarcoma resection (especially in chemotherapy-sensitive tumors) have increased long-term survival rates from 60 to 80%. Amputations, once a dominant treatment for malignant bone tumors, now are rarely and very selectively used. Most patients with extremity-localized osteosarcoma are candidates for limb-sparing procedures because of the: effective chemotherapeutic agents and regimens, the improved imaging modalities, and advances in reconstructive surgery.

Application of neoadjuvant chemotherapy improves survival rates and functional outcome in patients with non-metastatic, high-grade osteosarcoma of the extremities (Wittig et al., 2002).
Before consideration of limb preservation, the patient needs to be appropriately staged and assessed through a multidisciplinary approach. Some elements of the disease may warrant concern, including relative contraindications to such procedures. However, surgical treatment associated with a limb-sparing operation is also associated with a significant number of complications and requires extensive rehabilitation. The main risk of limb-salvage procedures is that complications sometimes may cause a delay of chemotherapy (Sæter al., 1996).

2. Osteosarcoma subtypes and characteristics

Depending on cytological or histo-pathological features of the tumor matrix or tumor cells, osteosarcomas are divided into two groups. In the first group there are patients with *low-grade osteosarcoma* and surgery alone has the primary role of treatment. In the second group there are patients with *high-grade osteosarcoma*. In this group of patients "sandwich therapy" is strongly preferred (neoadjuvant chemotherapy - surgery - adjuvant chemotherapy) (Enneking, 1975; Bacci et al., 1993; Messerschmitt et al., 2009).

2.1 Intramedullary osteosarcoma

Conventional or "classic" osteosarcoma is the most prevalent type in children and adolescents (up to 80% of all cases). This type of osteosarcoma originates from the intramedullary cavity and is typically high-grade (Fig. 1a). An osteoblastic and/or osteolytic lesion with vast cortical destruction and various amount of soft tissue extension dominates on X-rays. Histo-pathologic examination demonstrates malignant mesenhimal cells, spindle to polyhedral in shape, with pleomorphyc nuclei and occasional mitotic figures. Evidence of direct bone or osteoid production from the mesenhim is crucial for diagnosis (Fig. 1b, 1c). World Health Organization has further subcategorized high-grade intramedullary osteosarcoma since 2002, depending on the predominant extra cellular matrix on: *osteoblastic* (approximately 50% of cases), *chondroblastic* (25% of cases) or *fibroblastic* (25% of cases). (Fletcher et al., 2002).
Teleangiectatic osteosarcoma is a rare variant accounting for approximately 4% of all osteosarcoma cases in children and adolescents. Very often they are associated with pathological fracture of the first presentation. Eccentric osteolytic lesion on the metaphysis, with destruction and expansion of the eroded cortex dominates on x-ray (Fig. 1b). Histo-pathologic examination reveals a malignant tumor with multiple dilated hemorrhagic sinuses as well as a scarce amount of high-grade osteosarcoma cells and rare osteoid formation within the septa. These radiographic and histo-pathologic features resemble an aneurismal bone cyst which is cdaracteristic.
Low-grade intramedullary osteosarcoma constitutes 1 to 2% of all osteosarcoma cases and generally affects patients in the third or fourth decade. Lesions most commonly affect the distal femur and proximal tibia, with relatively unaggressive radiographic appearance, resembling fibrous dysplasia ("fibrous dysplasia-like" osteosarcoma). Histo-pathological features consist of well-differentiated cells dispersed within woven microtrabeculae of bone and fibrous stroma. Small amounts of osteoid, mitotic atypia and mitoses can also be seen (Fletcher et al., 2002).

Small-cell osteosarcoma is a rare variant constituting <1.5% of all osteosarcoma cases. This subtype is similar to the high-grade osteosarcoma, with the same site or age distribution and aggressive biologic behavior. The lesion is osteolytic with destruction of cortex and variable sclerosis. MRI reveals large spindle or circumferential tumor mass, similar to Ewing sarcoma. Small, round, malignant cells within an osteoid matrix make the histo-pathological diagnosis problematic. To differentiate this osteosarcoma from Ewing sarcoma, direct mesenhimal production of osteoid must be found, because this osteosarcoma is positive for CD 99 immuno-histochemical stains (Fletcher et al., 2002).

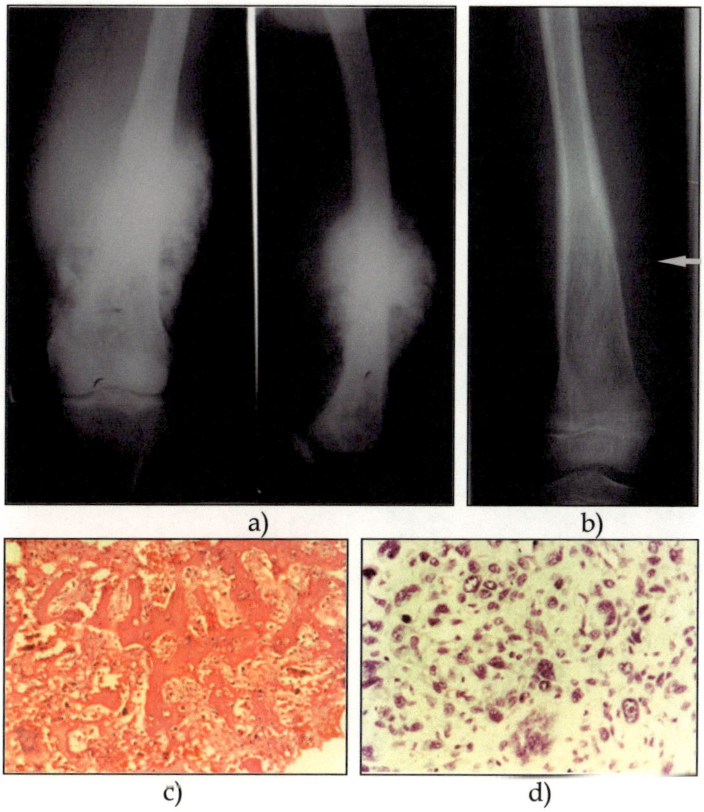

Fig. 1. **a)** X-ray of conventional intramedullary osteosarcoma (osteoblastic lesion with vast cortical destruction and soft tissue edema visible on x-rays); **b)** X-ray of teleangiectatic osteosarcoma with osteolytic lesion on the metaphysis of distal femur, destruction, expansion of the eroded cortex and Codman's periosteal reaction (arrow); **c)** Typical histo-pathological feature of osteosarcoma is osteoid formations directly from the mesenhime; **d)** Atypical osteoid formation in high-grade anaplastic osteosarcoma typifies the diagnosis.

A few osteosarcomas (less than 1% of all cases) have so many giant cells that they can be mistaken for giant cell tumors. Cytological atypia of the mononuclear cells can be very subtle and rare. It is important to remember the possibility of a *giant cell-rich osteosarcoma* when giant cell tumor-like lesion occurs in an unusual location and age, such as the metaphysis in children (Unni, 1998).

2.2 Surface osteosarcoma

Parosteal osteosarcoma arises on the outer surface of the long bone metaphysis, sparing the medullary canal (Fig. 2a). The peak incidence is in the second and third decade, affecting more females than males.[10] Parosteal osteosarcoma is most commonly seen as a juxtracortical variety and constitutes 1 to 6% of all osteosarcoma cases. Radiographs classically show densely ossified and lobulated mass on the posterior surface of the femur. Sometimes slow-growing tumors may encircle the bone. A low-grade, well differentiated fibrous stroma with osseous components is regularly seen on the histo-pathologic examination. Parallel orientation of trabeculae with additional cartilaginous differentiation is very common (Fig. 2d).

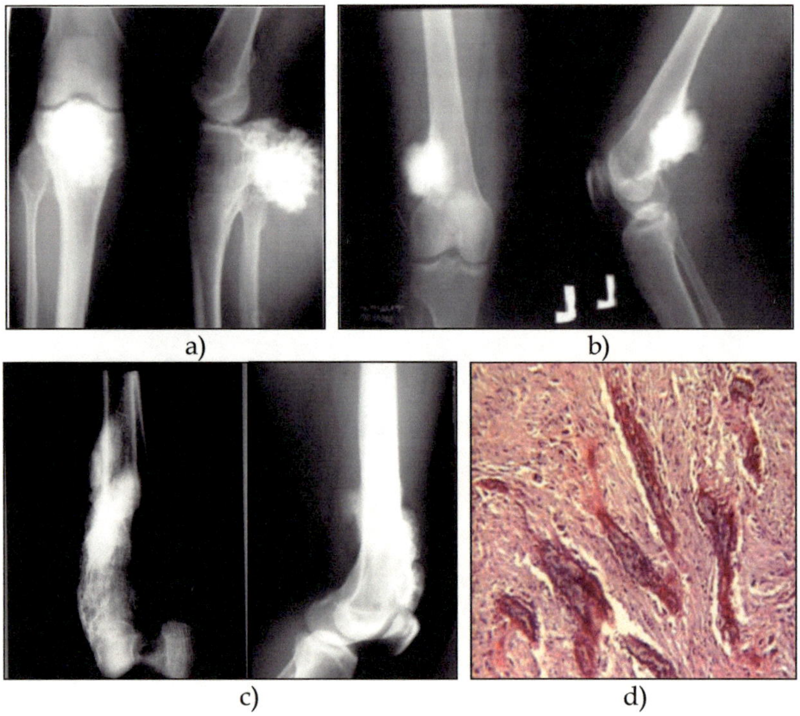

a) b) c) d)

Fig. 2. **a)** Frontal and lateral x-ray of the periosteal osteosarcoma of right distal femur; **b)** X-ray in frontal and lateral view of parosteal osteosarcoma of the proximal tibia; **c)** Frontal and lateral x-ray of high-grade surface osteosarcoma on the right distal femur; **d)** Parosteal osteosarcoma showing parallel osteoid trabeculae embedded in fibroblastic stroma (HE, x100).

Periosteal osteosarcoma constitutes 1 to 2% of all osteosarcoma cases and is usually more aggressive than the parosteal variant. A radiolucent lesion is located on the distal femur or proximal tibia, sparing the medullar cavity (Fig. 2b). Codman triangle and "sunburst" periosteal reaction are common radiographic features. Histo-pathologic evaluation demonstrates an intermediate-grade tumor, rich with cartilaginous matrix and rare osteoid fields.

High-grade surface osteosarcoma constitutes <1% of all osteosarcomas with the predominant site around the knee. Radiographic analysis shows surface lesion with partial mineralization and tumor extension into surrounding soft tissues. In earlier stages of the disease, destruction of the underlying cortex is absent, but with advanced lesions involvement of the medullary cavity is possible (Fig. 2c). The histological features are those of high-grade osteosarcoma, demonstrating spindle cells with atypia and a varying amount of osteoid. A high-grade surface osteosarcoma cannot be differentiated from a conventional osteosarcoma in histological findings alone (Fletcher et al., 2002; Samardziski et al., 2009).

3. Imaging

There are various radiological imaging techniques available to achieve an accurate diagnosis and staging of osteosarcoma and to detect local recurrence or distant metastases. Most commonly used are: plain-film radiographs (as "gold" standard), Tc-99m bone scintigrapy, CT of the affected site or of the lungs and CT or conventional angiography. Positron emission tomography (PET-scan) and Thallium scintigraphy have been seldom used due to questionable results in evaluating early osteosarcoma metastases or due to their high-cost (Messerschmitt et al., 2009).

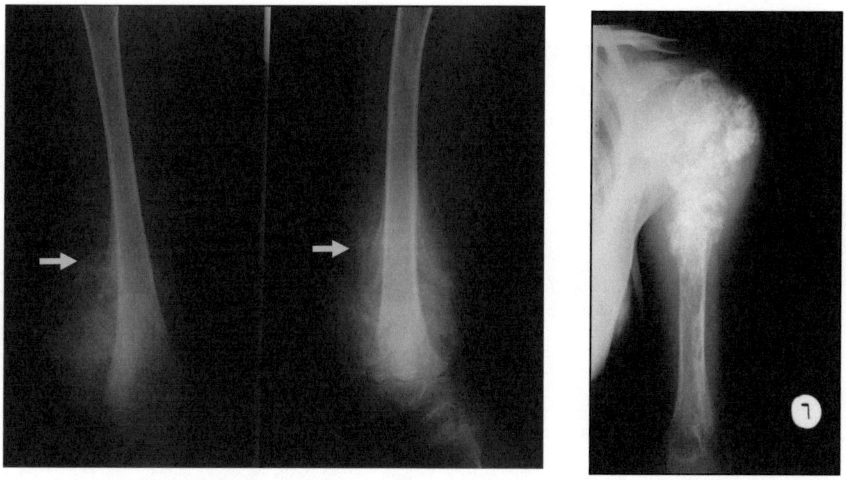

a) b)

Fig. 3. **a)** X-ray in two orthogonal planes of typical mixed sclerotic end lytic osteosarcoma of the distal femur. Tumor has penetrated bone and formed a soft tissue mass with Codman's triangles. **b)** Frontal plane X-ray of osteosarcoma situated on proximal humerus with small, confluent cloud-like densities, destroing the bone completely.

Plain-film radiographs in two ortogonal plains show mixed osteosclerotic and osteolytic tumor, affecting the metaphysis of the bone (although primarily sclerotic or lytic osteosarcomas can occur). The lesion is ill defined from the surrounding bone, affecting and destroing the cortex, with typical small, irregular, confluent, cloud-like densities. If the cortex is completely eroded the lesion forms a soft tissue mass extruding from the bone into the surrounding tissue and may demonstrate ossification detectable on the radiographs (Fig. 3). The destruction may be so advanced that pathological fractures or complete bone erosion could be present (Fig. 3b). There is a typical periosteal reaction due to aggressive expansion of the tumor, forming hairy, sun-ray or velvet-like specula of neoplastic bone. In some cases "Codman's triangles" (arrows on Fig. 3a) are present. Plain-film radiographs are used in correlation with bone scintigraphy and CT to detect local recurrence or bone and lung metastases. Additional data for diagnosis and decision-making process can be obtained using a "computer assisted diagnosis" in analysis of the x-rays (Lodwick et al., 1963; Samardziski et al., 2004).

Computer tomography (CT) scann of the affected extremity is useful in visualization of the intra and extra-osseous extent of the tumor, especially when extensive necrosis and surrounding edema are present. In this case CT may be superior to MRI. High-definition CT scans can obtain a three dimensional view of the tumor in relation to adjacent neurovascular structures, especially when contrast medium is used (Fig. 4a). All patients with osteosarcoma should undergo CT scanning of the chest and lungs for detection of pulmonary metastases, for diagnosis and staging. After surgery has been performed in patients with non-metastatic osteosarcoma, CT scans of the lung should be repeated every three to six months for two years (Wittig et al., 2002).

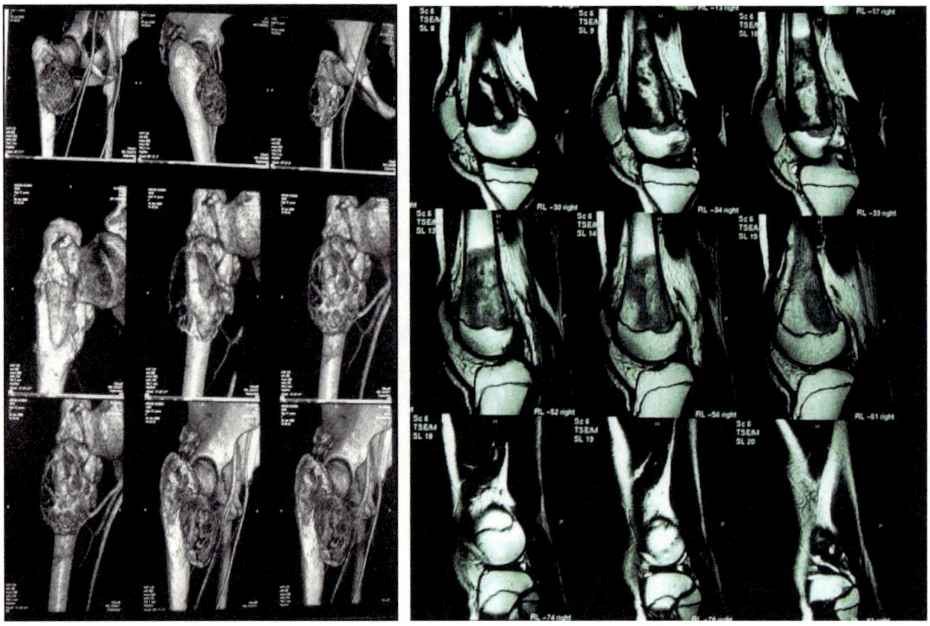

a) b)

Fig. 4. **a)** CT scans of proximal femur osteosarcoma, with visualization of the superficial and deep femoral artery **b)** T_2-weighted MRI image of distal femur osteosarcoma with no extra-osseous extension.

With magnetic resonance imaging (MRI), standard T_1 and T_2-weighted and fat-suppressed images are obtained to visualize the affected bone and surrounding tissue with osteosarcoma. Based on MRI studies, the intra-osseous and extra-osseous extent of the tumor is visible as well as reactive zone and tissue edema (Fig. 4b). Neurovascular structures and especially neurovascular encasement can be determined and it can help in the process of planning the definite method of treatment. (If encasement is present, amputation or wide resection with vascular reconstruction is obligatory).

Obtaining an MRI prior to surgical resection permits accurate planning of the osteotomy and gross tumor excision (together with the reactive zone) for achieving a "wide" surgical margin. Skip metastases on MRI are easily detectable in the same bone or in the adjacent joint and then a more extensive resection is required. MRI studies are inferior to high-definition CT scans for lung metastases detection (Di Caprio & Friedlander, 2003, 2003).

4. Biopsy and histo-pathological diagnosis

In spite of the risk for tumor spreading, biopsy is the key step in the diagnosis and treatment of osteosarcoma. Improperly performed biopsy may compromise the treatment plan. It is mandatory to place the biopsy in the line of definite surgical approach for osteosarcoma resection. A specimen taken from the necrotic tissue or from reactive zone (around the osteosarcoma) may be non informative. A large needle biopsy is sometimes preferable, because it is less invasive, with lower risk for skin necrosis, infection and pathological fracture. If no representative osteosarcoma tissue is obtained, an open biopsy will increase the risk of complications or local spreading of the tumor. The best results are achieved when all the biopsy samples are obtained by the same orthopedic oncologist (surgeon) who will perform the definite surgical procedure (Mankin et al., 1982; Campanacci, 1999). One must state that obtaining an accurate histo-pathological diagnosis of the tumor (especially of osteosarcoma) may be very delicate task (Fletcher et al. 2002).

Stadium	Grade	Localisation	Metastases
IA	G_1 - Low-grade	T_1 - Intraosseus	M_0 - No metastases
IB		T_2 - Extraosseus	M_0 - No metastases
IIA		T_1 - Intraosseus	M_0 - No metastases
IIB	G_2 - High-grade	T_2 - Extraosseus	M_0 - No metastases
IIIA	G_{1-2}	T_1 - Intraosseus	M_1 - With metastases
IIIB	G_{1-2}	T_2 - Extraosseus	M_1 - With metastases

Table 1. Enneking's surgical staging system: **G_1**-Low-grade; **G_2**-High-grade; **T_1**-Intraosseus; **T_2**-Extraosseus; **M_0**-No metastases; **M_1**-With metastases.

5. Staging

The American National Comprehensive Cancer Network recommends plain radiographs of the lesion and lungs, MRI scan of the extremity, CT scan of the tumor site and of the lungs, and radionuclide bone scan. Technetium Tc-99 methylene diphosphonate scintigraphy will reveal increased metabolic activity at the site of the tumor, but also at the site of distant skip or bone metastases. Thallium (Tl-201) is a potassium analog, actively transported by the sodium-potassium adenosine triphosphatase (ATP) pump. This radioisotope is well accumulated in benign or malignant tumors, reflecting tumor activity. Nevertheless,

Thallium scanning is mostly used for monitoring the response to neoadjuvant chemotherapy (especially when MRI is not helpful).
Osteosarcoma can be divided into high-grade or low-grade variants, depending of cellularity, pleomorphism, anaplasia and number of mitoses (Fletcher et al. 2002). This fact and the data for presence or absence of osteosarcoma metastases will be enough to do the Enneking's surgical staging (Table 1). This staging system, first used by the American Musculoskeletal Tumor Society and International Symposium on Limb-Salvage is widely accepted. An alternative system, established by the American Joint Committee on Cancer, can be used with Enneking's staging system (Enneking et al., 1980).

6. Treatment

A multidisciplinary approach is obligatory in the diagnosis and treatment of osteosarcoma. To achieve high standards in treatment there is a need for specialized radiologists, pathologists, orthopedic and other surgeons (specialized in oncology surgery), pediatric oncologists, specialized physical therapist and often social workers (Wittig et Al., 2002). When a proper chemotherapy and surgery protocol are followed, survival rates surpass 70%. High-grade osteosarcoma patients without clinically detectable lung metastases are presumed to have micro metastases. For these patients treatment consists of preoperative (neoadjuvant) chemotherapy, wide or radical surgical resection and postoperative (adjuvant) chemotherapy i.e. "sandwich therapy". Parosteal osteosarcoma or low-grade intra-medullar osteosarcoma patients are treated with wide or radical surgical resection alone. Chemotherapy is reserved only for cases with high-grade transformation. Periosteal osteosarcoma patients may be treated with preoperative (neoadjuvant) chemotherapy similar to that used for conventional osteosarcomas (Bacci et al., 1993; Bruland & Phil, 1999).

6.1 Chemotherapy

Advances in poly-chemotherapy protocols in the last 30 years have been responsible for improved survival rates and a possibility for limb salvage surgery. Since the beginning of the "odyssey" with Rosen and Jaffe, until now, chemotherapy has been shown to reduce the number of pulmonary metastases or to delay their appearance, facilitating surgical treatment (Rosen et al., 1976).
Standard modern regimens include drugs that have been shown to be the most effective against osteosarcoma: doxorubicin (Adriamycin), cisplatin (Platinol) ifosfamide (Ifex) with mesna (Mesnex) and high-dose methotrexate (Rheumatrex) with Leucoverin calcium rescue. Most standard protocols use doxorubicin and cisplatin with or without high-dose methotrexate for both neoadjuvant (preoperative) and adjuvant (postoperative) chemotherapy. The postoperative (adjuvant) chemotherapy is mostly dependent on the extent of tumor necrosis evaluated after surgical removal. The postoperative chemotherapy regimen is typically the same as the preoperative regimen when tumor necrosis is found to be ≥ 90% at the time of surgery. "Poor responders" to preoperative chemotherapy, defined as those with <90% tumor necrosis at the time of surgery, may benefit from postoperative chemotherapy. In these patients a salvage therapeutic regime is attempted with an increased dose of chemotherapy, an increased length of chemotherapy, or a change in chemotherapeutic agent. Recent trials have incorporated ifosfamide after conventional

chemotherapeutic drugs to improve patient survival rates (Jaffe et al., 1989; Sæter et al., 1996; Bacci et al., 2001; Messerschmitt et al., 2009).

6.2 Surgery

The two primary surgical options are tumor resection with limb-salvage, and amputation. Surgical margins in excision should encompass resection of tumor, pseudo capsule, and a cuff of normal tissue en block. Meticulous preoperative planning before the biopsy and definitive surgery will ensure better results. Prior to the emergence of limb-salvage surgery in the 1970s, amputation of the affected limb was considered the definitive surgical intervention. Amputation remains the indicated treatment when disease-free marginal resection leaves a nonfunctional limb.

The limb-salvage surgery for osteosarcoma patients is possible due to the use of preoperative (neoadjuvant) chemotherapy and to advancement in musculoskeletal imaging, prosthetic implant design and surgical technique (Fig. 5). Today limb sparing surgery is possible for >85% of patients with extremities localized osteosarcomas (Bacci et al., 2006; Di Caprio & Friedlander, 2003; Longhi et al., 2006).

Surgical treatment has to be planed keeping in mind four basic principles of limb-salvage procedures: local recurrence should be no greater and survival no worse than by amputation; the procedure, or treatment of its complications, should not delay adjuvant therapy; reconstruction should be enduring and not associated with a large number of local complications requiring secondary procedures and frequent hospitalizations; function of the limb should approach that obtained by amputation, although body image, patient preference and life style may influence the decision (González-Heranz et al. 1995).

There are a few relative contraindications to be taken in the consideration for limb-salvage surgery: wrong site or ill-planed biopsy; massive encasement of neurovascular bundles; extensive tumour involvement in soft tissue, muscles or skin; complex or complicated (i.e. with infection) pathological fractures; expected inequalities of the extremities more than 8 cm; and exceptionally poor effect of the neoadjuvant chemotherapy. In the process of decision making for limb-salvage surgery versus amputation the "rule of three" can be very helpful. For extremity survival the bone (1), nerves (2), blood vessels (3), and muscle and skin (4) are necessary to be preserved. If osteosarcoma involves one or two of the former structures, limb preserving is possible. If any three of the former are involved, amputation must be taken in consideration (Di Caprio & Friedlander, 2003).

When "negative" tumor margins are obtained, a large skeletal defect is often present, requiring reconstruction of the bone, muscles, other soft tissues, and the skin. Patient age, tumor location and extent of resection, determine the appropriate surgical alternatives. The extent of the disease, anatomical location of the tumor and the patient's age and psychological profile define the most appropriate surgical procedures. Several options for limb-sparing are available: resection arthrodesis and other similar techniques with special indications (Fig. 7c), modular or special expanding endoprostheses (Fig. 5), cortico-spongious or bulk auto graft.

For the patients who can't satisfy the principles of limb preservation, ablative surgery has to be taken into consideration. For these patients disarticulation of the hip or shoulder griddle, rotationplasty, femoral or below knee, humeral or other amputations are far more appropriate (González-Heranz et al., 1995; Sæter et al., 1996; Wittig et al., 2002; Samardziski et al. 2009).

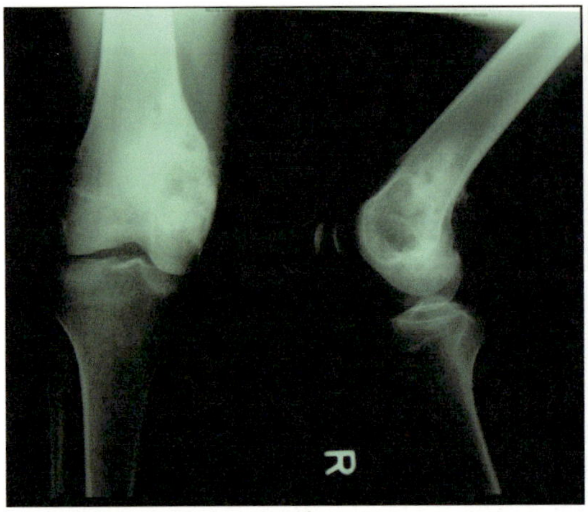

a)

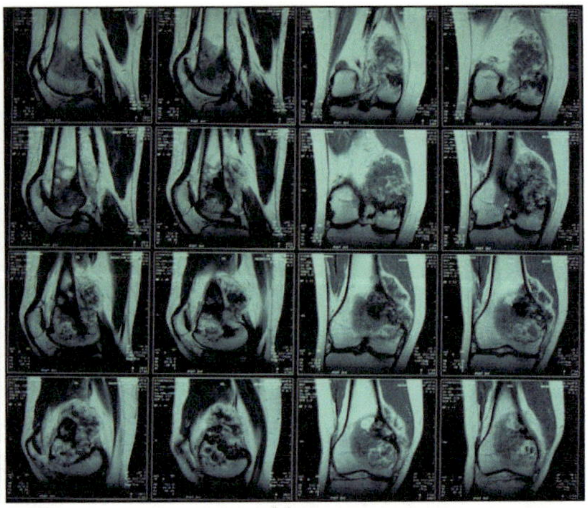

b)

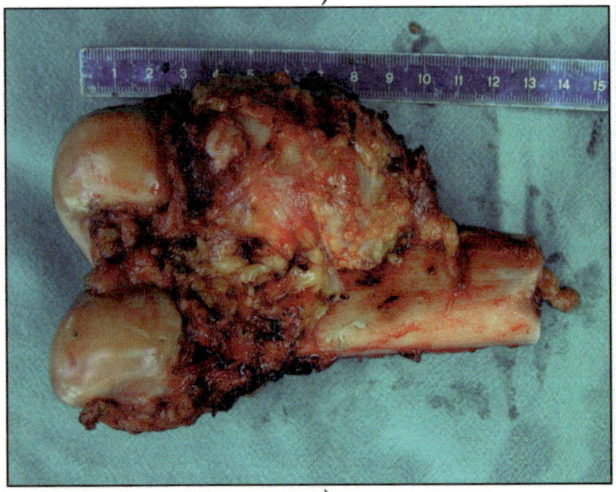

a)

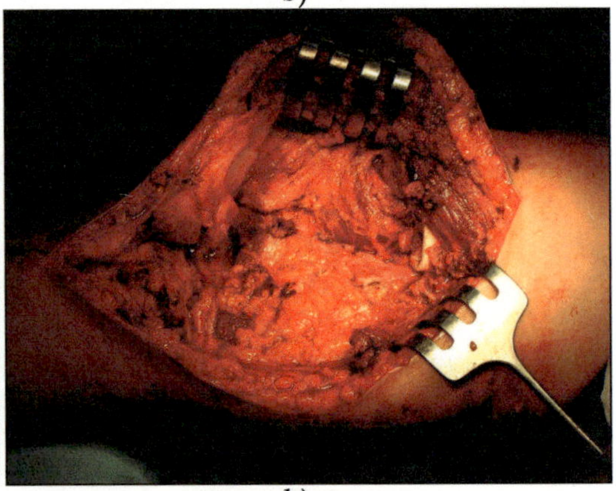

b)

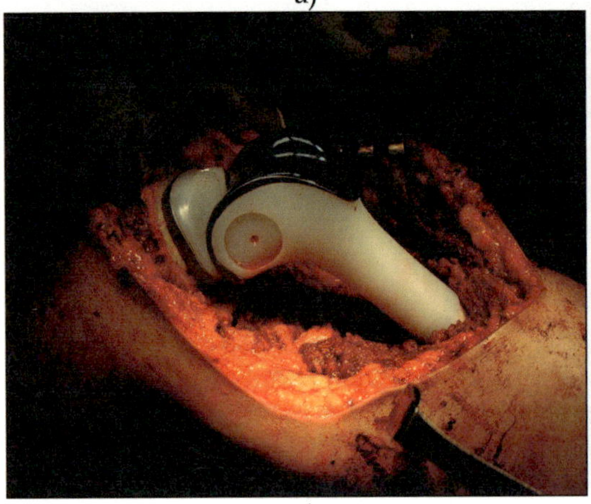

c)

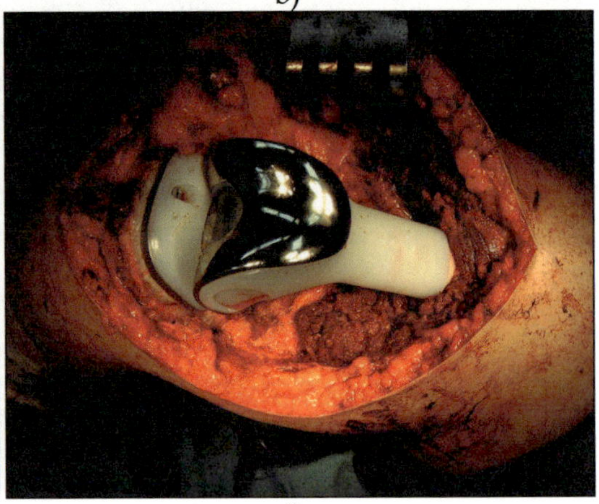

d)

Fig. 5. **a)** x-ray of high-grade chondroblastic osteosarcoma of right distal femur in a girl of 17; **b)** anterior and lateral MRI view of the lesion; **c)** photo of the resected tumor; **d)** tumor site ready for reconstruction; **e, f)** reconstructed right femur and knee (Link modular endoprosthesis).

The current recommendation for detectable metastases is to excise as many lesions as technically feasible following surgical treatment of the primary tumor. The survival rate for patients can be as high as 60%-75% when both the primary tumor and the solitary lung metastasis are adequately resected (Yonemoto et al., 1997; Bacci et al., 2006).
The rate of surgical site recurrence is 4% to 6% for both limb-salvage and amputations. Complications following limb-salvage reconstructions include wound complications, infections, mechanical failure, and nonunion. The reported incidence of complications with limb-salvage surgical techniques is 4% to 38% (Kotz et al., 2002).

6.3 Postoperative follow-up

After chemotherapy, the patient should be closely followed by the orthopedic oncology surgeon and the medical oncologist. The patient should be monitored for local recurrence, distant or systemic metastases and complications related to reconstruction of the extremity. CT scanning of the chest, plain film radiographs of the reconstructed extremity and meticulous physical examinations are recommended every three months for the first two years and at least every six months from the second year through to the fifth year, and subsequently on a yearly basis. Also, annual bone scintigraphy is mandatory for the first two years after completion of the chemotherapy.

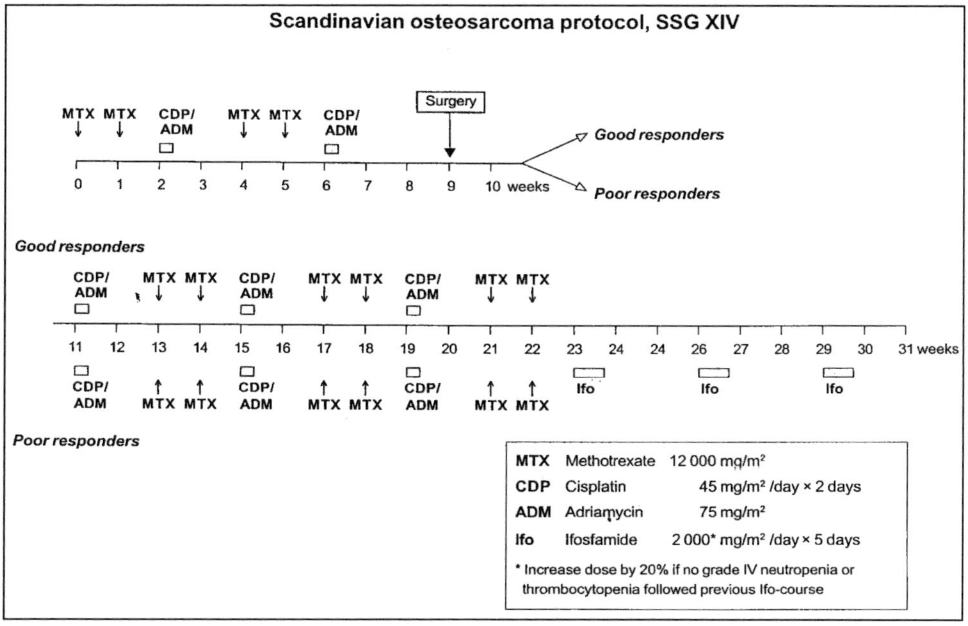

Fig. 6. Scandinavian Sarcoma Group Protocol XIV

7. Neoadjuvant chemotherapy

Dramatic changes over the past few decades have occurred with neoadjuvant (preoperative) and adjuvant (postoperative) poly chemotherapy protocols. This improved the ability to perform safe limb-sparing resection of the tumor in more than 85% of the osteosarcoma patients. Today, as reported in the literature, 60-80% of the patients with extremity localized non metastatic osteosarcomas are long term survivors.

Multidrug neoadjuvant chemotherapy, popularized for patients with osteosarcoma by Rosen and later by Jaffe in the late 1970's, is usually initiated as appropriate after histo-pathological diagnosis and staging. Neoadjuvant chemotherapy protocols with high-dose methotrexate, and cisplatin and doxorubicin dramatically improved long-term survival rates in patients with osteosarcoma sensitive to chemotherapy. Using high dose ifosfamide or different additional and more aggressive therapeutic agents for less sensitive in postoperative chemotherapy (as in: Cooperative Osteosarcomstudiengruppe 96 protocol, Scandinavian Sarcoma Group Protocol XIV and European bone over 40 sarcoma study) improved the results and overall survival of these patients (Kotz et al., 2002). Because of the aggressive nature of the protocols, rescue with Leucoverin (as antidote), bone marrow stimulation with Neupogen and renal protection with Uromitexan are essential. Maximal hydration followed by diuretic forced renal clearance further improves patient's chemotherapy tolerance. During chemotherapy, antiemetics, including: dexamethasone, diphenylhydramine and lorazepam are routinely used in all patients (Bacci et al., 1993; Bruland, 1999; Messershmitt et al., 2009).

7.1 Various neoadjuvant chemotherapy protocols

There are various poly-chemotherapy protocols (some in regular practice, other in experimental phase). Basic science is making continuous advance that may yield more specific, less-toxic drugs that will further improve survival rates. The use of high dose Ifosfamide or different, additional and more aggressive, therapeutic agents for less sensitive osteosarcoma patients in postoperative modern chemotherapy becomes a rule. There are many chemotherapy regimens, but most commonly reported are: Cooperative Osteosarcomstudiengruppe 96 protocol (COSS 96), Scandinavian Sarcoma Group Protocol (SSG) XIV, European bone over 40 sarcoma study (EURO-B.O.S.S/COSS), Italian Sarcoma Group protocol (ISG), Sloan-Kettering Center protocol T-10 (SSG III), American Society of Clinical Oncology (ASCO) protocol, etc. Introducing more aggressive chemotherapy for poor responders, improved the results and overall survival of these patients (Brulnad, 1999; Di Caprio & Friedlander, 2003).

7.2 Effects of neoadjuvant chemotherapy in high-grade non-metastatic osteosarcoma of extremities

Various effects of neoadjuvant therapy, such as: remission of pain, reduction of the size of the tumor, sclerosation, pseudo capsule formation, decreasing of neo-vascularisation, tumor necrosis and decrease of the elevated alkaline phosphathase and lactate dehydrogenase levels are widely reported. After neoadjuvant chemotherapy a clinical and radiological response of the tumor has been observed (Bacci et al., 1993). There was reduction, or more often complete remission of pain. This was usually followed with normalization of serum alkaline phosphathase and lactate dehydrogenase levels (if elevated). Bacci further reported an increased density (as seen on Fig. 7b) by the bone lesion on plain radiographs associated with decreased vascularity on angiograms.

Clinical and radiographic reduction in tumor size was observed in more than half of the patients. This was more due to a decrease of the surrounding inflammatory and reactive tissue than to an actual reduction in tumor size. Bacci reported that reduction in vascularity, was the one, most predictable criterion to assess the response of the tumor after neoadjuvant chemotherapy. Neoadjuvant chemotherapy may also decrease the size of the primary tumor

(Fig. 7) by reducing its neo-vascularity and promoting tumor demarcation from surrounding tissue with pseudo-capsule (Fig 5b). This makes limb-salvage surgery technically more feasible, even if a marginal resection is obtained (Messershmitt et al., 2009).

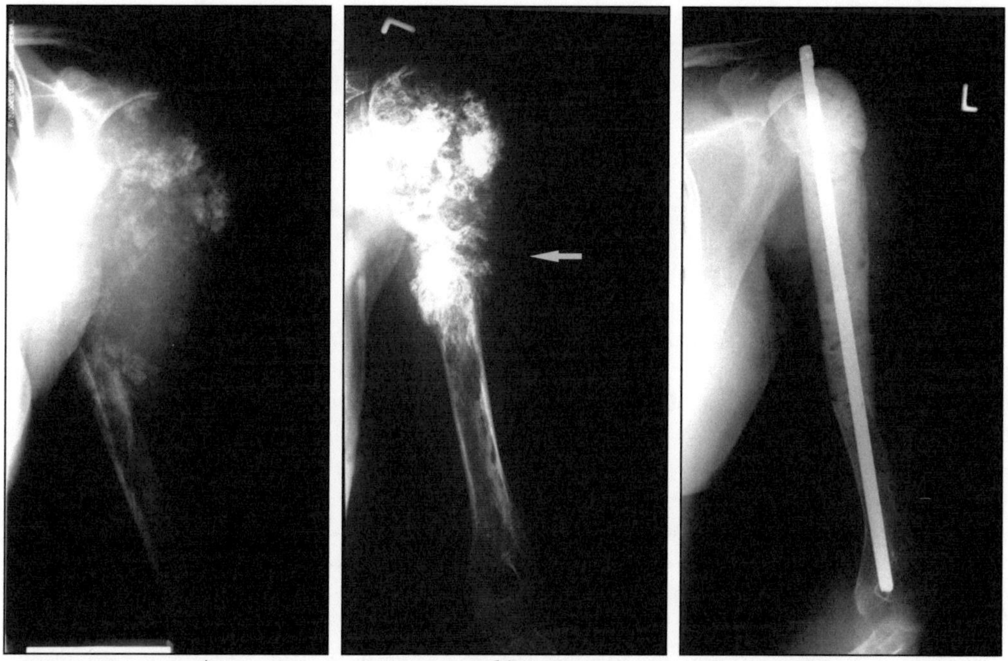

a) b) c)

Fig. 7. **a)** Fifteen years old female osteosarcoma patient with pathological fracture of the left proximal humerus at the first presentation. The patient had preoperative (neoadjuvant) chemotherapy with Swedish Sarcoma Protocol XIV. **b)** Excellent response (>90% tumor necrosis) with sclerosation after neoadjuvant chemotherapy (arrow shows the site of the pathological fracture). **c)** Radiograph of the humerus after wide resection of the osteosarcoma, and first stage reconstruction of the bone with intramedullary rod and bone cement.

The primary goal of neoadjuvant chemotherapy is to treat undetectable (or micro) metastases. It is reasonable to believe that neoadjuvant chemotherapy may decrease the risk of spreading viable tumor cells after biopsy, and therefore, decrease the possibility of distant metastases and of local recurrence. This is only possible with optimal serum concentration of methotrexate (at least 1000 μM) at the end of a 6 hour infusion. All of these advantages of neoadjuvant chemotherapy enables more options for wide or near-marginal resection of the tumor and for a limb-sparing surgery (Bruland & Phil, 1999).

7.3 Macedonian long-term follow-up experiences with the effects of neoadjuvant chemotherapy in patients with extremity localized high-grade osteosarcoma

Following the "wave of modern" poly-chemotherapy, in the period 2000-2008, a prospective study was done at the University Clinic for Orthopedic Surgery and Institute of Radiology

and Oncology in Skopje. In this period, 47 patients with high-grade osteosarcoma, were treated (Samardziski et al., 2009a).
Selection of patients for neoadjuvant chemotherapy and limb-salvage surgery was based on the following criteria:
Inclusion criteria:

- histopathologically proven high-grade osteosarcoma (grade III or IV);
- primary localization on the extremities, with no evidence of lung or other metastases;
- patient age between 8 and 65 years; normal hepatic and renal function;
- leukocyte count over 3.0×109/L and platelet count over 100×109/L;
- neoadjuvant chemotherapy was introduced no longer than 1 month after histological diagnosis of osteosarcoma.

Exclusion criteria:

- patients with central localization of osteosarcoma (e.g. pelvis, vertebra);
- evidence of lymphatic or haematogenous metastases at the time of diagnosis;
- patients under 8 years or older than 65 years;
- pregnant or nursing women.

According to the exclusion criteria, 8/47 patients were excluded, owing to lung metastases at first presentation or pelvic localization. Another 10/39 patients were excluded from the study due to primary indication for ablative surgery (amputation or disarticulation). Seventy five percent of the patients (29/39) were treated with limb-sparing surgery (Table 2). Fourteen (48%) patients were male and 15 (52%) were female. The mean age was 23.4 ± 14.5 years (range 8-63). Mean follow-up was 49.9 ± 23.1 months (range 23-108).
All patients received to the Scandinavian Sarcoma Group XIV neoadjuvant chemotherapy protocol (SSG XIV). Patients received 2 cycles of preoperative chemotherapy (high dose methotrexate 1200 mg/m^2, cisplatin 45 $mg/m^2/day$ ×2 days, and doxorubicin 75 mg/m^2), (Fig. 6).
After resection, a detailed histopathological assessment of the specimen was done to determine the extent of necrosis of the tumor tissue. Considering the percentage of necrotic tumor tissue, patients were classified into two groups. The first group experienced good response to chemotherapy (>90% necrosis of the tumor). The second group had a poor response to chemotherapy (>10% viable tumor). Regarding good or poor response of the tumor to chemotherapy, patients followed different branches of the protocol (Fig. 6). All 29 patients received 3 courses of postoperative chemotherapy (the same as preoperative). Patients with poor response received 3 more cycles of chemotherapy with high dose ifosfamide (2000 $mg/m^2/$ day ×5 days plus Mesna) every 3 weeks (Fig. 6). Histopathological assessment of the specimen did not only identify the extent of tumor necrosis, but information on tumor-free margins, too.
We have analyzed the following parameters of the clinical and radiological data after neoadjuvant chemotherapy: age, gender, time of follow-up, necrosis of the resected tumor after neoadjuvant chemotherapy (poor or good response), decrease of pain, decrease in tumor diameter, tumor pseudo-capsule seen on MRI, sclerosis seen on radiographs or CT, local recurrence and metastases (Table 2).
Response to neoadjuvant chemotherapy was good (more than 90% necrosis of the tumor) in 16/29 patients (55.2%). The examinees with good response to neoadjuvant therapy had significantly longer overall survival time than the patients with poor response (fig. 8). Ten percents of the patients with poor response survived for more than 65 months, while 58% of the patients with good response survived for more than 100 months (Log-Rank test=3,74 p=0.0002).

Patient No.	Age (y.)	Gender	Follow-up (m.)	Response to neoa-d. chemoth.	Decrease of pain	Decrease in diameter	Pseudo-capsule	Sclerosis	Recurrence (m.)	Metastases (m.)	Deceased after (m.)
1	25	M	30	P	0	1	0	0	0	22	30
2	13	M	32	P	1	1	1	0	0	27	32
3	23	M	50	G	1	1	U	1	0	29	-
4	16	F	44	P	1	1	1	1	0	38	44
5	15	F	68	G	1	1	1	1	50	57	68
6	14	M	51	G	1	1	1	1	0	0	-
7	8	F	50	G	1	1	1	1	29	43	50
8	13	M	45	G	1	1	1	1	0	0	-
9	16	F	54	P	1	1	1	1	0	36	54
10	17	F	23	P	0	0	0	0	6	12	23
11	54	F	38	P	1	1	U	1	0	0	38
12	14	F	98	G	1	1	1	1	0	0	-
13	63	M	106	G	1	1	1	1	96	100	106
14	17	M	67	P	1	0	1	1	54	60	67
15	16	M	59	G	1	1	1	0	0	0	-
16	20	F	54	P	1	1	1	0	0	46	54
17	20	F	47	G	1	1	1	1	0	0	-
18	16	M	10	P	0	0	0	0	2	4	10
19	39	F	61	P	1	0	1	1	53	57	61
20	14	M	26	P	0	0	0	0	19	19	26
21	8	M	40	G	1	1	1	0	0	0	-
22	44	F	59	G	1	1	U	1	0	0	-
23	14	M	40	G	1	1	1	1	0	30	40
24	44	F	35	P	0	1	0	0	21	28	35
25	15	F	108	G	1	1	1	0	0	0	-
26	15	M	27	P	0	0	0	0	2	11	27
27	48	F	43	G	1	1	1	1	0	0	-
28	24	F	33	G	1	1	1	1	18	0	-
29	34	M	51	G	1	1	0	1	35	45	51

M: male; **F:** female; **G:** good response after neoadjuvant chemotherapy (necrosis >90% of the tumor); **P**: poor response after neoadjuvant chemotherapy (>10% viable tumor); **U** -unknown or missing data; **1**-yes; **0**-no or none.

Table 2. Clinical data of patients with high-grade osteosarcoma of the extremities, treated with neoadjuvant chemotherapy.

Local recurrence appeared in 17/29 patients (58.6%). The examinees without local relapse had significantly longer overall survival time than the examined persons with no relapse. Ten percent of the patients with relapse survived more than 100 months, while 48% of the examined with no local relapse were alive even after 100 months (Log-Rank test p=0.0002).

Most of the tumor relapses were seen in the patients by 22 months after surgery. The 3 patients with early local recurrences had secondary extirpation of the relapsed tumor and one of them had to be amputated.

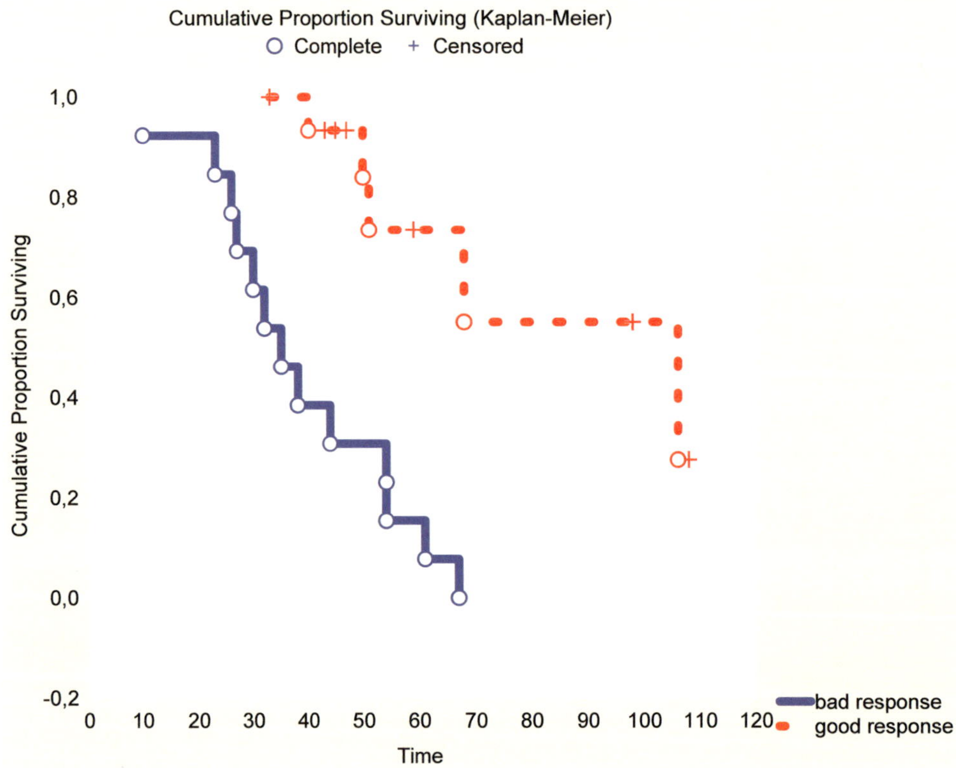

Fig. 8. Response of the patients after neoadjuvant chemotherapy treated with SSG XIV chemotherapy protocol.

Lung metastases appeared in 18/29 patients or 62.1%. The examinees with metastases had significantly shorter overall survival time than the metastasis-free patients. Four percent of the examined patients with metastases survived longer than 100 months, while 90% of the examined with no metastases were alive even after 100 months (Log-Rank test p=0.0002).

Plain radiograph or CT-scan sclerosis of the tumor after neoadjuvant chemotherapy was seen in 18/29 patients (62.1%). Pseudo-capsule was seen in 19/29 patients (65.5%), but in 3/29 (10.3%) MRI imaging showed inconclusive data. Cystic necrosis after neoadjuvant chemotherapy was seen in 14/29 patients (48.3%). Inconclusive results for cystic necrosis were found in 3 and data was missing for 1 patient.

Up to date 10/29 patients (34.5%) are disease or event free. Mean survival time of the patients was 53 months, and 20% of the examinees survived longer than 60 months (Fig. 9).

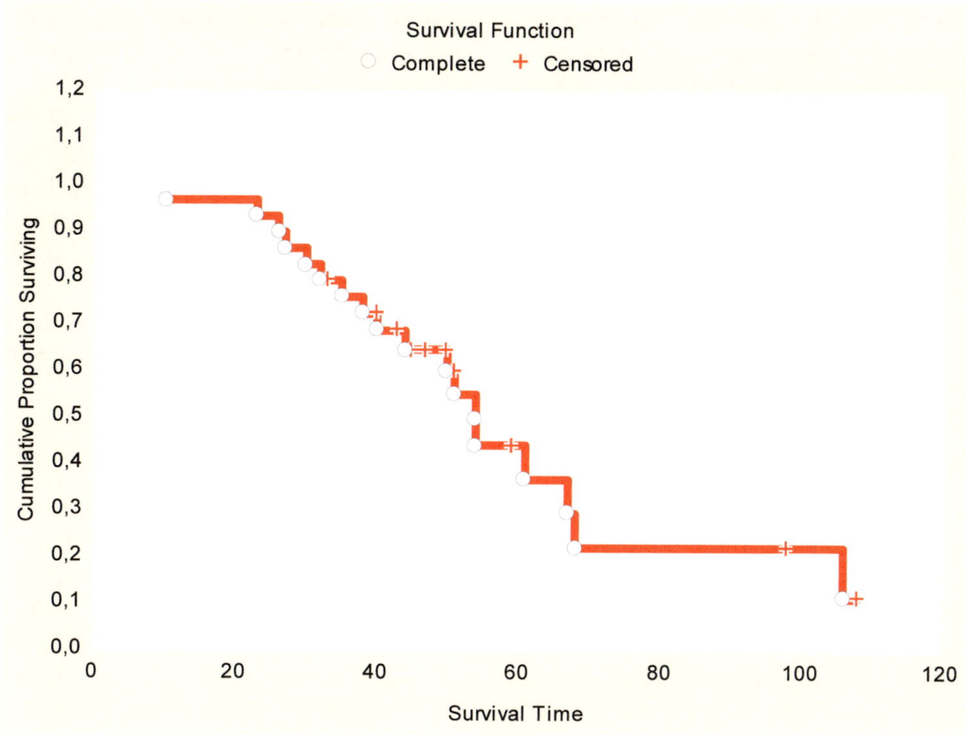

Fig. 9. Disease and event free survival time of the patients with extremity localized high-grade osteosarcoma treated with SSG XIV neoadjuvant chemotherapy protocol and surgery.

Using high dose ifosfamide for poor responders in postoperative chemotherapy should improve the results and overall survival time of these patients. If treatment and management principles of high-grade osteosarcoma are followed, limb-sparing with 60-80% survival rates could be achieved. Our preliminary results are slightly different from those published in the literature. There was a significantly different overall survival time in our study between the group of patients with good response to neoadjuvant chemotherapy compared to the group of patients with bad response. Furthermore, overall survival time in our group of patients was shorter than the time reported in the literature. In spite of the recorded differences in the results, the treatment regimen with neoadjuvant chemotherapy is promising and encouraging.

7.4 Toxic effects of neoadjuvant chemotherapy regimen

Most often hematologic toxicity is seen after chemotherapy. Various authors report Grade 3 or Grade 4 hematologic toxicity in 10-15% of the treated patients. Severe leucopenia and/or thrombocytopenia are the two conditions for readmitting patients in hospital. In that case Neupogen or Leucoverin rescue treatment is beneficial (Bacci & Picci, 1994).

Most of these patients with myelotoxicity have fever and microbiologically proven bacteremia during their granulocytopenic phase. Wide spectrum antibiotics in the beginning and specific antibiotics after microbiological assessment are necessary.

Cardiotoxicity is less often reported in patients with neoadjuvant chemotherapy. Unfortunately this side effect of the treatment is most serious and cardiopathy following the treatment may become a chronic life treating condition.
Due to general toxic effects to the human body and profound systemic reaction of all organs and systems to chemotherapeutics, sickness, malaise and weakness are general side effects. A common problem is abdominal pain associated with mild asscites, easily visualised on ultrasonography. Therefore antiemetics and corticosteroids, including dexamethasone, diphenylhydramine and lorazepam are routinely used in all patients (Bacci et al., 1993; Bruland, 1999; Messershmitt et al., 2009).
Skin necrosis, tender local swelling, inflammation, due to local intra-arterial cisplatin or venous trombophlebitis occurres in some patients. This lesions usually do not cause a major problem and usually heal in 2-3 weeks with pigmented scars.

8. Discussion

Prior to the introduction of chemotherapy, when amputation was the primary treatment for patients with osteosarcoma, the predicted long-term survival was 15-20%. Dismal survival rates were presumably attributable to pulmonary metastatic disease, whether clinically obvious or occult (Enneking, 1975). Survival rates dramatically increased during 1970's and 1980's with the pioneering work of Rosen and Jaffe. Currently, long-term survival rates are 60% to 70% for patients with localized osteosarcoma and for extremity localized up to 80% (Meyers et al., 2008). Despite the use of modern neoadjuvant chemotherapy the 10-year survival rates decline significantly to 20% in patients with clinically detectable metastases. Most of the patients ultimately die because of respiratory failure caused by the metastatic burden (Bacci et al., 2008; Messerschmitt et al., 2009; Samardziski et al., 2009a). Excluding high-grade surface osteosarcoma, which has similar prognosis to that of conventional osteosarcoma, the surface (parosteal and periosteal) osteosarcoma variants have the best prognosis of all. The 10-year survival rates for this group of patients is up to 85% (Samardziski et al., 2009b).
The site of the lesion has prognostic importance. The best survival rates are expected in patients with appendicular localization of the osteosarcoma. Central localization (pelvis, ribs and vertebrae) are less common sites of osteosarcoma, and have poorest prognosis. Osteosarcoma of the jaw is associated with an especially good prognosis, whereas osteosarcoma involving the skull has a very poor prognosis (Unni, 1998; Yu & Wang, 2009). Badly planned and ill preformed biopsy can complicate the final surgery and may decrease survival rates due to local spreading or risk for early metastatic disease (Mankin et al., 1982; Campanacci, 1999).
The overall treatment results in high-grade osteosarcoma are less impressive than widely presumed. Whereas classical osteosarcoma survival has indeed increased, in other subgroups, comprising more than 40% of the entire osteosarcoma population , the prognosis has been modestly improved. Today still more than half of an unselected osteosarcoma population eventualy succumbs to the disease, despite the current multimodal primary treatment as well as second-line chemotherapy and surgical metastatectomies (Bruland, 1999).
Neoadjuvant chemotherapy enables limb-sparing in the majority of patients with extremity localised ostesarcoma. During the past 20 years dramatic advances have been made in the

treatment of non-metastatic osteosarcoma in terms of cure rate and quality of life for survivors. These advances are due mainly to the development of effective adjuvant and neoadjuvant chemotherapeutic regimens. Reports on the progress and controversies in the treatment of osteosarcoma occurred with respect to the construct, expirimental design and interpretation of the studies. Never the les, this sdudyes led to remarkable results (Bacci, 2008).

8.1 Prognosis

Poor prognostic factors for patients with osteosarcoma include metastases at first presentation, extremely large primary tumor, increased alkaline phosphatase and lactate dehydrogenase levels, poor response to neoadjuvant chemotherapy, tumor discontinuous from bone, pathologic fractures and lymph node involvement (Longhi, et al. 2006). Despite current surgical and chemotherapeutic treatment regimens, 30% to 40% of osteosarcoma patients experience relapse within 3 years of treatment. Pulmonary recurrence is most common secondary to micro-metastatic disease. Regardless of poor prognosis, repeated tumor excisions can be performed (of primary site or metastatic one), because many studies have shown improved survival rates (Yonemoto, 1997; Bacci et al., 2001). The role of "second-line" chemotherapy regimen remains controversial because no standard regimen exists for the recurrence of the tumor.

The evaluation variables influencing systemic and local recurrence and final outcome are extremely important in defining risk-adapted treatments for patients with nonmetastatic osteosarcoma of the extremity. Upon multivariate analysis, age ≤ 14 years, high serum levels of alkaline phosphatase, tumor volume >200 mL, a dual-drug regimen chemotherapy, inadequate surgical margins, and poor histologic response to treatment maintained independent prognostic values on the outcome of nonmetastatic osteosarcoma of the extremities. These factors must be considered when deciding risk-adapted treatments for osteosarcoma patients (Pochanugool, 1997; Bacci, 2006; Yu & Wang, 2009). Amputation remains the indicated treatment when these factors are taken into consideration or tumor resection to disease-free margins leaves a nonfunctional limb (Enneking, 1975; Di Caprio & Friedlander, 2003).

8.2 Future considerations

A logical development of chemotherapy was introduction of local (or loco-regional) intra-arterial methods of chemotherapy. The obvious limitations are complicated intra-arterial techniques of application of chemotherapeutics and uncontrolled risk of tissue necrosis. Intra-arterial administration of cisplatin has been investigated for achieving improved histological response following chemotherapy. Since the originalr attempts to administer intra-arterial cisplatin from the 1980's, major advance in imaging and surgical techniques have improved the results and made it easier and safer. Reported studies demonstrate an increase in long-term survival up to 93%. Thus, a consensus on the routine use of intra-arterial chemotherapy does not exist (Jaffe, 1989; Bacci et al., 2001; Messershmit et al., 2009).

Basic science is making continuous advance in molecular mechanisms and biologic pathways that may yield more specific, less-toxic drugs that will further improve survival rates. Inhibition of tyrosine kinase signaling is known to regulate cell growth, cell proliferation, angiogenesis, and apoptosis and is an area of current interest (Messershmit et al., 2008). Liposomal muramyl tripeptide phosphatidilethanolamine (L-MTP-PE) is a promising drug in clinical trial that functions to stimulate the formation of tumoricidal macrophages (Meyers et al., 2008).

9. Conclusion

With advances in neoadjuvant chemotherapy, radiographic imaging, and reconstructive surgery, most patients with osteosarcoma can now be offered limb-sparing treatment. A multidisciplinary approach in diagnosis and treatment is mandatory. Surgical resection with wide margins after neoadjuvant and adjuvant chemotherapy after surgery is a current standard of care. Osteoarticular allografts, modular prostheses, or composites of these two approaches form the basis for most current reconstructions. However, amputation still plays an important role and offers a standard to which other approaches must be compared. Basic science is making continuous advance in molecular mechanisms and more specific, less-toxic drugs will further improve survival rates. Current research into the cell biology of osteosarcoma may lead to improved and more target-selective treatment with the intent of improved overall survival.

Applying neoadjuvant chemotherapy followed by appropriate surgery requires responsible, trained and highly engaged medical staff. If treatment and management principles of high-grade osteosarcoma with neoadjuvant therapy are followed, long-term 60-80% overall survival rates could be easily achieved.

10. Acknowledgement

Special thanks to Mrs. Marija Tanevska-Pulios for English language editing of the paper.

11. References

Bacci, G. et al. (1993). Primary chemotherapy and delayed surgery for non-metastatic osteosarcoma of the extremities. *Cancer*, Vol. 72, No.11, pp. (3227-3238), DOI: 10.1002/1097-0142(19931201)72:11<3227::AID-CNCR2820721116>3.0.CO;2-C.

Bacci, G. & Picci, P. (1994). Analysis of Factors Influencing Treatment Options in Osteosarcoma. Review. *Forum*, Vol. 4, No.1,(1994), pp. (52-64).

Bacci, G. et al. (2001). A comparison of methods of loco-regional chemotherapy combined with systemic chemotherapy as neoadjuvant treatment of osteosarcoma of the extremity. *Eur J Surg Oncol*, Vol. 27, (2001), pp. (98-104), PMID: 11237499.

Bacci, G. et al. (2006). Prognostic factors for osteosarcoma of the extremity treated with neoadjuvant chemotherapy: 15-Year experience in 789 patients treated at a single institution. *Cancer*, Vol. 106, No. 5, (2006), pp. (1154-1161), ISSN 0008-543X.

Bacci, G. et al. (2008). High-grade osteosarcoma of the extremities with lung metastases at presentation: Treatment with neoadjuvant chemotherapy and simultaneous resection of primary and metastatic lesions. *J Surg Oncol*, Vol. 98, (2008), pp. (415-420) PMID: 18792969.

Bruland, ØS. & Phil, A. (1999) On the current management of osteosarcoma. A critical evaluation and a proposal for modified treatment surgery. *Eur J Cancer*, Vol. 33, pp. (1725-1731), PMID: 9470825.

Campanacci, M. (1999). Errors in the diagnosis and treatment of the musculoskeletal tumors: What must not be done. *Chir Organi Mov*, Vol. 84, (1999), pp. (1-17).

Di Caprio, MR. & Friedlander, GE. (2003). Malignant Bone Tumours: Limb Sparing Versus Amputation. *J Am Acad Ort Surg*, Vol.11, No.1, pp. (125-129), PMID: 12699369 .

Enneking, WF. (1975). Osteosarcoma (editorial comment). *Clin Orthop Rel Research*, Vol. 111, (1975), pp. (2-4).

Enneking, WF. et al. (1980). A surgical staging of musculoskeletal sarcomas. *J Bone Joint Surg (Am)*, Vol. 62, (1980), pp. (1027-1030), PMID: 7449206.

Fletcher, CDM. et al. (2002). Classification of Tumours. Pathology and Genetics of Tumours of Soft Tissue and Bone. IARC Press, Lyon, ISBN: 92 832 2413 2.

González-Heranz, P. et al. (1995). The Management of Limb-Length Discrepancies in Children after Treatment of Osteosarcoma and Ewing's Sarcoma. *J Ped Orthop*, Vol. 15, (1995), pp.(561-565), PMID: 7593562.

Jaffe, N. et al. (1985). Analysis of efficacy of the intra-arterial cis-Diammine-dichlorplatinum-II and high dose methotrexate with citrovorum factor rescue in the treatment of primary osteosarcoma. *Reg Cancer Treat*, (1985). Vol. 2, pp. (157-63), PMID: 3874932.

Kotz, R. et al. (2002). Advances in bone tumor treatment in 30 years with respect to survival and limb salvage. A single institution experience. *Intern Othoped*, Vol. 26, (2002), pp. (197-206), DOI: 10.1007/s00264-002-0365-1.

Lodwick, GS. et al. (1963). Computer Diagnosis of Primary Bone Tumours, A Preliminary Report, *J Bone Joint Surg Am*, Vol. 80. (1963), pp. (273-275), DOI: 10.1148/80.2.273.

Longhi, A. et al. (2006). Primary bone osteosarcoma in the pediatric age: State of the art. *Cancer Treat Rev*,Vol. 32, (2006), pp. (423-436), DOI:10.1016/j.ctrv.2006.05.005.

Mankin, HJ. et al. (1982). The Hazards of Biopsy in Patients with Malignant Primary Bone and Soft-Tissue Tumours. *J Bone Joint Surg Am*, Vol. 64 (1982), pp. (1121-1127), PMID: 7130225.

Messershmitt, PJ. Et al. (2008). Specific tyrosine kinase inhibition regulated human osteosarcoma cells in vitro. *Clin Orthop Rel Res*, Vol. 466, (2008), pp. (2168-2175), DOI: 10.1007/S11999-008-0338-9.

Messerschmitt, PJ. et al. (2009). Osteosarcoma. *J Am Acad Ort Surg,;* Vol. 17, (2009), pp. (515-527), PMID: 19652033.

Meyers, PA. et al. (2008). Osteosarcoma: The addition of muramyl tripeptide to chemotherapy improves overall survival. A report from Children's Oncology Group. *J Clin Oncol*, Vol. 26, (2008), pp. (633-638), PMID: 18235123.

Price, CH. & Jeffree, GM. (1977). Incidence of bone sarcoma in SW England, 1946-74, in relation to age, sex, tumour site and histology. *Br J Cancer*. Vol.36, No.4, (October 1977), pp. (511-522), PMCID: PMC2025376.

Pochanugool, L. et al. (1997). Prognostic Factors Among 130 Patients With Osteosarcoma. *Clin Orthop Rel Res*. (1997). Vol. 345, pp.(206-214), PMID: 9418642.

Rosen, G et al., (1976). Chemotherapy, en bloc resection, and prosthetic bone replacement in the treatment of osteogenic sarcoma. *Cancer*, Vol. 37, No.1, (1976), pp. (1-11), PMID: 1082364.

Sæter, G. et al. (1996), Extremity and non-extremity high-grade osteosarcoma, *Acta Oncol,* Vol. 35, (1996), pp. (129-134), PMID: 9073059 .

Samardziski, M. et al. (2004). Computer assisted diagnosis of benign bone tumors. *Radiol Oncol,*Vol. 38, (2004), pp. (165-169), ISSN: 1581-3207.

Samardziski, M. et al. (2009a). Limb-sparing in patients with non-metastatic high-grade osteosarcoma. *J. BUON,* Vol. 14, (2009) pp. (63-69), PubMed ID: 19373949.

Samardziski, M. et al. (2009b). Parosteal Osteosarcoma. *Bratisl Lek Listy.* Vol. 110, (2009), pp. (240-244), PubMed ID: 19507652.

Unni, KK. (1998). Osteosarcoma of bone. *J Orthop Sci,* Vol. 3, (1998), pp. (287-294), DOI: 10.1007/s007760050055.

Wittig, JC. et al. (2002). Osteosarcoma: A Multidisciplinary Approach to Diagnosis and Treatment. *Am Fam Physician,* Vol. 65, No. 6, (2002), pp. (1123-1132), PMID: 11925089.

Yonemoto, T. et al. (1997). Prognosis of Osteosarcoma with Pulmonary Metastases at Initial Presentation is not Dismal. *Clin Orth Rel Res,* Vol. 349, (1997), pp. (194-199), PMID: 9584383.

Yu, XC & Wang, W. (2009). Multivariate analysis of factors influencing on preoperative chemotherapy response for osteosarcoma. *Cancer Research on Prevention and Treatment,* Vol. 36, No.10, (2009) pp. 863-868, ISSN 1000-8578.

15

Chemotherapy and Mechanisms of Resistance in Breast Cancer

Andre Lima de Oliveira[1], Roberto Euzebio dos Santos[1] and Fabio Francisco Oliveira Rodrigues[2]
[1]*DOGI General Gynecology Clinic, Brotherhood of the Santa Casa de São Paulo*
[2]*DOGI Pelvic Oncology Clinic, Brotherhood of the Santa Casa de São Paulo*
Brasil

1. Introduction

1.1 Adjuvant

In the mid 1950s, we started to have a much better understanding of the biological mechanisms of establishment of metastases and the role of regional lymph nodes as an effective barrier to tumor spread, because malignant cells have been observed in the bloodstream (Fisher, Turnbull, 1955).

Early studies with adjuvant chemotherapy after surgery in solid tumors (breast adenocarcinoma implanted in mice) began in 1957 (Shapiro, Fugman, 1957). Based on these findings, Bernard Fisher and colleagues began in 1958, the first collaborative study with the objective of evaluating the response to systemic administration of perioperative chemotherapy in patients with operable breast cancer (Fisher et al, 1958). Good results were obtained in relation to disease-free interval and overall survival in premenopausal women (Fisher et al, 1968). Similar results were also observed by other authors, with the use of multidrug therapy (cyclophosphamide, methotrexate and fluorouracil (CMF) with or without prednisone) in advanced breast cancer (BC)(Canellos et al, 1974 and 1976, Bonadonna et al, 1976). Therefore, the addition of adjuvant polychemotherapy in BC showed gain by controlling survival of micrometastases in patients with lymph nodes affected by cancer or not (Fisher et al, 1975; Bonadonna et al, 1976; Early Breast Cancer Trialists Collaborative Group (EBCTCG), 1988; Bonadonna, Valagussa, 1983,1985,1987, Henderson, 1987, Fisher et al, 1989; Bonadonna et al, 1995; Mansour et al, 1998, Carlson et al, 2000 and NIH 2000).

1.2 Neoadjuvant therapy

Neoadjuvant chemotherapy is defined as a treatment option where chemotherapy is introduced before local treatment, either surgery or radiotherapy (Bear, 1998). This was introduced by De Lena et al (1978) who administered adriablastin and vincristine in 110 women with advanced BC, achieving response rates of 70% partial.

The biological rationale for using neoadjuvant chemotherapy was based on observations in animal models where the removal of primary tumor growth accelerated due to changes in metastatic tumor kinetics, suggesting that growth factors derived from tumor influence the development of micrometastases. The prior addition of chemotherapy such as cyclophosphamide in mice transplanted with murine mammary tumor cells showed a significant reduction in the proliferation rate of residual tumor and metastases, and prolonged their survival (Gunduz et al, 1979, Fisher et al, 1989b; Fisher et al, 1989c).

The use of neoadjuvant chemotherapy has additional advantages in patients with locally advanced carcinoma, enhancing the possibility of performing conservative surgery due to the reduction of tumor size, as well as providing evidence in vivo of sensitivity to therapy and providing early treatment of micrometastases (Bonadonna et al. 1990; Wolff, Davidson, 2000, Kafka et al 2003, Hutcheon, Heys, 2004).

Studies demonstrated a significant increase in survival in patients with stage III breast carcinoma, influenced by neoadjuvant chemotherapy associated with local therapy (Canellos, 1976; Jacquillat et al, 1987 Valagussa et al, 1990). Six randomized trials compared the use of adjuvant and neoadjuvant therapy with the aim of measuring the survival of patients with complete clinical response rates from 6.6 to 41% and pathological complete rates of 3 to 29%, with high rates of breast conservation in patients undergoing neoadjuvant chemotherapy (Mauriac et al, 1991; Semiglazov et al, 1994; Scholl, 1994; Powles et al, 1995, van der Hage et al, 2001; Wolmark et al, 2001). One of the major studies related to neoadjuvant chemotherapy was the National Surgical Adjuvant Breast and Bowel Project B18 (NSABP B18), which showed no significant difference between the rates of disease-free survival and survival free of distant disease (among those who received neoadjuvant chemotherapy and those who received postoperative adjuvant chemotherapy). However, neoadjuvant chemotherapy allowed higher rates of conservative surgery and the study in vivo of tumor biology (Fisher et al, 1998). Further analysis, with a follow up of nine years, showed that patients under 49 years experienced a significant advantage in terms of survival rates and disease-free survival when they were submitted to primary chemotherapy in relation to patients 50 years or more, suggesting that age could influence the indication of neoadjuvant chemotherapy, continuing the strong correlation between the clinical primary tumor response to chemotherapy and prognosis (Wolmark et al, 2001).

The neoadjuvant therapy was extended for the treatment of patients with operable breast tumors initially with different chemotherapy regimens and variable rates of clinical response (Scholl et al, 1994; Ragaz et al, 1997, Fisher et al, 1997, Fisher et al, 1998). The clinical response to neoadjuvant administration of chemotherapy, namely the reduction of tumor size, was 10 to 75% in several studies (Kafka et al, 2003).

1.3 Mechanisms of resistance to chemotherapeutic agents

The main reasons responsible for treatment failure in cancer patients are the mechanisms of drug resistance and emergence of disseminated disease (Terek et al, 2003). We identified two types of resistance most relevant to BC: primary resistance, which corresponds to the clinical situation where the patient showed no response to therapy, and secondary or acquired resistance in which, initially, there is an observed response and a subsequent failure of the treatment regimen (Kroger et al, 1999).

Several mechanisms may cause the phenotype of multidrug resistance to chemotherapy drugs and are well characterized in in vitro experiments, including alterations in systemic pharmacology (pharmacokinetics and metabolism), extracellular mechanisms (tumor environment, multicellular drug resistance), and cellular mechanisms (cellular pharmacology, activation and inactivation of drugs, modification of specific targets and regulatory pathways of apoptosis) (Leonessa et al, 2003, Riddick et al, 2005). Identification of factors that affect cell metabolism, which are related to drug resistance, will enable the identification of which patients are at particular risk of treatment failure.

Among the biochemical and molecular mechanisms of drug resistance, we stress: changes in the activity of topoisomerase II, alterations in the DNA repair mechanism, overexpression of P-glycoprotein; high intracellular concentrations of enzymes purification of cellular metabolism - among them enzymes the family of glutathione S-transferases (GSTs) and changes in the mechanisms of signaling via c-Jun N-terminal kinase 1 (JNK1) -and "apoptosis signal-regulating kinase (ASK1) required for activation of the" mitogen-activated protein (MAP kinases) in apoptosis and cellular restoration. These pathways are also mediated by proteins encoded by genes of GSTs (O'Brien, Tew, 1996; Burg, Mulder, 2002, L'Ecuyer et al, 2004).

Different response rates to particular chemotherapy regimens, as observed in patient groups with the same biological characteristics and stage, suggest the existence of different mechanisms of drug resistance, probably induced by genetic alterations (Hayes, Pulford, 1995; O'Brien , Tew, 1996; Pakunlu et al, 2003).

Among the mechanisms of purification of cellular metabolism involved in the inactivation of toxic substances to the cell there is the action of the enzyme family of GSTs in phase II metabolism of cell purification. The first evidence of their involvement in resistance to drugs used in chemotherapy have emerged from research published by scientific groups Schisswelbauer et al (1990), Tew (1994) and Hayes, Pulford, (1995). However, the relationship between GSTs and resistance to chemotherapy remains inconsistent (Riddick et al, 2005). This mechanism of resistance is related to the ability to regulate the action of enzymes involved in catalyzing electrophilic compounds harmful to cells from activation by cytochrome P-450 1A1 and 1B1 (Phase I). These compounds in turn are substrates for phase II enzyme systems, represented here by the family of GSTs, which are involved on two fronts in the process of drug resistance: production of protective enzymes of metabolism and cellular apoptotic processes via inhibition of JNK1 and ASK1 (Townsed, Cowan, 1989, Hamada et al, 1994; Tew, 1994; O'Brien, Tew, 1996; Gaudiano et al, 2000, O'Brien et al, 2000; Tashiro et al, 2001; Harbottle et al, 2001; Townsend, Tew, 2003b).

1.3.1 Glutathione S-transferases (GSTs)

The family of GSTs consists of eight classes termed cytosolic and symbolized by the Greek alphabet: Alpha, Kappa, Mu, Omega, Pi, Sigma, Theta and Zeta. They are highly polymorphic, with about 30% homology between their base sequences. Each of these classes has several alleles that reach 50% similarity between their base sequences, and are able to produce enzymes of phase II cell purification.

Cellular purification occurs through the ability to regulate the action of protein kinases involved in the catalysis of electrophilic compounds harmful to cells (xenobiotics) from the activation by cytochrome P-450 1A1 and 1B1, such as genotoxic chemical carcinogens and cytotoxic agents chemotherapeutic drugs and their metabolites by means of connection to glutathione (Fig. 1) (Townsed, Cowan, 1989, Shea et al, 1990; Tew, 1994, Shimada et al, 1996; Townsend, Tew, 2003a, b; Daly, 2003). The enzymes of the GST family represents about 5 to 10% of all cellular proteins (Burg, Mulder, 2002).

Studies have shown that the GST enzyme complex participates in the JNK1 and ASK1 pathways necessary for activation of MAP kinase signaling processes involved in apoptosis and cellular restoration. They also participate in and catalyze the conjugation of electrophilic compounds and free radicals to the tri-peptide glutathione (γ-glu-cys-gly, or GSH), produced by GSH-reductase. Thus, they become less chemically reactive and more soluble, and its excretion facilitated by membrane enzyme complexes, among which stands out the GP1 enzyme encoded by the MRP1 gene family of ABC transporters (Arrick, Nathan, 1984; Townsed Cowan, 1989, Hamada et al, 1994; Tew, 1994; O'Brien, Tew, 1996, Morrow et al, 1998, Gaudiano et al, 2000; Harbottle et al, 2001; Burg, Mulder, 2002; Townsend, Tew, 2003a, b; Parl, 2005).

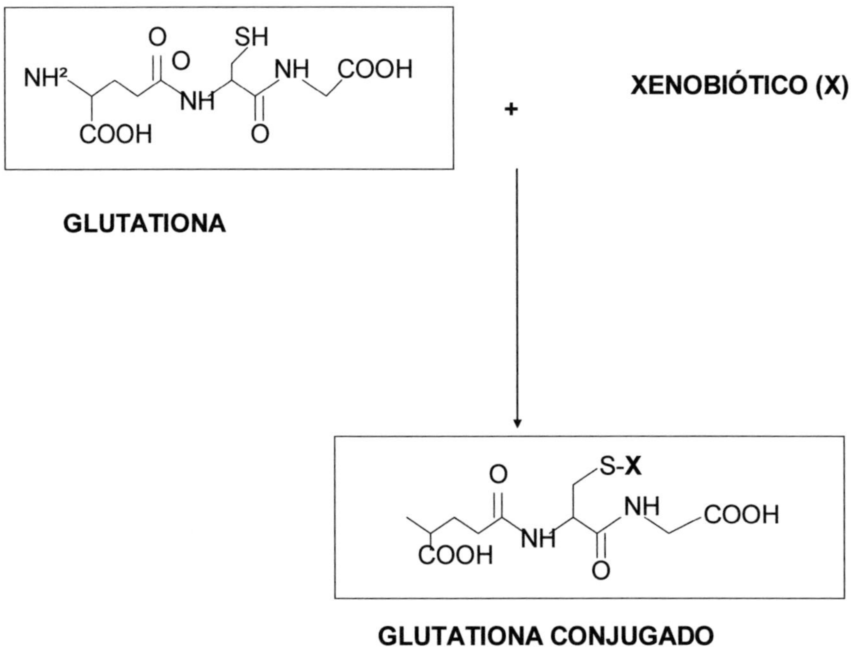

Fig. 1. Conjugation of glutathione to a generic xenobiotic (X) via catalysis by GSTs to form a conjugate of GST.

Glutathione (GSH) is a major intracellular non-protein substance present in the process of activation and inactivation of toxic substrates to the cell cycle. These reactions begins in the presence of free radicals and products released by the oxide-reactive phenomena of stress and inflammation than healthy and tumor cells are subjected (Arrick, Nathan, 1984; Russo, Mitchell, 1985, Asakura et al, 1999, Adler et al, 1999; Burg, Mulder, 2002; McIlwain et al, 2006). Thus, GSH plays an important role in cell survival and can be found in high concentrations in tumor tissue, where the highest enzyme activity of GSTs family exists (O'Brien, Tew, 1996, O'Brien et al, 2000).
GSH may present itself in several ways, most commonly its reduced sulfhydryl which is related to reactions with substances or reduced-oxide reactions with electrophilic substances. These reactions may be reversible or irreversible, spontaneous or mediated by

the enzymes of the family of GSTs (Arrick, Nathan, 1984; O'Brien, Tew, 1996; Burg, Mulder, 2002).
GSH has four functions in the anti-cancer therapy: cell protection by blockade of toxic substances to the cell, mediating the formation of toxic to cells, cellular targeting, allowing the efflux and influx of substances through association with enzyme systems membrane and therapeutic interaction through changes in the effectiveness of certain drugs (Arrick, Nathan, 1984). Among the substrates for the cytosolic enzymes of the family of GSTs are anti-neoplastic drugs such as melphalan, chlorambucil, adriamycin, cyclophosphamide, and platinum salts among others (Table 1), which, in the presence of these enzymes, have a lower intracellular concentration (Dirven, 1994; Paumi et al, 2001; Townsend, Tew, 2003a, b).

Direct substrates of GSTs
Chlorambucil
Melphalan
Nitrogen mustard
Mustard Phosphoramide
Acrolein
Carmustine
Hidroxialquilantes
Ethacrynic acid
Steroids
Substances not characterized as direct substrates of GSTs
Antimetabolites *
Antitubulin drugs *
Inhibitors of topoisomerases I and II *
Bleomycin
Hepsulfan
Mitomycin C *
Adriamycin *
Cisplatin *
Carboplatin

* Requires activation of JNK for cytotoxicity
(Adapted from Townsend, Tew, 2003b)

Table 1. Nonsteroidal anti-neoplastic agents associated with increased levels of GST and cellular resistance.

Cytotoxic and carcinogenic substances from the environment such as tobacco, alcohol and red meat, which are possibly related tocarcinogenesis in various organs such as breast, bladder and colon are also substrates for the enzymes of the GST family of

1.3.1.1 The glutathione S-transferases (GSTs) and breast cancer

The classes of GSTs are related to the BC classes Alpha, Theta, and Pi Mu. In this review we approach the last three, as they are most frequently studied and their analysis has provided further information in relation to adjuvant chemotherapy and CM.
The proteins that belong to the Mu class are encoded by a group of genes located on chromosome 1 (GSTM 1-5). These genes are related to various diseases and susceptibility to

various forms of cancer (Townsend, Tew, 2003a). The GSTM1 gene (Genbank access number AY532926) is the most studied and has four different allelic forms (GSTM 1 * A, B 1 * 1 * 1 * 0 null and Ax2 that are related to a variety of malignancies, as lung, colorectal, oropharyngeal, bladder and breast cancers (Bell et al, 1993; Ambrosone et al, 1995; Saarikoski et al, 1998; Helzlsouer et al, 1998; Jourenkova-Mironova et al, 1999, Dunning et al, 1999; Ambrosone et al, 2001; Loktionov et al, 2001 and Sgambati et al, 2002; Townsend, Tew, 2003a). However, some authors failed to demonstrate such a relationship (Bailey et al, 1998; Lizard-Nacolia et al , 1999; Garcia-Close et al, 1999).

The enzymes encoded by the gene GSTM1 catalyze the conjugation of electrophilic compounds and free radicals by GSH and still exert an inhibitory effect on apoptosis via ASK1, independent of its catalytic action. This inhibition occurs while the enzyme complexes of GSTM1/ASK1 are related. In the presence of high concentrations of oxide-reactive substances, this complex dissociates, releasing enzymes to ASK1 phosphorylation and signaling of apoptosis (Fig. 2) (Cho et al, 2001).

The GSTM1 null genotype polymorphism results from the absence of the two alleles that determine gene expression. Thus, individuals with this genotype do not have the capacity to produce the enzymes necessary to catalyze the conjugation with GSH. Moreover, they also do not synthesize the proteins that coalesce to the ASK1 pathway proteins necessary for the inhibition of this pathway of apoptosis (Cho et al, 2001; McIlwain et al, 2006). The null genotype is present in 40 to 50% of the population (Tew, 1994), ranging from 22% in Nigeria, 58% among Chinese, 45% in Western Europe and up to 67% in Australia, and it is related to better response to some classes of chemotherapeutic agents against various types of cancer (Alpert et al, 1997; Ambrosone et al, 2001; Sgambati et al, 2002; Autrup et al, 2002; Townsend, Tew, 2003a; Khedhaier et al, 2003; Parl , 2005).

The proteins of the class Theta are encoded by two genes (T1 and T2), which are located on chromosome 22. The class GSTT1 (accession number AB057594 in Genbank) has three allelic forms: * The T1, T1 and T1 * B * 0 or null, but the latter is present between 10 and 30% in African populations, 10% in European and American populations, and 64% in Asian populations (Townsend, Tew, 2003a). The T1 null allele is associated with a predisposition to some cancers (Townsend, Tew, 2003a; Saarikoski, 1998; Helzlsouer et al, 1998; Jourenkova-Mironova et al, 1999 and Ambrosone et al, 2001), among them breast cancer in postmenopausal women, users of large quantities of alcoholic and longtime smokers, as well as in premenopausal women or nulliparous women who gave birth after age 30 (Park et al, 2000, Zheng et al, 2002, Zheng et al, 2003; Park et al, 2003), although some studies have not shown this relationship (Bailey et al, 1998; Garcia-Close et al, 1999; Millikan et al, 2000). The presence of the GSTT1 null form, in which there is not production of the enzymes, was associated with a better response to chemotherapy in patients with BC and the greater toxicity of some chemotherapeutic agents (Howells et al, 2001;Naoe et al, 2002; Khedhaier et al, 2003).

The class Pi, in turn, consists of only one protein encoded by a gene located on chromosome 11 and called GSTP1 (GenBank access number AY324387). The GSTP1 gene has three allelic forms. The wild GSTP1 * A (Ile105Ile/Ala113Ala) genotype results in the replacement of Ile by Val at least one amino acid at codon 105 and\) and two polymorphic forms, GSTP1 * B (Val 105Ile Val/113 Val) where, in addition to the alteration observed in GSTP1B * there is also replacement of Ala by Val in at least one amino acid codon 113.\ \GSTP1 * C (105 Ile Ala. These forms are represented, respectively, in 68%, 26% and 7% of the Caucasian population (Townsend, Tew, 2003a).

The enzymes produced by gene GSTP1 * A prevails as a marker of carcinogenesis, since they are present in many tumor cells (Townsend, Tew, 2003a). Their relationship with cell protection is more related to performance in the apoptotic process. While the proteins encoded by the form "wild" GSTP1 * A are related to proteins of the JNK pathway, which inhibits apoptosis. This action will cease as the intensity of the phenomena of stress to which the cell is subjected to increase (fig 2), a phenomenon that occurs independently of its catalytic action. Since the polymorphic forms do not have the capacity to synthesize proteins that coalesce to JNK pathway enzymes and therefore do not have the ability to inhibit this pathway of apoptosis (Adler et al, 1999, Dang et al, 2005).

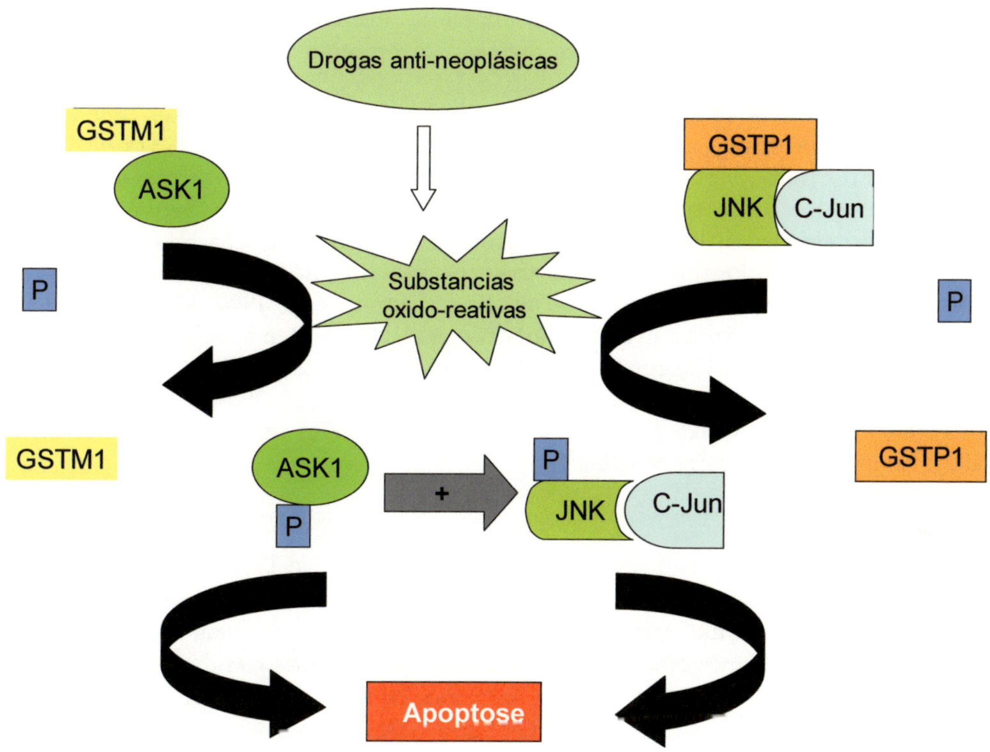

ASK1: "Apoptosis Signal-Regulating Kinase"
JNK / Cjun: "c-Jun N-terminal Kinase 1"
P: phosphorus atom

Fig. 2. Action of GSTM1 and GSTP1 on pathways of apoptosis. While related enzymes ASK1 and JNK1, the proteins encoded by the genes GSTM1 and GSTP1 exert an inhibitory effect of the corresponding pathways of apoptosis. Once exposed to substances oxide - reactive is the dissociation of the complex and phosphorylation of enzymes ASK1 and JNK1 pathways that pass the signal to the apoptosis pathway.

The involvement of enzymes encoded by the gene GSTP1 * A in cell survival processes by catalyzing GSH seems to be a secondary response or consequence of the phenomena of stress to which the cells are submitted and occur in two ways of acting. The first one is mainly related to anthracycline chemotherapy drugs and their substrates when associated with the ABC membrane transporters, responsible for one of the mechanisms of complex cellular efflux of GSH / drug. The second route of action would be on inhibitory complexes GSH / drugs on the enzymes of class GSTP1 * A, stimulating the process of apoptosis (Nakagawa et al, 1988.1990; Tew, 1994; Helzlsouer et al, 1998, Adler et al , 1999, Sweeney et al, 2000; Tashiro et al, 2001, Wang et al, 2001; Autrup et al, 2002; Townsend, Tew, 2003a, Huang et al, 2003; McIlwain et al, 2006).

The presence and distribution of genes encoding the synthesis of enzymes of the family of GSTs in humans are variable. Some individuals do not express the genes GSTM1 and GSTT1, which determine the production of the enzyme purification. It is said that these people have "deleted" these alleles, known as GSTs null. These in turn are unable to promote catalysis of toxic substances with GSH and unable to promote inhibition of protein kinases required for the apoptotic process. Since the class Pi presents a substitution of amino acid isoleucine (Ile) by valine (Val) at codon 105 (GSTP1 * A → GSTP1 * B) This change, either in a strand of DNA (heterozygous) or both strands (homozygous) also makes cells unable to produce their own enzymes catalyzing GSH, which was similar to the GSTs null, and no longer inhibit the JNK apoptosis 1 (McIlwain et al, 2006).

Comparable studies have shown varying results on the correlation between GSTs and chemotherapy response in various fields of oncology, including CM. Some authors have found a positive relationship between the presence of these enzymes and increased chemotherapeutic resistance (Hamada et al, 1994; Dirven et al, 1994, Morrow et al, 1998, Sweeney et al, 2000, O'Brien et al, 2000; Harbottle et al, 2001; Allan et al, 2001; Ambrosone et al, 2001; Naoe et al, 2002, Dasgupta et al, 2003, Huang et al, 2003, Yang et al, 2005), while others failed to demonstrate such a relationship (Moscow et al, 1989; Leyland-Jones et al, 1991, Peters et al, 1993, Morrow et al, 1998, Alpert et al, 1997, Konishi et al, 1998; Osmak et al, 1998; Allan et al, 2001;Yang et al, 2005).

1.3.2 P-glycoprotein

The phenomenon of multi-drug resistance was first described in 1970 in ovarian cancer cells derived from Chinese hamsters exposed to increasing concentrations of various chemotherapeutic agents like actinomycin D, anthracyclines, vinca alkaloids and etoposide, until chemo resistant clones emerged (Bield, Riehm, 1970). Subsequently, Riordan and Ling (1979) showed the phenotype of multidrug resistance by measuring a deficit accumulation of cytotoxic drugs in the intracellular environment due to the action of a specific glycoprotein.

One of the proteins responsible for determining this resistance phenotype is the P-glycoprotein (Pgp), first described by Juliano and Ling (1976), responsible for the permeation and elimination of substances through the cell membrane (Carlsen et al, 1976; Riordan, Ling, 1979). This transmembrane protein has a molecular weight of 170 kd, 1280 amino acids, is encoded by the gene MDR-1 and depends on energy coming from the metabolism of adenosine triphosphate (ATP) (Sauna et al, 2001). The MDR -1 gene in humans is located on the long arm of chromosome 7 (7 q 21) consisting of a central promoter region and 29 exons ranging from 6.3 to 210 kilobases (Bodor et al, 2005).

Pgp is the most investigated of a superfamily called ATP - binding cassette transporters, or ABC multidrug transporters. It is encoded by some genes as MRP-1, MRP- 2, MRP-3, MRP-4, MRP- 5,MRP-6, MRP-8, BSPE, BCRP (Goldstein, 1996; Scotto, 2003) ABC transporters are characterized functionally by their ability to eliminate antiblastic hydrophilic drugs from the intracellular environment , as shown below (Fig.3), (Sauna et al, 2001).

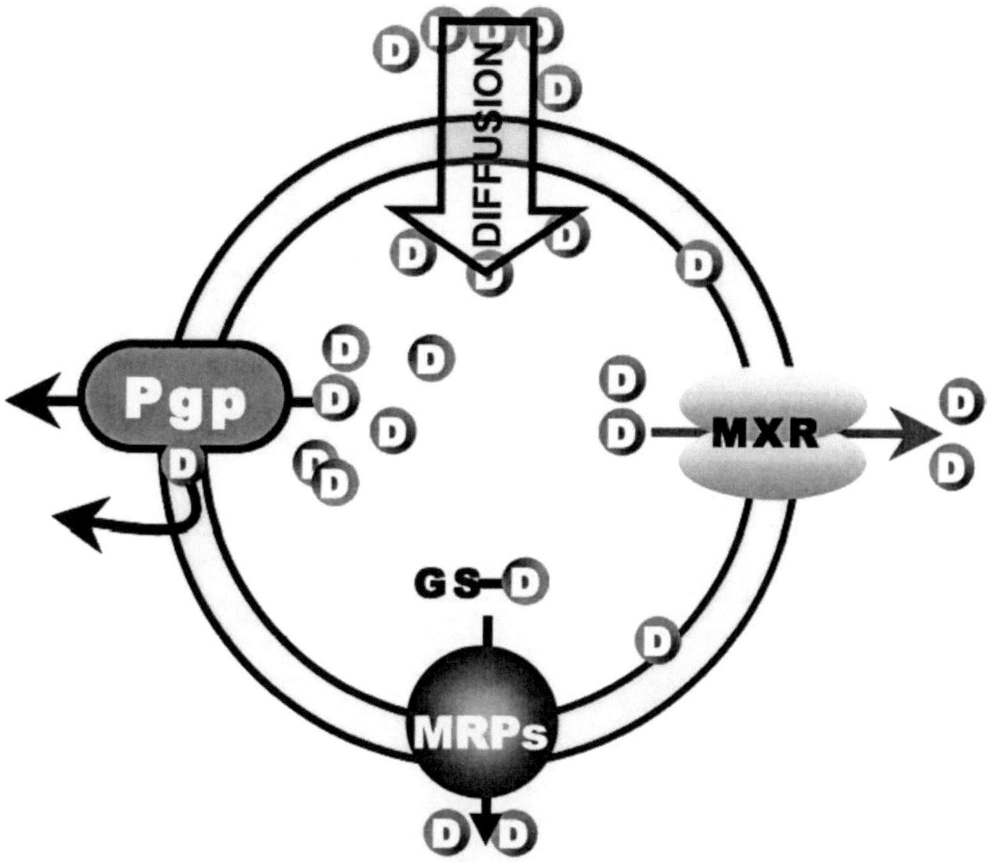

Fig. 3. Schematic representation of several proteins belonging to the superfamily multidrug ABC transporters, including Pgp. (Adapted from Sauna et al, 2001).

Several drugs are substrates to the protein encoded by MRP's as anthracyclines agents, vinca's alkaloid, taxanes, actinomycin D, among others (Goldstein, 1996). It consists of a basic structure composed of two transmembrane domains (TMD) associated with two helical domains attached to nucleotides, in a conical shape of 10 nm depth, oriented perpendicular to the cell membrane, as visualized in Fig. 4 (Leonessa, Clarke, 2003).

The three-dimensional shape of Pgp consists of a conical shape with a central pore, with its base open to the extracellular medium and its apex toward the intracellular region, virtually closed when this protein is not active (Leonessa, Clarke, 2003). The substrates of Pgp diffuse into the inner layers of the cell membrane along the propeller of their domains. With binding of the substrate on Pgp, ATP hydrolysis occurs after the conformational rearrangement of the protein obliterates the internal pore. Simultaneously, there is rotation of the helix, contributing to the decrease in the affinity between substrate and protein, eliminating it from the external environment. (Leonessa, Clarke, 2003). The mechanism by which Pgp interacts with this wide variety of substrates is still unclear. However, all substrates have in common that they are hydrophobic, have a molecular weight from 300 to 2000 Da; and some carry a positive charge at neutral pH (Sauna et al, 2001).

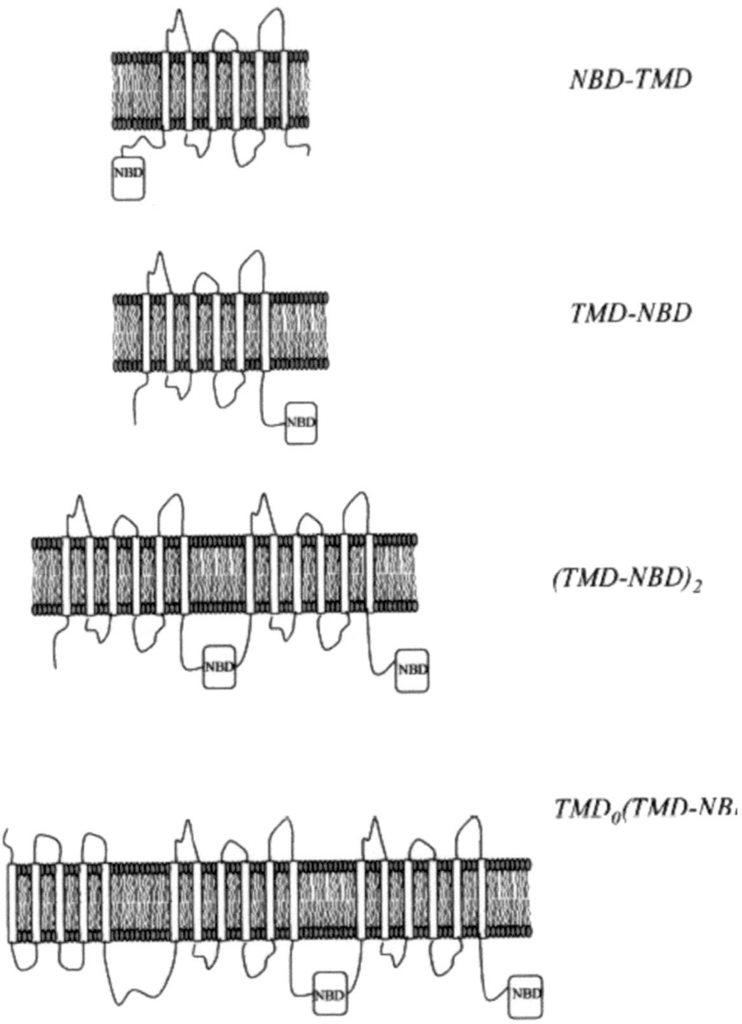

Fig. 4. Schematic representation of Tansmembranas domains (TMD) that make up the various ABC multidrug transporters, including Pgp. (Adapted from Leonessa, Clarke, 2003)

The expression of Pgp is not uniform across tissues, occurring both in normal and neoplastic tissues (Goldstein, 1996; Sauna et al, 2001) and is expressed physiologically in the blood-brain barrier, liver, kidneys, intestine, adrenal glands and testicles, functioning to control the absorption, distribution and excretion of xenobiotics (Gottesmann, Pastan, 1993; Ambudkar et al, 1999). High levels of Pgp are found in renal tumors, liver and colon, low concentrations are identified in bladder tumors, breast cancer and stomach cancer. In tumors that have failed initial treatment, its expression is particularly high, as in breast, ovarian and non-Hodgkin lymphoma (Goldstein, 1996). Tumors that initially show resistance to drug infusion (primary resistance) to anthracycline derivatives also express high concentrations of P-glycoprotein (Goldstein, 1996).

Pgp expression is and adverse prognostic factor on multivariate analysis, in patients with neuroblastoma and childhood sarcomas (Chan et al, 1990, Chan et al 1991), although this has not been consistent association (Goldstein, 1996). The expression of Pgp associated with bcl-2 in acute lymphoblastic leukemia in adults is an independent prognostic factor for disease-free survival (Del Principe et al, 2003). In endometrial carcinoma, the immunohistochemical overexpression of Pgp is seen especially in premenopausal patients compared to patients of advanced age (Terek et al, 2003). In ovarian cancer, overexpression of MDR-1 gene is associated with decreased disease-free survival and tumor progression during chemotherapy (Kavallaris et al, 1996; Raspollini et al, 2005). In breast carcinoma, the expression of Pgp shows great heterogeneity due to the detection methods and different degrees of their induction by the use of multiple chemotherapeutic agents (Trock et al, 1997; Leonessa, Clarke, 2003). The expression of Pgp may be quantified by immunohistochemical analysis (IHC) or by use of polymerase chain reaction reverse transverse (RT-PCR) to identify the levels of ribonucleic acid type (mRNA) in order to identify its protein expression (Ro et al, 1990; Leonessa, Clarke, 2003). In patients with previously untreated breast carcinoma, the detection rates observed by IHC ranged from 0% (Yang et al, 1999) to 100% (Del Vecchio et al, 1997) with average rates of 45.9% (Leonessa, Clarke, 2003). We verified the expression of Pgp mRNA by RT-PCR ranging from 0 to 100% with average rates of 63% (Leonessa, Clarke, 2003). The comparison between the methods of evaluation shows sensitivity of detection comparable between the two methods, with agreement rates of about 73% between IHC and RT-PCR (Chevillard et al, 1996; Filipits et al, 1996).

1.3.2.1 Polymorphism C3435T of the MDR-1 gene

The single nucleotide polymorphism (SNP) is a substitution of bases, with sporadic occurrence in the population, which may or may not alter the function of the protein encoded by this codon (Hoffmeyer et al, 2000; Banhomme-Faivre et al, 2004). About 20 SNPs of the MDR-1 gene have been described by Hoffmeyer et al (2000) and Tanabe et al (2001). Brinkmann and Eichelbaum (2001) described 28 polymorphisms related to this gene, but the most studied polymorphism in these reports, with functional and clinical implications, is what happens C3435T in exon 26. In this SNP, the CC allele is considered as wild and replacing one or two of the nitrogen bases by T (CT or TT) represents the polymorphic genotype (Hoffmeyer et al 2000).

Hoffmeyer et al (2000), assessed by RT-PCR the distribution of this polymorphism in 21 healthy volunteers and showed that its occurrence was 23.9% homozygous and heterozygous, 48.3%. Cavaco et al (2003) reported that genotyping by using polymerase chain reaction linked to research the size polymorphism of restriction fragments (PCR-RFLP) in a sample of 100 healthy Caucasian Portuguese, demonstrated frequencies of 64.5% for the 3435T SNP and 35.5% for the C3435 SNP, resulting in the incidence in this population of the following genotypes: CC 12%, CT 47% and 41% TT. Balram et al. in 2003 described the incidence of the SNP C3435T using the methodology of PCR-RFLP in an Asian population comprised of 290 individuals (98 Chinese, 99 Malays and 93 Indians) and found that the CC genotype was present in 24% of Chinese, 25% of Malays, and 18% of Indians; the CT genotype was found in 44% of Chinese, Malays 46%, and 39% of Indians; the TT genotype was found in 32% of Chinese, 28% of Malays, and 43% of Indians. Hamdy et al (2003), using PCR-RFLP, described the following allele frequency distribution in 200 individuals of Egyptian origin: 34% genotype CC, 51.50% CT and 14.50%.

Experimental studies with cultured cell lines of breast and ovarian carcinomas subjected to the technique of RT-PCR showed that the basal expression of MDR-1 gene was absent or weakly present when associated with the TT genotype polymorphisms (Sauer et al,

2002). Hoffmeyer et al (2000) using the genotype represented by the SNP, determined the different forms of action of Pgp. These authors found, by sequencing the gene MDR-1 in 21 healthy volunteers, there was a significant correlation between the C3435T polymorphism in exon 26 and the function of Pgp where individuals with the TT genotype had lower protein function as compared to normal CC heterozygotes; and CT showed intermediate levels of Pgp function. This differential protein function resulted in different phenotypes associated with serum concentrations of several known substrates of Pgp, such as oral digoxin, These authors found a significant inverse correlation between the polymorphism of exon 26 and plasma levels of digoxin, which reflects its activity in vivo. Individuals with the TT genotype in the intestinal epithelium had significantly higher blood levels of digoxin than individuals with the CC and CT genotype, demonstrating functional differences in their activity and in their expression (Hoffmeyer et al, 2000). Other authors such as Kim et al (2001), confirmed these findings through research of this functional polymorphism using the technique of single-strand conformation polymorphism (SSCP) in peripheral blood samples of different populations of Euro-American individuals and African Americans. These authors, using another Pgp substrate, fexofenadine, reported that CC homozygotes had higher rates of serum concentration of this substrate when compared with the TT genotype, also demonstrating functional differences between different polymorphisms of the MDR-1 gene and consequently the expression of Pgp.

This scenario has clear implications when considering the therapeutic use of drugs that are substrates related to Pgp and may, depending on the functional action determined by this polymorphism, have different rates of clinical response. Kafka et al. (2003), showed a significant correlation between the C3435T polymorphism of the MDR-1 gene and partial and complete response to primary chemotherapy with anthracyclines, in patients with locally advanced breast carcinoma. These authors found that the presence of genotype TT was significantly correlated with clinical response, suggesting that the demonstration of this polymorphism could identify tumors sensitive and resistant to anthracyclines, and allow better individualization of therapy.

2. Summary

Different response rates suggest the existence of different mechanisms of drug resistance. Identification of factors which are related to drug resistance will enable the identification of which patients are at particular risk of treatment failure.

Pgp, encoded by the gene MDR-1, is the most investigated of a superfamily called ATP - binding cassette transporters, or ABC multidrug transporters. It has been involved as one of the drug-resistance's mechanisms since 1976. On the other hand, the action of GSTs family as cellular enzymes purification as signaling apoptosis has been studied since 1990's. The whole involvement of these enzymes is not totally clear yet, but seems that together represents a very important resistant mechanism to the chemotherapy treatments. More research is needed in this line of research to better understand these mechanisms.

3. References

[1] Adler V, Yin Z, Fuchs SY, Benezra M, Rosario L, Tew KD, et al. Regulation of JNK signaling by GSTp. EMBO J. 1999; 18:1321-34.

[2] Allan JM, Wild CP, Rollinson S, Willett EV, Moorman AV, Dovey GJ, et al. Polymorphism in glutathione S-transferase P1 is associated with susceptibility to chemotherapy-induced leukemia. Proc Natl Acad Sci U S A. 2001; 98:11592-7.

[3] Alpert LC, Schecter RL, Berry DA, Melnychuk D, Peters WP, Caruso AJ, et al. Relation of Glutathione S-Transferase α and μ isoforms to response to therapy in human breast cancer. Clin Cancer Res. 1997; 3:661-7.

[4] Ambrosone CB, Freudenhein JL, Graham S, Marshall JR, Vena JE, Brasure JR, et al. Cytochrome P4501A1 and Glutathione S-Transferase (M1) genetic polymorphisms and postmenopausal breast cancer risk. Cancer Res. 1995; 55:3483-5.

[5] Ambrosone CB, Sweeney C, Coles BF, Thompson PA, Mcclure GY, Korourian S, et al. Polymorphism in glutatione S-transferases (GSTM1 and GSTT1) and survival after treatment for breast cancer. Cancer Res. 2001; 61:7130-5.

[6] Ambudkar SV, Dey S, Hrycyna CA, Ramachandra M, Pastan I, Gostesman MM. Biochemical, cellular, and pharmacological aspects of the multi drug transporter. [Review] Annu Rev Pharmacol Toxicol 1999; 39: 361-98.

[7] Arrick BA, Nathan CF. Glutatione metabolism as a determinant of therapeutic efficacy: a review. Cancer Res. 1984; 44:4224-32.

[8] Asakura T, Sawai T, Hashidume Y, Ohkawa Y,Yokoyama S, Ohkawa K. Caspase-3 activation during apoptosis caused by glutathione-doxorubicin conjugate. Br J Cancer. 1999; 80:711-5.

[9] Autrup JL, Hokland P, Pedersen L, Autrup H. Effect of glutathione S-transferases on the survival of patients with acute myeloid leukaemia. Eur J Pharmacol. 2002; 438:15-8.

[10] Bailey LR, Roodi N, Verrier CS, Yee CJ, Dupont WD, Parl FF. Breast cancer and *CYPIA1, GSTM1, and GSTT1* polymorphisms: evidence of a lack of association in Caucasians and African Americans. Cancer Res. 1998; 58:65-70.

[11] Balram C, Sharma A, Sivathasan C, Lee EJD. Frequency of C3435T single nucleotide MDR-1 genetic polymorphism in an Asian population: phenotypic-genotypic correlates. Br J Clin Pharmacol 2003;56:78-83.

[12] Banhomme-Faivre L, Devocelle A, Saliba F, Chatled S, Maccario J, Farinotti R, et al MDR-1 C3435T Polymorphism influences cyclosporine A dose requirement in liver-transplant recipientes. Transplantation 2004;78:21-5.

[13] Bear HD. Indications for neoadjuvante chemotherapy for breast cancer. Semin Oncol. 1998; 25(2 Suppl. 3):3-12.

[14] Bell DA, Taylor JA, Paulson DF, Robertson CN, Mohler JL, Lucier GW. Genetic risk and carcinogen exposure: a commom inherited defect of the carcinogen-metabolism gene glutathione S-transferase M1(GSTM1) that increases susceptibility to bladder cancer. J Nat Cancer Inst. 1993; 85:1159-64.

[15] Biedler JL , Riehm H. Cellular resistance to actinomycin D in Chinese hamster cells in vitro: cross-resistance, radioautographic, and cytogenetic studies. Cancer Res 1970; 30:1174-84.

[16] Bodor M, Kelly EJ, Ho RJ. Characterization of the human MDR-1 gene. AAPS J 2005; 7:E1-5.

[17] Bonadonna G, Brusamolino E, Valagussa P, Rossi A, Brugnatelli L, Brambilla C, et al. Combination chemotherapy as an adjuvant treatment in operable breast cancer. N Engl J Med. 1976; 294:405-10.

[18] Bonadonna G, Valagussa P, Moliterni A, Zambetti M, Brambilla C. Adjuvant cyclophosphamide, methotrexate, and fluorouracil in node-positive breast cancer- the results of 20 years of follow-up. N Engl J Med 1995; 332:901-6.

[19] Bonadonna G, Valagussa P. Adjuvant systemic therapy for resectable breast cancer. [Review] J Clin Oncol 1985; 3: 259-75.

[20] Bonadonna G, Valagussa P. Chemotherapy of breast cancer: current views and results. [Review] Int J Radiat Oncol Biol Phys 1983; 9:279-97.

[21] Bonadonna G, Valagussa P. Current status of adjuvant chemotherapy for breast cancer. [Review] Semin Oncol 1987; 14: 8-22.

[22] Bonadonna G,Veronesi U, Brambilla C, Ferrari L, Luini A, Greco M, et al. Primary Chemotherapy to avoid mastectomy in tumors with diameters of three centimeters or more. J Natl Cancer Inst 1990;82:1539-45.Burg D, Mulder GJ. Glutatione conjugates and their synthetic derivates as inhibitors of glutatione-dependent enzymes involved in cancer and drug resistance. Drug Metab Rev. 2002; 34:821-63.

[23] Brinkmann U, Eichelbaum M. Polymorphisms in ABC drug transporter gene MDR-1. Prospective comparison of multiple drug therapy with L-phenylalanine mustard. [Review] Pharmacogenomics J 2001; 1:59-64.

[24] Canellos GP, DeVita VT, Gold GL, Chabner BA, Schein PS, Young RC. Cyclical combination chemotherapy for advanced breast carcinoma. Br Med J. 1974; 1:218-20.

[25] Canellos GP, DeVita VT, Gold GL, Chabner BA, Schein PS, Young RC. Combination chemotherapy for advanced breast cancer: response and effect on survival. Ann Intern Med. 1976; 84:389-92.

[26] Carlsen SA, Till JE, Ling V. Modulation of membrane drug permeability in Chinese hamster ovary cells. Biochim Biophys Acta 1976; 455:900-12.

[27] Carlson RW, Anderson BO, Bensinger W, Cox CE, Davidson NE, Edge SB, et al. NCCN Practice Guidelines for Breast Cancer. Oncology. (Williston Park) 2000; 14:33-49.

[28] Cavaco I, Gil JP, Gil-Berglund E, Ribeiro V. CYP3A4 and MDR-1 Alleles in a Portuguese Population. Clin Chem Lab Med 2003; 41(10): 1345-50.

[29] Chan HSL, Thorner PS, Haddad G, Ling V. Immunoistochemical detection of P-glycoprotein prognostic correlation in soft tissue sarcoma of childhood J Clin Oncol 1990; 8: 689-704.

[30] Chan HSL, Haddad G, Thorner PS. P-glycoprotein expression as a predictor of the outcome of therapy for neuroblastoma. New Engl J Med 1991; 325: 1608-1614.

[31] Chevillard S, Pouillart P, Beldjord C, Asselain B, Belzeboc P, Magdelenat H et al. Sequential assessment of multidrug resistance phenotype and measurement of S-phase fraction as predictive markers of breast cancer response to neoadjuvante chemotherapy. Cancer 1996; 77:292-300.

[32] Daly A K. Pharmacogenetics of the major polymorphic metabolizing enzymes. Fundam Clin Pharmacol. 2003; 17:27-41.

[33] Dang DT, Chen F,Kohli M, Rago C, Cummins JM, Dang LH Glutathione S- transferase π1 promotes tumorigenicity in HCT116 colon cancer cells. Cancer Res. 2005; 65:9485-94.

[34] Dasgupta RK, Adamson PJ, Davies FE, Rollinson S, Roddam PL, Ashcroft AJ, et al. Polymorphic variation in GSTP1 modulates outcome following therapy for multiple myeloma. Blood. 2003; 102:2345-50.

[35] De Lena M, Zucali R, Viganotti G, Valagussa P, Bonadonna G Combined chemotherapy-radiotherapy approach in locally advanced (T3b – T4) breast cancer. Cancer Chemother.Pharmacol.1978; 1:53-9.

[36] Del Principe MI, Del Poeta G, Maurillo L, Buccisano F, Venditti A, Tamburini A, et al. P glycoprotein and BCL-2 levels predict outcome in adult acute lymphoblastic leukaemia. Br J Haematol 2003; 121:730-8.
[37] Del Vecchio S, Ciarmiello A, Pace L, Potena MI, Carriero MV, Mainolfi C et al. Fractional retention of technetium-99m-sestamibi as na index of P-glycoprotein expression in untreated breast câncer patients. J Nucl Med 1997; 38:1348-51.
[38] Dirven HA, van Ommen B, van Bladeren PJ. Involvement of human glutathione S-transferase isoenzymes in the conjugation of cyclophosphamide metabolites with glutathione. Cancer Res. 1994; 54:6215-20.
[39] Dunning AM, Healey CS, Pharaoah PD, Teare MD, Ponder BA, Easton DF. A systematic review of genetic polymorphisms and breast cancer risk. Cancer Epidemiol Biomarkers Prev. 1999; 8:843-4.
[40] Early Breast Cancer Trialists Collaborative Group. Effects of adjuvant tamoxifen and of cytotoxic therapy on mortality in early breast cancer: an overview of 61 randomized trials among 28,896 women. N Engl J Med. 1988; 319:1681-92.
[41] Filipits M, Suchomel RW, Dekan G, Haider K, Valdimarsson G, Depisch D et al. MRP and MDR-1 gene expression in primary breast carcinomas. Clin Can Res 1996; 2:1231-7.
[42] Fisher ER, Turnbull RB Jr. The cytolologic demonstration and significance of tumor cells in the mesenteric venous blood in patients with colorectal carcinoma. Surg Gynecol Obstet. 1955; 100:102-8.
[43] Fisher B, Ravdin RG, Ausman RK, Slack NH, Moore GE, Noer RJ. Surgical adjuvant chemotherapy in cancer of the breast: results of a decade of cooperative investigation. Ann Surg. 1968; 168:337-56.
[44] Fisher B, Carbone P, Economou SG, Lerner H, Frelick R, Glass A, et al. 1-Phenylalanine mustard (L-PAM) in the management of primary breast cancer. A report of early findings. N Engl J Med 1975; 292:117-22.
[45] Fisher B, Bauer M, Margolese R, Poisson R, Pilch Y, Reymond C, et al. Five year results of a randomized clinical trial comparing total mastectomy and segmental mastectomy with or without radiation in the treatment of breast cancer. N Engl J Med. 1985; 312:665-73.
[46] Fisher B, Redmond C, Dimitrov NV, Bowman D, Legault-Poisson, S, Wickerham DL, et al. A randomized clinical trial evaluating sequential methotrexate and fluorouracil in the treatment of patients with node-negative breast cancer who have estrogen-receptor negative tumors. N Engl J Med. 1989; 320:473-8.
[47] Fisher B, Anderson S, Redmond CK, Wolmark N, Wickerham DL, Cronin WM. Reanalysis and results after 12 years of follow-up in a randomized clinical trial comparing total mastectomy with lumpectomy with or without irradiation in the treatment of breast cancer. N Engl J Med 1995; 333:1456-61.
[48] Fisher B, Bryant J, Wolmark N, Mamounas E, Brown A, Fisher ER, et al. Effect of preoperative chemotherapy on the outcome of women with operable breast cancer. J Clin Oncol. 1998; 16:2672-85.
[49] Garcia-Closas M, Kelsey KT, Hankinson SE, Spiegelman D, Springer K, Willett WC, et al. Glutathione S-transferase mu and theta polymorphisms and breast cancer susceptibility. J Natl Cancer Inst 1999; 91:1960-4.
[50] Gaudiano G, Koch, TH, Lo Bello M, Nuccetelli M, Ravagnan G, Serafino A, et al. Lack of glutathione conjugation to adriamycin in human breast cancer MCF-7/DOX cells. Biochem Pharmacol. 2000; 60:1915-23.

[51] Goldstein LJ.MDR1 gene expression in solid tumors. [Review] Eur J Cancer 1996; 32A:1039-50.

[52] Gottesmann MM, Pastan I. Biochemistry of multidrug resistance mediated by the multidrug transporter. [Review] Annu Rev Biochem 1993; 62:385-427.

[53] Gunduz N, Fisher B, Saffer EA. Effect of surgical removal on the growth and kinetics of residual tumor. Cancer Res 1979; 39:3861-5.

[54] Hamada S, Kamada M, Furomoto H, Hirao T, Aono T. Expression of Glutatione S-transferase-п in human ovarian cancer as an indicator of resistance to chemotherapy. Gynecol Oncol. 1994; 52:313-9.

[55] Hamdy SI, Hiratsuka M, Narahara K, Endo N, El-Enany M, Moursi N, et al. Genotype and allele frequencies of TPMT, NAT2, GST, SULTIA1 and MDR-1 in the Egyptian population.Br J Clin Pharmacol 2003;55:560-9.

[56] Harbottle A, Daly AK, Atherton K, Campbell FC- Role of glutathione S-transferase P1, P-glycoprotein and multidrug resistance-associated protein 1 in acquired doxorubicin resistance. Int J Cancer. 2001; 92:777-83.

[57] Hayes JD, Pulford DJ The glutathione S-transferase supergene family: regulation of GST* and the contribution of the isoenzymes to cancer chemoprotection and drug resistence. Crit Rev Biochem Mol Biol. 1995; 30:445-600.

[58] Helzlsouer KJ, Selmin O, Huang H, Strickland PT, Hoffman S, Alberg AJ, et al. Association between glutatione S-transferase M1, P1, and T1 genetic polymorphism and development of breast. J Natl Cancer Inst. 1998; 90:512-8.

[59] Henderson IC. Adjuvant systemic therapy for early breast cancer. Curr Probl Cancer 1987;11:125-207

[60] Hoffmeyer S, Burk O, von Richter O, Arnold HP, Brockmöller J, Johne A et al. Functional polymorphisms of the human multidrug-resistance gene: Multiple sequence variation and correlation of one allele with P-glycoprotein expression and activity *in vivo.* Proc Natl Acad Sci 2000; 97(7):3473-8.

[61] Howells RE, Holland T, Dhar KK, Redman CW, Hand P, Hoban PR, et al. Glutathione S-transferase GSTM1 and GSTT1 genotypes in ovarian cancer: association with p53 expression an survival. Int J Gynecol Cancer. 2001; 11:107-12.

[62] Huang J, Tan PH, Thiyagarajan J, Bay B. Prognostic significance of glutathione S-transferase-Pi in invasive breast cancer. Mod Pathol. 2003; 16:558-65.

[63] Hutcheon AW, Heys SD. Primary systemic chemotherapy of large and locally advanced breast cancer. ASCO 2004; 63-79.

[64] Jacquillat C, Weil M, Baillet F. Results of neoadjuvant chemotherapy (NEOAD CHEM) with or without hormonotherapy and external and interstitial radiation in 98 locally advanced breast cancer (LABC). Proc Am Soc Clin Oncol 1987;6:A257.

[65] Jourenkova-Mironova N, Voho A, Bouchardy C, Wikman H, Dayer P, Benhamou S, et al. Glutathione S-transferase GSTM1, GSTM3, GSTP1 and GSTT1 genotypes and the risk of smoking-related oral and pharyngeal cancers. Int J Cancer. 1999; 81:44-8.

[66] Juliano RL, Ling V. A surface glycoprotein modulating drug permeability in Chinese hamster ovary cell mutants. Biochim Biophys Acta 1976; 455:152-62.

[67] Kafka A, Sauer G, Jaeger C, Grundmann R, Kreienberg R, Zeillinger R, et al. Polymorphism C3435T of the MDR-1 gene predicts response to preoperative chemotherapy in locally advanced cancer. Int J Oncol 2003;22:1117-21.

[68] Kavallaris M, Learey JA, Barrett JA, Frielander ML.MDR-1 and multi drug resistance-associated protein(MRP) gene expression in epithelial ovarian tumors. Cancer Lett 1996;102:7-16.

[69] Khedhaier A, Remadi S, Corbex M, Ahmed SB, Bouaouina N, Mestiri S, et al. Glutathione S-Transferases (GSTT1 and GSTM1) gene deletions in tunisians: susceptibility and prognostic implications in breast carcinoma. Br J Cancer. 2003; 89:1502-7.

[70] Kim RB, Leake BF, Choo EF, Dresser GK, Kubba SV, Schwarz UI, et al. Identification of functionally variant MDR-1 alleles among European Americans and African Americans. Clin Pharm Ther 2001;70:189-99.

[71] Konishi I, Nambu K, Mandai M, Tsuruta Y, Kataoka N, Nagata Y, et al. Tumor response to neoadjuvant chemotherapy correlates with the expression of P-glycoprotein and PCNA but not GST-п in the tumor cells of cervical carcinoma Gynecol Oncol. 1998; 70:365-71.

[72] Kroger N, Acterrath S, Hegewisch-Becker K, Mross K, Zander AR. Current options in treatment of anthracycline-resistant breast cancer. Cancer Treat Rev. 1999; 25:279-91.

[73] L'Ecuyer T, Allebban Z, Thomas R, Vander Heide RV. Glutathione S-transferase over expression protects against anthracycline-induced H9C2 cell death. Am J Physiol Heart Circ Phisiol. 2004; 286:H2057-64.

[74] Leonessa F, Clarke R. ATP binding cassette transporters and drug resistance in breast cancer. Endocr Relat Cancer. 2003; 10:43-73.

[75] Leyland-Jones BR, Towsend AJ, Tu CD, Cowan KH, Goldsmith ME. Antineoplastic drug sensitivity of human MCF-7 breast cancer cells stably transfected with a human α class glutathione S-transferase gene. Cancer Res. 1991; 51:587-94.

[76] Lizard-Nacol S, Coudert B, Colosetti P, Riedinger JM, Fargeot P, Brunet-Lecomte P. Glutathione S-transferase M1 null genotype: lack of association with tumour characteristics and survival in advanced breast cancer. Breast Cancer Res. 1999;1:81-7.

[77] Loktionov A, Watson MA, Gunter M, Stebbings WS, Speakman CT, Bingham SA. Glutathione-S-transferase gene polymorphisms in colorectal cancer patients: interaction between GSTM1 and GSTM3 allele variants as a risk-modulating factor. Carcinogenesis. 2001; 22:1053-60.

[78] Mansour EG, Gray R, Shatila AH, Tormey DC, Cooper MR, Osborne CK, et al. Survival advantage of adjuvant chemotherapy in high-risk node-negative breast cancer: ten-year analysis--an intergroup study. J Clin Oncol. 1998;16:3486-92.

[79] McIlwain CC, Townsend DM, Tew KD. Glutathione S-transferase polymorphisms: cancer incidence and therapy. Oncogene. 2006; 25:1639-48.

[80] Mauriac L, Durand M, Avril A, Dilhuydy JM. Effects of primary chemotherapy in conservative treatment of breast cancer patients with operable tumors large than 3 cm. Results of a randomized trial in a single centre. Ann Oncol 1991;2: 347-54.

[81] Millikan R, Pittman G, Tse CK, Savitz DA, Newman B, Bell D. Glutathione S-transferases M1, T1, and P1 and breast cancer. Cancer Epidemiol Biomarkers Prev. 2000; 9:567-73.

[82] Morrow CS, Smitherman PK, Diah SK, Schneider E, Townsend AL. Coordinated action of glutathione S-transferases (GSTs) and multidrug resistance protein 1 (MRP1) in antineoplastic drug detoxification. Mechanism of GST A1-1- and MRP1-associated resistance to chlorambucil in MCF7 breast carcinoma cells. J Biol Chem. 1998; 273:20114-20.

[83] Moscow JA, Townsend AJ, Cowan KH. Elevation of п class glutathione S-transferase activity in human breast cancer cells by transfection of the GSTп gene and its effect on sensitivity to toxins. Mol Pharmacol. 1989; 36:22-8.

[84] Nakagawa K, Yokota J, Wada M, Sasaki Y, Fujiwara Y, Sakai M, et al. Levels of glutathione S-transferase п mRNA in human lung cancer cell lines correlate with the resistance to cisplatin and carboplatin. Jpn J Cancer Res; 1988; 79:301-4.

[85] Nakagawa K, Saijo N, Tsuchida S, Sakai M, Tsunokawa Y, Yokota J, et al. Glutathione-S-transferase п as a determination of drug resistance in transfectant cell lines. J Biol Chem. 1990; 265:4296-301.

[86] Naoe T, Tagawa Y, Kiyoi H, Kodera Y, Miyawaki S, Asou N, et al. Prognostic significance of the null genotype of Glutathione S-Transferase-T1 in patients with acute myeloid leukemia: increased early death after chemotherapy. Leukemia. 2002; 16:203-8.

[87] O'Brien ML, Tew KD. Glutathione and related enzymes in multidrug resistance. Eur J Cancer. 1996; 32A:967-78.

[88] O'Brien M, Kruh GD, Tew KD. The influence of coordinate overexpression of glutathione phase II detoxification gene products on drug resistance. J Pharmacol Exp Ther. 2000; 294:480-7.

[89] Osmak M, Brozovic A, Ambriovic-Ristov A, Hadzija M, Pivcevic B, Smital T. Inhibition of apoptosis is the cause of resistance to doxorubicin in human breast adenocarcinoma cells. Neoplasma. 1998; 45:223-30.

[90] Pakunlu R, Cook T, Minko T. Simultaneous modulation of multidrug resistance and antiapoptotic cellular defense by MDR-1 and BCL-2 targeted antisense oligonucleotides enhances the anticancer efficacy of doxorubicin. Pharm Res 2003; 20:351-9.

[91] Parl FF. Glutathione S-transferase genotypes and cancer risk. Cancer Lett. 2005; 221:123-9.

[92] Park SK, Yoo KY, Lee SJ, Kim SU, Ahn SH, Noh DY, et al. Alcohol consumption, glutathione S-transferase M1 and T1 genetic polymorphisms and breast cancer risk. Pharmacogenetics. 2000; 10:301-9.

[93] Paumi CM, Ledford BG, Smitherman PK, Townsend AJ, Morrow CS. Role of multidrug resistance protein 1 (MRP1) and glutathione S-transferase A1-1 in alkylating agent resistance. Kinetics of glutathione conjugate formation and efflux govern differential cellular sensitivity to chlorambucil versus melphalan toxicity. J Biol Chem. 2001; 276: 7952-6.

[94] Peters WH, Roelofs HM, van Putten WL, Jansen JB, Klijn JG, Foekens JA. Response to adjuvant chemotherapy in primary breast cancer: no correlation with expression of glutathione S- transferases. Br J Cancer. 1993; 68:86-92.

[95] Powles TJ, Hickish TF, Makris A, Ashley SE, O'Brien MER, Tidy VA, et al. Randomized trial of chemoendocrine therapy started before or after surgery for treatment of primary breast cancer. J Clin Oncol 1995;13:547-52.

[96] Ragaz J, Baird R, Rebbeck P, Trevisan C, Goldie J, Coldman A, et al. Preoperative versus postoperative chemotherapy for stage (I&II) breast cancer: long-term analysis of British Colombia randomized trial. [Abstract] Proc Am Soc Clin Oncol 1997; 16:142a.

[97] Raspollini MR, Amunni G, Villanucci A, Boddi V, Taddei GL. Increased Cyclooxygenase-2(COX-2) and P-glycoprotein-170(MDR-1) expression is associated with chemotherapy resistance and poor prognosis. Analysis in ovarian carcinoma patients with low and high survival. Int J Gynecol Cancer 2005; 15:255-60.

[98] Riddick DS, Lee C, Ramji S, Chinje EC, Cowwen RL, Willians KJ, et al. Cancer chemotherapy and drug metabolism. Drug Metab Dispos. 2005; 33:1083-96.
[99] Riordan JR, Ling V. Purification of P-glycoprotein from plasma membrane vesicles of Chinese hamsters ovary cell mutants with reduced colchicine permeability. J Biol Chem 1979; 254:12701-5.
[100] Ro J, Sahin A, Ro JY, Fritsche H, Hortobagyi G, Blick M. Immunohistochemical analysis of P-glycoprotein expression correlated with chemotherapy resistance in locally advanced breast cancer. Human Pathol 1990; 21:787-91.
[101] Russo A, Mitchell JB. Pontentiation and protection of doxorubicin cytotoxicity by cellular glutathione modulation. Cancer Treat Rep. 1985; 69:1293-96.
[102] Saarikoski ST, Voho A, Renikainen M, Antilla S, Karjalainen A, Malaveille C, et al. Combined effect of polymorphic GST genes on individual susceptibility to lung cancer. Int J Cancer. 1998; 77:516-21.
[103] Sauer G, Kafka A, Grundmann R, Kreinberg R, Zeillinger R, Deissler H. Basal expression of the multidrug resistance gene 1 (MDR-1) is associated with the TT genotype at the polymorphic site C3435T in mammary and ovarian carcinoma cells lines. Cancer Lett 2002;185:79-85.
[104] Sauna ZE, Smith MM, Müller M, Kerr KM, Ambudkar SV. The mechanism of action of multidrug-resistance linked P-glycoprotein. [Review] J Bioenerg Biomembr 2001; 33:481-91.
[105] Schisselbauer JC, Silber R, Papadopoulos E, Abrams K, LaCreta FP, Tew KD. Characterization of glutathione S-transferase expression in lymphocytes from chronic lymphocytic leukemia patients. Cancer Res. 1990; 50:3562-8.
[106] Semiglazov VF, Topuzov EE, Bavli JL, Moiseyenko VM, Ivanova OA, Seleznev IK, et al. Primary (neoadjuvant) chemotherapy and radiotherapy compared with primary alone in stage IIB-IIIA breast cancer. Ann Oncol 1994;5:591-5.
[107] Shapiro DM, Fugmann RA. A role for chemotherapy as an adjunct to surgery. Cancer Res. 1957; 1098-101.
[108] Shea TC, Claflin G, Comstok KE, Sanderson BJ, Burstein NA, Keenan EJ, Glutathione transferase activity and isoenzyme composition in primary human breast cancer Cancer Res. 1990; 50:6848-53.
[109] Shimada T, Hayes, CL, Yamazaki H, Amin S, Hecht SS, Guengerich FP, et al. Activation of chemically diverse procarcinogens by human cytochrome P-450 1B1. Cancer Res. 1996; 56:2979-84.
[110] Scholl SM, Fourquet A, Asselain B, Pierga JY, Vilcoq JR, Durand JC, et al. Neoadjuvant versus adjuvant chemotherapy in premenopausal patients with tumors considered too large for breast conserving surgery: preliminary results of a randomized trial: S6. J Eur J Cancer 1994; 30A:645-52.
[111] Scotto KW. Transcriptional regulation of ABC drug transporters. Oncogene 2003;22:7496-7511.Swenney C, McLure GY, Fares MY, Stone A, Coles BF, Thompson PA, et al. Association between survival after treatment for breast cancer and Glutathione S-transferase P1 Ile105Val polymorphism Cancer Res. 2000; 60:5621-4.
[112] Tanabe M, Ieiri I, Nagata N, Inoue K, Ito S, Kanamoru Y, et al. Expression of P-glycoprotein in human placenta relation to genetic polymorphism of the multidrug resistance (MDR)-1 gene. J Pharmacol Exp Ther 2001; 297:1137-43.

[113] Tashiro K, Asakura T, Fujiwara C, Ohkawa K, Ishibashi Y. Glutathione-S-transferase-π expression regulates sensitivity to Glutathione-doxorubicin conjugate. Anti-Cancer Drugs. 2001; 12:707-12.
[114] Terek MC, Zekioglu O, Sendag F, Akercae F, Ozsaran A, Erhan Y. MDR-1 Gene expression in endometrial carcinoma. Int J Gynecol Cancer. 2003; 13:673-7.
[115] Tew KD. Glutahione-associated enzymes in anticancer drug resistance. Cancer Res. 1994; 54:4313-20.
[116] Townsend AJ, Cowan KH. Glutathione S-transferases and antineoplastic drug resistance. Cancer Bull. 1989; 41:31-6.
[117] Townsend D, Tew K. Cancer drugs, genetic variation and the glutathione-S-transferase gene family. Am J Pharmacogenomics. 2003a; 3:157-72.
[118] Townsend D, Tew KD. The hole of glutathione-S-transferase in anti-cancer drug resistance. Oncogene. 2003b; 22:7369-75.
[119] Trock DJ, Leonessa F, Clarke R. Multidrug resistance in breast cancer: a meta-analysis of MDR-1/gp170 expression and its possible functional significance. J Nat Cancer Inst 1997; 89:917-931.
[120] Valagussa P, Zambetti M, Bonadonna G, Zucali R, Mezzanotte G, Veroneso U. Prognostic factors in locally advanced noninflammatory breast cancer. Long-term results following primary chemotherapy. Breast Cancer Res Treat 1990; 15:137-47.Van der Hage JA, van de Velde CJH, Julián JP, Tubiana-Hulin M, Vandervelden C, Duchateau L et al. Preoperative chemotherapy in primary operable breast cancer: results from The European Organization for research and treatment of cancer trial 10902. J Clin Oncol 2001;19: 4224-37.
[121] Yang G, Shu XO, Ruan ZX, Cai QY, Jin F, Gao YT, et al. Genetic polymorphisms in glutathione-S-transferase genes (GSTM1, GSTT1, GSTP1) and survival after chemotherapy for invasive breast carcinoma. Cancer. 2005; 103:52-8.
[122] Yang X, Uzely B, Groshen S, Lukas J, Israel V, Russell C et al. MDR-1 gene expression in primary and advanced breast cancer. Lab Invest 1999; 79:271-280.
[123] Wang T, Arifoglu P, Ronai Z, Tew KD. Glutathione S-transferase P1-1 (GSTP1-1)Inhibits c-Jun N-terminal Kinase (JNK1) Signaling through Interaction with the C Terminus. J Biol Chem. 2001; 276:20999-1003.
[124] Wolff AC, Davidson NE. Primary systemic therapy in operable breast cancer. [Review] J Clin Oncol 2000; 18:1558-69.
[125] Wolmark N, Wang J, Mamounas E, Bryant J, Fisher B. Preoperative chemotherapy in patients with operable breast cancer: nine-year results from National Surgical Adjuvant Breast and Bowel Project B-18. J Natl Cancer Inst Monogr 2001;30:96-102.
[126] Zheng T, Holford TR, Zahm SH, Owens PH, Boyle P, Zhang Y, et al. Cigarette smoking, glutathione-S-transferase M1 and T1 genetic polymorphisms, and breast cancer risk(United States). Cancer Causes Control. 2002; 13:637-45.
[127] Zheng W, Wen WQ, Gustafson DR, Gross M, Cerhan JR, Folsom AR. GSTM1 and GSTT1 polymorphisms and postmenopausal breast cancer risk. Breast Cancer Res Treat. 2002; 74:9-16.
[128] Zheng T, Holford TR, Zahm SH, Owens PH, Boyle P, Zhang Y, et al. Glutathione S-transferase M1 and T1 genetic polymorphism, alcohol consumption and breast cancer risk. Br J Cancer. 2003; 88:58-62.